OXFORD MEDICAL PUBLICATIONS

Oxford Handbook of
Clinical Pharmacy

Published and forthcoming Oxford Handbooks

Oxford Handbook for the Foundation Programme 3e
Oxford Handbook of Acute Medicine 3e
Oxford Handbook of Anaesthesia 3e
Oxford Handbook of Applied Dental Sciences
Oxford Handbook of Cardiology 2e
Oxford Handbook of Clinical and Laboratory Investigation 3e
Oxford Handbook of Clinical Dentistry 5e
Oxford Handbook of Clinical Diagnosis 2e
Oxford Handbook of Clinical Examination and Practical Skills
Oxford Handbook of Clinical Haematology 3e
Oxford Handbook of Clinical Immunology and Allergy 2e
Oxford Handbook of Clinical Medicine—Mini Edition 8e
Oxford Handbook of Clinical Medicine 8e
Oxford Handbook of Clinical Pharmacy 2e
Oxford Handbook of Clinical Rehabilitation 2e
Oxford Handbook of Clinical Specialties 8e
Oxford Handbook of Clinical Surgery 3e
Oxford Handbook of Complementary Medicine
Oxford Handbook of Critical Care 3e
Oxford Handbook of Dental Patient Care 2e
Oxford Handbook of Dialysis 3e
Oxford Handbook of Emergency Medicine 4e
Oxford Handbook of Endocrinology and Diabetes 2e
Oxford Handbook of ENT and Head and Neck Surgery
Oxford Handbook of Expedition and Wilderness Medicine
Oxford Handbook of Gastroenterology & Hepatology 2e
Oxford Handbook of General Practice 3e
Oxford Handbook of Genitourinary Medicine, HIV, and Sexual Health 2e
Oxford Handbook of Geriatric Medicine
Oxford Handbook of Infectious Diseases and Microbiology
Oxford Handbook of Key Clinical Evidence
Oxford Handbook of Medical Dermatology
Oxford Handbook of Medical Imaging
Oxford Handbook of Medical Sciences
Oxford Handbook of Neonatology
Oxford Handbook of Nephrology and Hypertension
Oxford Handbook of Neurology
Oxford Handbook of Nutrition and Dietetics 2e
Oxford Handbook of Obstetrics and Gynaecology 2e
Oxford Handbook of Occupational Health
Oxford Handbook of Oncology 3e
Oxford Handbook of Ophthalmology 2e
Oxford Handbook of Oral and Maxillofacial Surgery
Oxford Handbook of Paediatrics
Oxford Handbook of Pain Management
Oxford Handbook of Palliative Care 2e
Oxford Handbook of Practical Drug Therapy 2e
Oxford Handbook of Pre-Hospital Care
Oxford Handbook of Psychiatry 2e
Oxford Handbook of Public Health Practice 2e
Oxford Handbook of Reproductive Medicine & Family Planning
Oxford Handbook of Respiratory Medicine 2e
Oxford Handbook of Rheumatology 3e
Oxford Handbook of Sport and Exercise Medicine
Oxford Handbook of Tropical Medicine 3e
Oxford Handbook of Urology 2e

UKMI specialist information centres

Specialist topic	Centre
Drugs in pregnancy	Wolfson Unit Regional Drugs and Therapeutics Centre (Newcastle)
Drugs in lactation	Trent and West Midlands MIC
Complementary medicine	Welsh MIC
Drugs in cardiothoracics	Royal Brompton and Harefield NHS Foundation Trust MIC
Drugs in dentistry	North West MIC
Medicines in children	Alder Hey Royal Liverpool Children's Trust MIC
Drugs in liver impairment	Leeds MIC
Drugs in renal impairment	South West MIC
Drugs in porphyria	Welsh MIC
Drugs in psychiatry	Pharmacy Department, Maudsley Hospital
Ophthalmic drugs	Moorfields Hospital MIC
HIV/AIDS	Chelsea and Westminster Hospital MI MIC
Toxicology and poisoning (not emergency enquiries)	Wolfson Unit Regional Drugs and Therapeutics Centre (Newcastle)/Regional Medicines and Poisons Information Centre, Northern Ireland

Contact details are on the UKMI website www.ukmi.nhs.uk

UK National Poisons Information Service

NPIS is comprised of four Poison Centres (Birmingham, Cardiff, Edinburgh, and Newcastle) with a single national telephone number: 0844 892 0111 (www.npis.org)

615.
1

WIF

Oxford Handbook of
Clinical
Pharmacy

Second edition

Edited by

Philip Wiffen

Director of Training, UK Cochrane Centre,
and Visiting Professor, Department of Pharmacy and
Pharmacology, University of Bath, UK

Marc Mitchell

Divisional Pharmacist
Surgery, Cancer, Neurosciences & Critical Care
Oxford Radcliffe Hospitals NHS Trust, UK

Melanie Snelling

Lead Pharmacist
HIV and Infectious Diseases
Oxford Radcliffe Hospitals NHS Trust, UK

Nicola Stoner

Lead Cancer Pharmacist
Cancer Directorate and Cancer Research UK
Oxford Radcliffe Hospitals NHS Trust,
and Principal Visiting Fellow, School of Pharmacy
University of Reading, UK

OXFORD
UNIVERSITY PRESS

OXFORD
UNIVERSITY PRESS

Great Clarendon Street, Oxford OX2 6DP

Oxford University Press is a department of the University of Oxford.
It furthers the University's objective of excellence in research, scholarship,
and education by publishing worldwide in

Oxford New York

Auckland Cape Town Dar es Salaam Hong Kong Karachi
Kuala Lumpur Madrid Melbourne Mexico City Nairobi
New Delhi Shanghai Taipei Toronto

With offices in

Argentina Austria Brazil Chile Czech Republic France Greece
Guatemala Hungary Italy Japan Poland Portugal Singapore
South Korea Switzerland Thailand Turkey Ukraine Vietnam

Oxford is a registered trade mark of Oxford University Press
in the UK and in certain other countries

Published in the United States
by Oxford University Press Inc., New York

© Oxford University Press, 2012

First edition published 2007
Second edition published 2012

British Library Cataloguing in Publication Data
Data available

Library of Congress Cataloging in Publication Data
Data available

Typeset by Cenveo, Bangalore, India
Printed in China on acid-free paper through
Asia Pacific Offset

ISBN 978-0-19-960364-0

10 9 8 7 6 5 4 3 2 1

Foreword

The world we live and work in has changed, and continues to change rapidly. Clinical pharmacy is one area where change is at its most rapid, and the extent and speed of change poses a major challenge. Although this book covers a huge amount of ground, perhaps three main areas stand out to a non-pharmacist looking over the pharmacist's shoulder.

The first is the interpretation of clinical evidence about efficacy (or effectiveness) and harm of medicines. The number of new medicines, and studies of existing medicines, is exploding, producing more information than we can handle. The key to handling it is often to have good systematic reviews of good randomized trials, when the results will be secure.

The second is to reassess how we look at harm. Adverse events that are rare, but serious, will hardly ever be uncovered in randomized trials because of insufficient numbers. The trend is to perform large observational database studies of clinical practice, often with millions of participants; some of these will make us think again about medicines we have always considered safe.

The third is the translation of knowledge into clinical practice. There are any number of different ways this can affect clinical pharmacists—from use of expert computer systems to halve the rates of adverse drug reactions, to the generation of care pathways to deliver better outcomes for patients with less hassle and at lower cost. This requires real management skills—not bureaucracy, let me emphasize, which is what most of us see badged as management.

All three of these demand that clinical pharmacists have a range of skills, and the key is that they know and understand the tools of evidence-based healthcare. This includes management as well as knowledge of clinical trials in order to convert efficacy into effectiveness.

The use of evidence is massively misunderstood. The most often used definition of evidence-based medicine is the *'conscientious, explicit and judicious use of current best evidence in making decisions about the care of individual patients'.*[1] It is interesting that this was in response to a critic of evidence-based medicine, John Grimley Evans, who made a very similar point: *'Managers and trialists may be happy for treatments to work on average; patients expect their doctos to do better than that'.*[2]

Both of these emphasize the point that each of us is an individual, and that we have to treat average results from trials or reviews with a degree of caution, both for efficacy and harm. Robert Temple, a thoughtful FDA researcher, has recently commented that *'whether accomplished by sophisticated genetic or receptor analyses or by empirical observation of response to treatment, there is growing recognition that people are not all the same in the way that they respond to treatment and that groups that might*

1 Sackett DL, Rosenberg WM, Gray JA, Haynes RB, Richardson WS (1996). Evidence based medicine: what it is and what it isn't. *British Medical Journal* **312**, 71–2.

2 Grimley Evans J (1995). Evidence-based and evidence-biased medicine. *Age and Ageing*, **24**, 461–3.

respond differently should be studied, a change from the established wisdom of conducting trials with broad entry criteria while eschewing subset analyses'.[3]

There are some intriguing results out there, relating differences in efficacy to genetic polymorphisms affecting drug absorption and metabolism, the way drugs pass the blood–brain barrier, as well as changes in receptors. Keeping up and coping with these changes is by no means going to be easy, let alone incorporating them into clinical pharmacy. All we can be sure of is that more change is on the way.

Andrew Moore
Chief Editor, *Bandolier*
2006

3 Temple RJ (2005). Enrichment designs: efficiency in development of cancer treatments. *Journal of Clinical Oncology* **23**, 4838–9.

Preface to the second edition

The second edition of this book sees some significant revisions following feedback on the first edition and also developments in therapeutics. We have been encouraged to see the use of the first edition and also the production of the *Oxford American Handbook of Clinical Pharmacy* which has borrowed extensively from our work.

Clinical pharmacy services are only as good as the pharmacists who provide them, and there are still battles to be fought and won. It remains a disappointment that clinical pharmacy in the UK has not embraced the academic rigour seen in some countries and that the research culture inbred into junior doctors has yet to infect pharmacists in the same way.

This book is the distillation of 60–70 years of combined experience between the authors with the hope that it will contribute to assisting clinical pharmacists fulfil their potential. The book is organized into chapters that follow, we hope, a logical layout, with additional information organized into chapters designed to provide additional know-how. This handbook was never perceived as a formulary, but hopefully it will provide wisdom that can be used at the bedside, in the department, or on call.

The Oxford Handbook series is well established and although pharmacists have used many of the volumes, this is the first is written specifically for pharmacists. We hope that it will prove useful to clinical pharmacy practitioners and teachers.

PW
MM
MS
NS
2011

Preface to the first edition

One of the authors began their clinical pharmacy career at a time when pharmacists entered a ward with trepidation and more than once was shouted at by a feisty ward sister protecting her territory. Since then, things have moved on a long way such that an internationally renowned surgeon stated recently that clinical pharmacy (provided by his capable clinical pharmacist) was one of the best things anyone had provided for him in his professional career.

This illustrates, perhaps, that clinical pharmacy services are only as good as the pharmacists who provide them and there are still battles to be fought and won. It remains a disappointment that clinical pharmacy in the UK has not embraced the academic rigor seen in some countries and that the research culture inbred into junior doctors has yet to infect pharmacists in the same way.

This book is the distillation of 60–70 years of combined experience between the authors with the hope that it will contribute to assisting clinical pharmacists fulfil their potential. The book is organized into chapters that follow, we hope, a logical layout with additional information organized into chapters designed to provide additional know-how. This handbook was never perceived as a formulary, but hopefully it will provide wisdom that can be used at the bedside, in the department, or for on-call.

The Oxford Handbook series is well established and although pharmacists have used many of the volumes, this is the first is written specifically for pharmacists. We hope that it will prove useful to clinical pharmacy practitioners and teachers.

PW
MM
MS
NS
2006

Acknowledgements

We are grateful to the following people who provided comments and help:
John Beale, Sarah Cripps, Mrudula Patel, Rhoda Welsh, and Rebecca White.

We are also grateful to the following reviewers:
Jon Hayhurst, Phil Rogers, and Nicola Walker.

Contents

Contributors *xiii*
Symbols and abbreviations *xiv*

1	Adherence	**1**
2	Adverse drug reactions and drug interactions	**13**
3	Anaphylaxis	**25**
4	Clinical pharmacy skills	**33**
5	Clinical trials	**107**
6	Controlled drugs	**119**
7	Evidence-based medicine	**125**
8	Herbal medicines	**149**
9	Medical gases	**161**
10	Patient management issues	**177**
11	Patient-specific issues	**205**
12	Pharmaceutical calculations	**235**
13	Pharmaceutical care	**243**
14	Medicines management	**255**
15	Research	**303**
16	Therapy-related issues: gastrointestinal system	**313**
17	Therapy-related issues: cardiovascular system	**337**
18	Therapy-related issues: respiratory system	**389**
19	Therapy-related issues: central nervous system	**395**
20	Therapy-related issues: infections	**411**
21	Therapy-related issues: endocrine system	**443**
22	Therapy-related issues: obstetrics, gynaecology, and urinary tract disorders	**459**
23	Therapy-related issues: malignant disease and immunosuppression	**465**

24 Therapy-related issues: nutrition and blood 497

25 Therapy-related issues: musculoskeletal diseases 547

26 Therapy-related issues: skin 559

27 Therapy-related issues: palliative care 577

28 Therapy-related issues: miscellaneous 591

Appendix: Supplementary data 627

Index 649

Contributors

Sarah Poole
Pharmacy Department,
Churchill Hospital,
Oxford, UK

Laura Watson
Pharmacy Department,
John Radcliffe Hospital,
Oxford, UK

Matthew White
Pharmacy Department,
John Radcliffe Hospital,
Oxford, UK

Scott Harrison
Pharmacy Department,
John Radcliffe Hospital,
Oxford, UK

Mark Borthwick
Pharmacy Department,
John Radcliffe Hospital,
Oxford, UK

Janet Hemingway
Lead Pharmacist,
Nuffield Orthopaedic Centre,
Oxford, UK

Rebecca White
Pharmacy Department,
Churchill Hospital,
Oxford, UK

Gwen Klepping
Pharmacy Department,
Churchill Hospital,
Oxford, UK

Elise Cockrum
Pharmacy Department,
John Radcliffe Hospital,
Oxford, UK

Symbols and abbreviations

↑	increased
↓	decreased
>	greater than
<	less than
♂	male
♀	female
°	degrees
A&E	accident and emergency
A&W	alive and well
AAA	abdominal aortic aneurysm
ABC	airway, breathing, and circulation
abdo	abdominal
ABPI	Association of the British Pharmaceutical Industry
ACE	angiotensin-converting enzyme
ACV	assist control ventilation
ADR	adverse drug reaction
AF	atrial fibrillation
AFB	acid-fast bacilli
ALP	alkaline phosphatase
ALT	alanine aminotransferase
APPT	activated partial thrombin time
AS	ankylosing spondylitis
AST	aspartate aminotransferase
AUC	area under the plasma concentration curve
AV	arteriovenous
BiPAP	bilevel positive airway pressure
BMI	body mass index
BMR	basal metabolic rate
BNF	*British National Formulary*
BP	blood pressure
BPH	benign prostatic hyperplasia
BSA	body surface area
C/O	complaining of
CAPD	continuous ambulatory peritoneal dialysis
CAVD	continuous arteriovenous haemodialysis

CAVH	continuous arteriovenous haemofiltration
CD	controlled drug
CHF	congestive heart failure
C-MRSA	community-acquired MRSA
CMV	continuous mandatory ventilation
CNS	central nervous system
CO_2	carbon dioxide
COC	combined oral contraceptive
COPD	chronic obstructive pulmonary disease
COSHH	Control of Substances Hazardous to Health
CPAP	continuous positive airway pressure
CSF	cerebrospinal fluid
CTC	common toxicity criteria
CVC	central venous catheter
CVP	central venous pressure
CVS	cardiovascular system
CVVHDF	continuous venovenous haemodiafiltration
CXR	chest X-ray
CYP450	cytochrome P450
Da	dalton
DBP	diastolic blood pressure
DDx, ΔΔ	differential diagnosis
DHx	drug history
DIC	disseminated intravascular coagulation
DM	diabetes mellitus
DOE	disease-orientated evidence
DTI	direct thrombin inhibitor
DUE	drug-use evaluation
DVT	deep vein thrombosis
Dx, Δ	diagnosis
E/C	enteric-coated
EBM	evidence-based medicine
ECF	extracellular fluid
ECG	electrocardiogram
eGFR	estimated glomerular filtration rate
ESBL	extended-spectrum β-lactamases
EU	European Union
FH	family history
G6PD	glucose 6-phosphate dehydrogenase
GABA	γ-aminobutyric acid

GCP	good clinical practice
GFR	glomerular filtration rate
GI	gastrointestinal system
GIT	gastrointestinal tract
GMP	good manufacturing practice
GOR	glucose oxidation rate
GORD	gastro-oesophageal reflux disease
GP	general practitioner
GSL	general sales list
GTN	glyceryl trinitrate
HbA_{1c}	glycosylated haemoglobin
HD	haemodialysis
HDL	high-density lipid
HDF	haemodiafiltration
HF	haemofiltration
HIT	heparin-induced thrombocytopenia
HIV	human immunodeficiency virus
HPA	Health Protection Agency
HPC	history of presenting complaint
HRS	hepatorenal syndrome
HRT	hormone replacement therapy
IA	intra-arterial
ICF	intracellular fluid
IM	intramuscular
IMP	investigational medicinal product
IMV	intermittent mandatory ventilation
INR	international normalized ratio
IO	intra-osseous
IPS	Institute of Purchasing Supply
ITU	intensive therapy unit
IV	intravenous
Ix	investigations
JVP	jugular venous pressure
K^+	potassium
KCCT	kaolin cephalin clotting time
LFT	liver function test
LMWH	low molecular weight heparin
LTOT	long-term oxygen therapy
M/R	modified-release
MAOI	monoamine oxidase inhibitor

MARS	molecular absorbent recirculating system
MCH	mean corpuscular haemoglobin
MCHC	mean corpuscular haemoglobin concentration
MCV	mean cell volume
MDA	Medical Devices Agency
MDI	metered-dose inhaler
MDS	monitored dose system
MHRA	Medicines and Healthcare Products Regulatory Agency
MI	myocardial infarction
MIC	minimum inhibitory concentration
MOAI	monoamine oxidase inhibitor
MRSA	meticillin-resistant *Staphylococcus aureus*
MSSA	meticillin-susceptible *Staphylococcus aureus*
NBM	nil by mouth
ng	nanogram
NGT	nasogastric tube
NHS	National Health Service
NICE	National Institute of Health and Clinical Excellence
NNH	number needed to harm
NNRTI	non-nucleoside reverse transcriptase inhibitor
NNT	number needed to treat
NPSA	National Patient Safety Agency
NSAID	non-steroidal anti-inflammatory drug
NSF	National Service Framework
NSTEMI	non-ST-segment elevation myocardial infarction
NYHA	New York Heart Assocation
O/E	on examination
O_2	oxygen
ortho	bones and joints
PA	psoriatic arthritis
PABA	para-amino benzoic acid
$PaCO_2$	partial pressure of carbon dioxide in arterial blood
PaO_2	partial pressure of oxygen in arterial blood
PC	presenting complaint
PCC	prothrombin complex concentrate
PCI	percutaneous coronary intervention
PE	pulmonary embolism
PEEP	Positive end-expiratory pressure
PEG	percutaneous endoscopic gastroscopy
PGD	patient group direction

PICC	peripherally inserted central catheter
PMCPA	Prescription Medicines Code of Practice Authority
PMH	past medical history
PMR	prescription medication records
PMS	pre-menstrual syndrome
PNS	peripheral nervous system
po	per os (by mouth)
POD	patient's own drug
POEM	patient-orientated evidence that matters
POM	prescription-only medicine
PONV	postoperative nausea and vomiting
POP	progestogen-only pill
PPI	proton pump inhibitor
ppm	parts per million
pr	per rectum (by the rectum)
prn	pro re nata (as required)
PSV	pressure support ventilation
PT	prothrombin time
PUD	peptic ulcer disease
QP	qualified person
RA	rheumatoid arthritis
RBC	red blood cell
Resp	respiratory system
RPSGB	Royal Pharmaceutical Society of Great Britain
SBOT	short-burst oxygen therapy
SBP	systolic blood pressure
SC	subcutaneous/ly
S/R	systems review
SH	social history
SIMV	synchronous intermittent mandatory ventilation
SOB	short of breath
SPC	summary of product characteristics
SR	sinus rhythm
SSRI	selective serotonin re-uptake inhibitor
stat	at once
STEMI	ST-segment elevation myocardial infarction
T_3	tri-iodothyronine
T_4	thyroxine
T_{max}	time to maximum drug concentration
TB	tuberculosis

TBC	to be confirmed/awaiting confirmation
TBG	thyroid-binding globulin
TDM	therapeutic drug monitoring
TENS	transcutaneous electronic nerve stimulation
TG	triglyceride
TIA	transient ischaemic attack
TPN	total parenteral nutrition
TNF	tumour necrosis factor
TPO	thyroid peroxidase
TRH	thyrotrophin-releasing hormone
TSH	thyroid-stimulating hormone
t-PA	tissue plasminogen activator
U&E	urea and electrolytes
UFH	unfractionated heparin
UKMI	UK Medicines Information
v/v	volume in volume
v/w	volume in weight
VAC	vacuum-assisted closure
VAS	visual analogue scale
VAT	value added tax
VF	ventricular fibrillation
VRE	vancomycin resistant enterococci
VRSA	vancomycin resistant MRSA
VT	ventricular tachycardia
VTE	venous thromboembolism
VV	venovenous
WCC	white cell count
w/v	weight in volume
w/w	weight in weight
WHO	World Health Organization

Adherence

Introduction to adherence 2
Assessing adherence 4
Strategies to improve adherence 6
Adherence counselling 8
Writing patient information leaflets 10

Introduction to adherence

What is adherence?

'To be taken as directed' is an instruction that frequently appears on medicine labels. It suggests that a patient will obey the doctor's 'orders' without question. However, as most pharmacists are well aware, patients frequently choose not to 'take as directed'.

'Compliance' is a term used to describe whether or not a patient takes their medicines as directed. It implies a paternalistic relationship between the doctor (or other healthcare professional) and the patient, with little, if any, discussion or negotiation.

'Concordance' is a two-way exchange between healthcare professional and patient. The patient participates in both the consultation and the decision-making process, and the patient's preferences and beliefs are taken into account. However, this rarely happens in full in a busy general practitioner's (GP's) surgery, hospital ward, or out-patient clinic.

'Adherence' is somewhere between compliance and concordance. The healthcare professional accepts that the patient's beliefs, preferences, and prior knowledge influence medicine-taking and attempts to address this. However, adherence interventions are frequently made after the prescription is written and the patient might not have had much influence on the choice of drug. Consequently, pharmacists and specialist nurses tend to have a bigger role in facilitating adherence than doctors.

Concordance requires a high level of resources and a multidisciplinary effort. However, adherence support can be carried out by pharmacists to some extent in their everyday practice. Thus this discussion will concentrate on adherence.

Why is adherence important?

It is estimated that, on average, 50% of patients on long-term therapy do not take their medicines 'as directed'. The costs of this are potentially significant on both personal and public levels. It is estimated that up to 30% of drug-related hospital admissions result from non-adherence. In one study, 91% of non-adherent renal transplant patients experienced organ rejection or death compared with 18% of adherent patients.[1] The cost of wasted medicines and ↑ health expenditure to treat uncontrolled disease represent a significant public cost.

Why do patients not take their medicines?

Numerous studies have attempted to identify the causes of non-adherence and many factors have been identified (Table 1.1). Different factors are relevant to different diseases or settings; for example, cost is an issue in the USA (because patients have to pay for medicines/health insurance) but rarely in the UK. The reasons for non-adherence generally fall into two categories:
- involuntary or behavioural (e.g. simply forgetting)
- voluntary or cognitive (e.g. concerns about side effects).

1 De Geest S *et al.* (1995). Incidence, determinants, and consequences of subclinical noncompliance with immunosuppressive therapy in renal transplant patients. *Transplantation* **59**: 340–7.

Pharmaceutical manufacturers tend to concentrate on behavioural factors—producing combination tablets or once-daily versions of their medicines, which are supposedly easier to take. There is evidence to suggest that adherence is reduced if the dose frequency is more than three times daily, but no data are available to support once-daily over twice-daily dosing. Patients might prefer combination products or once-daily dosing, but preference does not necessarily relate to adherence. Once-daily dosing could, in fact, lead to a worse therapeutic outcome because missing one dose means missing a whole day's therapy.

Many adherence strategies focus on cognitive issues. Intuitively it seems right that if patients do not adhere because of fears or misconceptions about their medicines, addressing these issues should improve adherence. However, it is not clear whether non-adherent patients lack knowledge and understanding or whether these are the patients who fail to seek advice.

Ultimately, it is the patient's, not the healthcare professional's, agenda that influences whether or not they take their medicines.

Table 1.1 Factors reported to affect adherence

Ability to attend appointments
Age
Beliefs about medicines
Chaotic lifestyle
Complexity of regimen
Concerns about confidentiality
Cost
Cultural practices or beliefs
Depression
Educational status
Frequency of doses
Gender
Health beliefs and attitudes (towards self and others)
Impact on daily life
Language (if the patient's first language is different from that of healthcare professional's)
Literacy
Manual dexterity
Past or current experience of side effects
Satisfaction with healthcare
Self-esteem
Side effects
Socioeconomic status

Assessing adherence

Various methods of measuring adherence have been developed, but none of them is entirely satisfactory.

- Treatment response—the most clinically relevant method of assessing adherence. If the patient has been taking their medicines, logically their health should improve (assuming that the choice of therapy was appropriate). A reasonably non-invasive and simple marker of treatment success is necessary (e.g. measuring blood pressure (BP) or cholesterol levels). However, some markers might only show recent adherence (e.g. blood glucose levels).
- Therapeutic drug monitoring (TDM)—this has limited use for assessing adherence. If serum levels are within the therapeutic range, recent, but not long-term, adherence can be assumed. Sub-therapeutic levels can be an indicator of erratic or recent non-adherence, but could also reflect malabsorption of the drug or a drug interaction.
- Medicines event monitoring systems (MEMSs)—these are special bottle caps that record each time the bottle is opened. The information can be downloaded so that each time and date the bottle was opened can be read. However, MEMS caps can only record whether the bottle has been opened, not whether any drug (or how much) was taken out of the bottle. Ideally, they should be used in conjunction with some form of patient diary so that if the bottle is opened or not opened for some reason (e.g. taking out two doses at once), this can be recorded. MEMS caps are expensive and are usually only used in clinical trials. Blister-packed medicines have to be popped into a suitable container, which can be time consuming and inconvenient.
- Pharmacy records (refills)—these can be used to check whether the patient collects the correct quantity of tablets each time, so that they do not run out if they have been taking their drugs correctly. However, this system cannot determine whether the patient actually takes the tablets.
- Patient self-report—the patient should be asked (in a non-judgemental way) whether they have missed or delayed any doses, and if so, how many. Patients tend to overestimate their level of adherence and could give the answer they feel the enquirer wants to hear rather than a true picture. However, patient self-report correlates well with other measures and is relatively cheap and easy to do.

Strategies to improve adherence

Numerous strategies have been used to attempt to improve adherence, but there is little evidence that any of them are effective in the long term. Interventions to support adherence are discussed here.

Monitored dose systems (MDSs)

MDSs ('dosette boxes') are useful for patients who might have difficulty understanding or following instructions—because of language, learning, or memory problems. Different types of box are available and it is important to ensure that the patient has the dexterity required to use them. There is no guarantee that the patient will actually take their tablets, but MDSs provide a useful check for whether or not a dose has been taken—if the tablets are still there, clearly the dose has been missed, but an absence of tablets doesn't necessarily mean that the tablets have been swallowed.

MDSs are time consuming to fill and pharmacists must ensure that if a patient starts to use an MDS in hospital, a continuing supply of filled MDSs can be ensured in the community. MDSs can only be used for solid-dose formulations and are not suitable for hygroscopic tablets (e.g. sodium valproate), 'as required' drugs (e.g. analgesics), or variable-dose medicines (e.g. warfarin).

Alarms

Alarms, bleeps, and phone calls have all been used to remind patients to take their medicines. Many patients find it useful to set the alarm on their mobile phone because this is less obvious than a special alarm. Text messaging has also been used to remind patients to take their tablets, but this requires a system to be set up to send the messages and should only be done with the patient's consent.

Refill/follow-up reminders

Patients who attend follow-up clinics and collect refill or repeat prescriptions are more likely to adhere to their medication regimen. Adherence support should not just concentrate on medicine-taking, but also ensure that the patient adheres to other therapies, out-patient appointments, etc. Keeping the patient engaged with the whole of their care could be the most important adherence intervention.

Regimen simplification

Patients who have to take their medicines more than three times daily are less likely to adhere fully to their regimen. Further complications, such as having to take medicines with food or on an empty stomach, make adherence even harder. Ideally, the regimen should be simplified to three times daily or less, with times that fit in with the patient's lifestyle.

Written and oral patient information

Bombarding the patient with drug information can be counterproductive, but well thought out advice is important. Much of this can be done when handing out the medicine. A simple explanation of the dosage schedule and probable side effects should be given with every prescription handover. Remember that patients might not understand terms that seem obvious to a healthcare professional. For example, 'take two tablets twice daily' could be interpreted as 'take one tablet morning and evening' (i.e. two tablets in 24h). Clearly stating that the patient should 'take two tablets in the morning and two tablets in the evening' helps to clarify exactly what is expected.

Manufacturers' patient information leaflets are frequently complex and beyond the reading ability of many patients. A list of side effects can scare patients and confirm the belief that the medicine could do more harm than good. A brief explanation of common side effects and what to do about them, in addition to reassurance that the patient is unlikely to experience other less common side effects listed, can be of considerable benefit.

For more complex or problematic therapies, it might be necessary to spend a substantial amount of time discussing treatment with the patient. This is often a task for specialist pharmacists (where available) in hospitals or GP's surgeries. The patient should be given time to express their fears and beliefs and to ask questions about therapy. Two-way communication between patient and healthcare professional has the following benefits.
- Improves patient satisfaction with care.
- Improves patients' knowledge of their condition and treatment.
- Increases the level of adherence.
- Improves health outcomes.
- Leads to fewer medication-related problems.

Verbal information should be backed up with written information. For many chronic diseases, there is a wealth of literature available from the Pharmaceutical Industry or self-help organizations (e.g. Diabetes UK). It might be appropriate to write tailor-made patient information for certain drugs or therapies.

Comprehensive management

This involves a multidisciplinary approach, which encompasses all the strategies outlined in this section. It is potentially complex, labour intensive (with associated costs), and not feasible or necessary in many situations. However, it is appropriate for some diseases and treatments (e.g. diabetes mellitus and antiretrovirals). Some schemes can be quite intensive and care must be taken that patients do not lose autonomy as a result of the scheme. Expert patient schemes are a good example of comprehensive disease self-management (alongside conventional care), whereby patients are taught by their peers. See ℜ http://www.nhs.uk/conditions/Expert-patients-programme-/Pages/Introduction.aspx. These schemes deal with complete management of the disease, not just drug therapy.

Adherence counselling

Pharmacists involved in adherence counselling should ideally employ the communication skills discussed in Chapter 4 (see 📖 p.94).

When discussing treatment with the patient for the first time, it is important to establish what they already know and any beliefs they hold. Possible questions to ask the patient include the following.

- Tell me anything you already know about the disease/treatment.
- What have the doctors already told you?
- Have you read/found any information about the disease/treatment (e.g. on the internet)?

Having established baseline knowledge, the pharmacist can then proceed to fill in gaps and attempt to correct any misconceptions. The latter must be done tactfully, in order not to undermine patient self-confidence and their confidence in others (bear in mind that the most cited sources of medicines information are family and friends). A checklist of information that could be provided is shown in Box 1.1, but this should be tailored according to the setting and patient's needs.

Sometimes it is useful to provide written information (to complement verbal information) at the beginning of the session so that you can go through the information with the patient, but sometimes it is better to supply written information at the end so that the patient is not distracted by what they have in their hand. Suggest other sources of information, such as self-help organizations and suitable websites, and provide your contact details for further questions.

When questioning the patient about the level of adherence, it is important to do so in a non-judgemental way. A reasonably accurate picture of adherence, and whether the patient's lifestyle affects it, can be obtained if the patient is asked how many doses they have missed or delayed:

- in the past month
- in the past week
- over a weekend.

This method tends to give a more realistic idea of adherence, but patients tend to underestimate how many doses they have missed. It is also important to confirm that the correct dose (e.g. number of tablets) has been taken and that any food restrictions have also been adhered to.

If the patient has been non-adherent, ask them why they think they missed doses and if they can think of ways to overcome this. Work together with the patient to find strategies to overcome non-adherence. Ask the patient to tell you in their own words why adherence is important and reflect this back, correcting any inaccuracies as you do so. Verify that the patient understands the regimen—e.g. ask the patient 'Tell me exactly how you take your medicines'. Try to find something positive to say about their adherence, even if this is saying something along the lines of 'I'm glad you've told me about these problems with taking your tablets . . .'.

Give positive reinforcement to patients who are fully adherent and encourage any improvements. Be careful not to be patronizing! If you have access to any results that could reflect adherence (e.g. BP readings and glycosylated haemoglobin (HbA$_{1c}$)), show the patient these results, and explain how they reflect improvement in control of the disease.

Box 1.1 Checklist of medication information for patients

Basic information
- Drug name (generic and trade name), strength, and formulation
- How it works—non-technical explanation
- Why it is important to keep taking the treatment correctly

Using the treatment
- How much to use—e.g. number of tablets
- How often to use—e.g. twice daily, about 12h apart
- Special information—e.g. with food or drink plenty of water
- Storage—e.g. in the original container, in the fridge, or expiry date

Side effects
- Common side effects—e.g. when they might occur and what to do about them
- Managing side effects (e.g. taking drugs with food might reduce nausea or using over-the-counter drug treatments for symptom control)
- Serious side effects—e.g. what to do and whether to contact clinic (provide a phone number, if appropriate), local doctor, or hospital

Drug interactions
Any drugs that the patient should avoid/be cautious with—in particular, mention over-the-counter medicines, herbal and traditional medicines and recreational drugs

Other
- Availability
- Cost (per month/per year)
- Monitoring—e.g. frequency of tests and costs of tests

Further reading

NICE guideline: Medicine adherence, http://guidance.nice.org.uk/CG76/NICEGuidance/pdf/English.
A competency framework for shared decision making with patients http://www.keele.ac.uk/pharmacy/
npcplus/medicinespartnershipprogramme/medicinespartnershipprogrammepublications/
acompetencyframeworkforshareddecision-making/.

Writing patient information leaflets

Written information is an important supplement to the verbal information on medicines and disease that pharmacists provide. Patient information leaflets help patients retain the information discussed and provide a source of information for future reference. In the European Union, pharmacists are required to distribute the patient information leaflets supplied by the pharmaceutical industry with each drug when it is dispensed, but additional information might also be required.

Pharmacy-generated patient information leaflets can be used to describe the following.
- The disease and how it could affect the patient's daily life.
- Disease prevention—e.g. stopping smoking.
- Treatment or treatment options if there is more than one.
- Details of drug therapy, including the following.
  - Dose and regimen.
  - The importance of continuing chronic therapy even if the patient feels well.
  - Side effects—e.g. risks and benefits, and what to do if they occur.
  - Drug interactions—e.g. over-the-counter and herbal medicines, food, alcohol, and recreational drugs.
  - Other special considerations—e.g. use in pregnancy and lactation.
  - Further sources of information and support—e.g. pharmacy contact details, self-help organizations, and websites.

Before you start
- Discuss the following with patients.
  - Do they feel they need additional information? What information would they like?
  - What are they worried about?
  - What type of leaflet design do they prefer?
- Don't reinvent the wheel! Check whether a leaflet covering the topic you intend to write about is already available—useful sources are the pharmaceutical industry and patient organizations.
- Look at other leaflets and see how they have been written.
  - Does the style and layout fit what you want to do?
  - Do you find it easy to read and understand?
  - What good/bad aspects of design and content can you learn from these?
- Check whether your hospital or primary care trust has guidelines on writing patient information leaflets. Some organizations require leaflets to be written in a standard format and the final version to be approved by a senior manager.
- Check what facilities there are for printing and distribution and what funding is available. There is no point spending hours producing a full-colour leaflet that requires professional printing if the funds will only stretch to a black and white photocopy.
- Talk to your organization's information technology adviser/medical illustration department—they might have access to computer programs that will make designing the leaflet much easier.

Content

- State the aim of the leaflet at the beginning—e.g. 'This leaflet is for people starting treatment for . . .'.
- Be relevant—decide on the scope of the information you are providing and stick to that. Don't get sidetracked into providing information that is not directly relevant to the aim. The leaflet should provide sufficient detail that the reader can understand the main points but not so much that it becomes confusing and the main points are lost.
- Be accurate—the leaflet must include the most up to date information available and should also address the following points.
  - Be consistent with current guidelines or best practice.
  - Give an honest description of risks and benefits.
  - Where there is a lack of clear evidence, explain that this is the case.
  - Be updated as new information becomes available or guidelines are updated.
- Be understandable, acceptable, and accessible to the audience.
  - Apply the rules for clear writing discussed in Chapter 4 (see 📖 p.86).
  - Consider the target group—are there any religious or cultural issues that could influence the content? How can you make the leaflet accessible to patients with visual impairment or who do not speak English? Be careful about getting leaflets translated because sometimes the meaning can be inadvertently changed.
  - Get patient's opinions on the content—check that they understand/ interpret the information correctly, tone and style are acceptable (see Box 1.2), layout and presentation are easy to follow, and they think that it covers all the relevant issues.

Box 1.2 Patient preferences for tone and style of written information

Likes	Dislikes
• Positive tone	• Negative tone
• Friendly	• Stress on what could go wrong
• Encouraging	• Unrealistic
• Reassuring	• Over-optimistic
• Non-alarmist	• Misleading
• Honest	• Patronizing
• Practical	• Childish
• Understanding	• Cold
• Not condescending	
• Talking to you personally	
• Using 'you' a lot	
• Warm	

Design and layout

Once you have drafted the text, think about how best it can be presented (Fig. 1.1). Use the guidance in Chapter 4 (see 📖 p.88) on font type and basic layout.

Large amounts of type on an A4-size sheet of paper is hard work for anyone to read. A5 size (ideally a single side) is the maximum size that should be used. If you have a lot of information to present, use an A5 or smaller booklet format or a three-fold A4 leaflet.

Graphics can be helpful to break up the text and 'signpost' new ideas, but be careful not to overdo it so that the graphics overwhelm the text. Graphics must be relevant to the text. Ensure that graphics are culturally acceptable and bear in mind that some stylized pictures or icons could be interpreted differently by people of different cultures (e.g. a crescent moon to indicate night time might be interpreted as a religious symbol).

Review and update regularly

The leaflet should state the author's name and job title, the date of production, and a future review date. Depending on what new information becomes available, it might be necessary to update the leaflet sooner than the review date. If the information is significantly out of date, the leaflet should be withdrawn from use until an updated version is available.

Fig. 1.1 Writing reports: design and layout.

Adverse drug reactions and drug interactions

Introduction to ADRs *14*
Classification of ADRs *15*
Adverse reactions: drug or disease? *16*
Helping patients understand the risk of ADRs *17*
Reporting ADRs *18*
Drug interactions *20*
Managing drug interactions *23*

Introduction to ADRs

Adverse drug reactions (ADRs), also known as 'side effects', 'adverse drug events', or 'drug misadventures', are a frequent cause of morbidity in hospital and the community. They have a significant cost both financially and in terms of quality of life. Few studies of ADRs have been carried out in the community so the effect on primary care is harder to assess, but studies in the hospital environment have shown the following.

- ADRs occur in 10–20% of patients in hospital.
- ADRs are responsible for 5% of admissions to hospital.
- ADRs might be responsible for 1 in 1000 deaths in medical wards.
- ADRs are the most common cause of iatrogenic injury in hospital patients.

The World Health Organization (WHO) defines an ADR as follows:
'a drug-related event that is noxious and unintended and occurs at doses used in humans for prophylaxis, diagnosis or therapy of disease or for the modification of physiological function.'

However, this definition does not take into account the following scenarios, all of which can also cause ADRs:

- overdose (including prescribing or administration errors)
- therapeutic failure
- drug interactions
- drug withdrawal.

Pharmacists have an important role in identifying, reporting, and preventing ADRs.

Classification of ADRs

A number of classification systems exist, but the most widely accepted is to group ADRs as either type A (predictable) or type B (unpredictable) reactions. This system is not ideal because some types of reaction (e.g. teratogenic effects) do not fit easily into either category. However, it is a useful system in most cases because immediate management of the ADR and future drug choices can be guided by the ADR type.

Type A reactions

An exaggerated, but otherwise normal, pharmacological action. Type A reactions have the following characteristics:
- largely predictable
- usually dose-dependent
- incidence and morbidity high
- mortality low.

Examples of type A reactions include respiratory depression with opioid analgesia, cough with angiotensin-coverting enzyme (ACE) inhibitors, and withdrawal effects with benzodiazepines or alcohol.

Type B reactions

Idiosyncratic, aberrant, or bizarre drug effects that are unrelated to the pharmacology of the drug. Type B reactions have the following characteristics:
- usually unpredictable
- might not be picked up by toxicological screening
- not necessarily dose-related
- incidence and morbidity low
- mortality high.

Type B reactions are most commonly immunological (e.g. penicillin allergy).

Adverse reactions: drug or disease?

Determining whether or not a symptom is an ADR can be difficult, especially if the patient has multiple pathologies. Experience has shown that pharmacists tend to blame the drug and doctors to blame the disease. Questions to ask are as follows.

- Is there another explanation for the symptom (e.g. disease-related)?
- Is this a previously reported side effect of this drug? How common is it? This is harder to assess for new drugs because there is less information available.
- Is the timing right? Most ADRs occur soon after starting a drug, although some ADRs (e.g. hepatotoxicity) might be delayed. The onset of some hypersensitivity reactions (e.g. penicillin rash) can be delayed for up to 10 days after starting the drug. This can cause confusion, especially if the antibiotic course has been completed before the rash appears.
- Is the dose excessive? Check serum levels if available. Check renal function—was the dose too high if renal function is impaired? If the symptom can be explained as a type A reaction and the dose is high for whatever reason, it is more probable that the reaction is drug-induced.
- Does the symptom resolve on stopping the drug or reducing the dose (de-challenge)? Type A reactions are usually dose-dependent and so will worsen on dose increase, but rapidly resolve or improve on dose reduction or drug withdrawal. Type B reactions are dose-independent and will rarely resolve with dose reduction. Drug withdrawal is necessary, but if symptoms are caused by immunological effects (rather than direct drug action) it could take some days or weeks for symptoms to resolve.
- Does the symptom recur on restarting the drug (re-challenge)? Remember that re-challenge can be especially hazardous for type B reactions and is usually not advised.

If the answer to the first question is 'no' and the answer to (most of) the other questions is 'yes', it is highly probable that the event is an ADR.

Factors predisposing to ADRs

Factors that predispose to ADRs are many and varied, and some are related only to specific disease–drug interactions, such as rash with amoxicillin in patients with glandular fever. However, the following factors are generally considered to ↑ patient risk:

- age
- renal impairment
- hepatic impairment
- 'frailty'
- polypharmacy
- ♀
- previous history of ADRs
- genetics.

The first four factors predispose to type A reactions because they are determinants of drug toxicity, but the remaining factors predispose to type A or type B reactions.

Helping patients understand the risk of ADRs

Terms such as 'common' and 'uncommon' are used to describe levels of risk of ADRs in patient information leaflets and summaries of product characteristics. The terms are standardized by the European Union according to the reported frequency found in clinical trials for example (Table 2.1), but patients routinely overestimate the level of risk that these terms are intended to imply.

The following strategies should help in communicating risk to patients.
- Avoid using verbal descriptors such as 'common'.
- Use frequencies rather than percentages—e.g. 1 person in every 1000 rather than 0.1%.
- Use the same denominator throughout—i.e. 1 in 1000 and 10 in 1000 rather than 1 in 1000 and 1 in 100.
- Give both positive and negative information—e.g. 95 out 100 patients did not get the side effect and 5 patients did.
- Give information about baseline risk—e.g.
  • The risk of deep vein thrombosis (DVT) in non-pregnant women who are not taking the combined oral contraceptive (COC) is 5 cases per 100 000 women per year.
  • The risk of DVT in pregnancy is 60 cases per 100 000 pregnancies.
  • The risk of DVT in women taking the COC is 15–25 cases per 100 000 per year.

Table 2.1 Terminology as standardized by the European Union according to reported frequency in clinical trials

EU terminology	Level of risk
Very common	>10%
Common	1–10%
Uncommon	0.1–1%
Rare	0.01–0.1%
Very rare	<0.015%

Reporting ADRs

Most ADRs are not reported and this can lead to delays in identifying important reactions. The reasons for failure to report ADRs have been called the 'seven deadly sins' (Box 2.1). Pharmacists should attempt to address these and encourage their medical and nursing colleagues to report ADRs, in addition to sending in their own reports.

The regulatory authorities in many countries have systems for reporting ADRs, and it is important to find out how ADRs are reported and whether pharmacists can submit reports. In the UK, doctors, dentists, pharmacists, nurses, and patients can report ADRs to the Medicines and Healthcare products Regulatory Agency (MHRA) through the yellow card scheme. New drugs are labelled with a black inverted triangle in the *British National Formulary* (*BNF*), and the MHRA requests that all ADRs to these drugs are reported. For established drugs, unusual or significant reactions should be reported. Yellow card data can be accessed online.[1]

Box 2.1 Failure to report ADRs: the 'seven deadly sins'

1 **Complacency**—a mistaken belief that only safe drugs are allowed onto the market and that these will not cause serious ADRs
2 **Fear** of involvement in litigation, or of a loss of patient confidence
3 **Guilt** that a patient has been harmed by a prescribed treatment
4 **Ambition**—to collect and publish a personal series of cases
5 **Ignorance** of what should be reported or how to make a report
6 **Diffidence**—a reluctance to report an effect for which there is only a suspicion that it is drug-related
7 **Lethargy**—this may include a lack of time or interest, inability to find a report card, etc.

Drug interactions

Drug interactions occur when the effect of a drug is altered by the co-administration of any of the following:
- another drug.
- food.
- drink.

The outcome of this is as follows:
- frequently clinically insignificant
- sometimes beneficial
- occasionally potentially harmful.

Mechanisms of drug interactions

Interactions can be caused by pharmacokinetic mechanisms (i.e. the handling of the drug in the body is affected) or pharmacodynamic mechanisms (i.e. related to the pharmacology of the drug). Sometimes the interaction can be caused by more than one mechanism, although usually one mechanism is more significant. The majority of interactions are caused by the following mechanisms.

Pharmacokinetic mechanisms

Absorption

One drug will ↑ or ↓ the absorption of another. This is most frequently due to one drug or compound interacting with another—by adsorption, chelation or complexing—to form a product that is poorly absorbed. This can be beneficial (e.g. activated charcoal adsorbs certain poisons) or problematic (e.g. antacids and tetracyclines).

Changes in gastric pH affect the absorption of certain drugs—e.g. ketoconazole and itraconazole require an acidic environment to be absorbed; thus proton pump inhibitors can ↓ absorption and an acidic drink such as fruit juice or soft drinks (especially Coca Cola®) will ↑ absorption.

Most drugs are absorbed from the upper part of the small intestine. Thus changes in gut motility potentially affect absorption. Usually the total amount absorbed is unaffected, but the rate of absorption might be altered. This effect is used in some combination migraine products—e.g. including metoclopramide (an antiemetic) speeds up the rate of absorption of the analgesic.

Distribution

Some drugs are bound to proteins in the serum. Only free (unbound) drug is active. Protein binding is a competitive effect, so one drug can displace the other from protein binding sites. This interaction is only an issue with highly protein bound drugs and is only significant if most of the drug remains in the plasma rather than being distributed into tissues (i.e. a low volume of distribution). Displacement of drug from protein binding sites often only causes a small 'blip' in drug levels before equilibrium is restored (because the free drug is also now available for metabolism and excretion), but it could be significant for drugs with a narrow therapeutic index (e.g. warfarin).

Metabolism

Accounts for the majority of clinically significant pharmacokinetic interactions. Induction or inhibition of the cytochrome P450 (CYP450) system leads to changes in drug levels. CYP450 represents a large group of isoenzymes; drugs are rarely metabolized by a single enzyme, although one usually predominates. Equally, drugs can induce or inhibit several enzymes and some drugs can induce some enzymes and inhibit others (e.g. efavirenz). In addition, some (but not all) enzyme inhibitors or inducers can induce or inhibit their own metabolism.

When only two drugs are involved, the effect is fairly easy to predict, even if each drug is likely to affect the metabolism of the other. However, if three or more drugs, all of which are inducers or inhibitors, are involved, the effect is almost impossible to predict, and this type of combination should be avoided if possible.

The full effects of enzyme induction and inhibition do not occur immediately.

- Enzyme induction takes about 2–3wks to develop and wear off.
- Enzyme inhibition takes only a few days.

Thus, it might be necessary to delay dose adjustment or TDM until a few days (inhibition) or at least a week (induction) after starting or stopping the offending drug(s).

An emerging area of study is drug interactions involving induction or inhibition of p-glycoprotein. This probably includes interactions involving ↑ in bioavailability because it affects drug metabolism in the gut wall—e.g. grapefruit juice ↑ levels of ciclosporin by inhibiting gut wall metabolism.

Excretion

Some drugs interfere with excretion (usually renal) of other drugs. If both drugs are excreted by the same active transport system in the kidney tubule, the excretion of each drug is ↓ by the other. This might be used as a beneficial effect—e.g. probenecid has been used to prolong the half-life of penicillin—or be problematic—e.g. methotrexate and non-steroidal anti-inflammatory drugs (NSAIDs).

Pharmacodynamic interactions

These occur if the pharmacological effects of two drugs are additive or opposing.

- Additive—the desired or adverse effects of the two drugs are the same. This can be beneficial or potentially harmful (e.g. ↑ sedation with alcohol plus hypnotics).
- Synergism—which is a form of additive effect. In this instance the combination of the two drugs has a greater effect than just an additive effect (e.g. ethambutol ↑ the effectiveness of other anti-tubercular drugs).
- Antagonism—at receptor level (e.g. a β-blocker should be prescribed with caution to an asthmatic patient who uses a β-agonist inhaler) or because of opposing effects (e.g. the desired effects of diuretics could be, at least partly, opposed by fluid retention caused by NSAIDs).

Predicting drug interactions

- Are the desired or adverse effects of the two drugs similar or opposing?
- If there is no information available for the drugs in question, are there reports of drug interactions for other drugs in the same class?
- Are both drugs metabolized by the liver and, if so, by which enzymes? Information on which drugs are metabolized by which CYP450 enzymes might be listed in the summary of product characteristics and can also be found on the following websites:
  - www.hiv-druginteractions.org
  - medicine.iupui.edu/flockhart/
- Drugs that are predominantly renally cleared are unlikely to interact with enzyme inducers and inhibitors.

Managing drug interactions

- Check whether or not the drug combination is new.
- If the patient has already been taking the drug combination, have they tolerated it? If yes, there is probably no need to change therapy, although monitoring might be required.
- Is the interaction potentially serious (e.g. significant risk of toxicity or ↓ drug effect)—in which case seek alternatives.
- Is the interaction potentially of low to moderate significance—in which case it might only be necessary to monitor side effects and therapeutic effect, or arrange TDM.
- Remember that some drugs in the same class can have different potentials to cause interactions (e.g. ranitidine versus cimetidine).
- Remember that not only do interactions occur when a drug is started, but unwanted effects can also occur when a drug is stopped.
- The elderly are at greater risk of drug interactions, because of polypharmacy and impaired metabolism and excretion. Additive side effects can be a particular problem.
- Be aware of high-risk drugs and always check for potential interactions with these drugs:
  - enzyme inhibitors and inducers (e.g. erythromycin, rifampicin, phenytoin, and protease inhibitors)
  - drugs with a narrow therapeutic index (e.g. warfarin, digoxin, lithium, phenytoin, theophylline, and gentamicin).
- Remember that interactions can occur with non-prescription drugs, which the patient might not tell you about:
  - herbal or traditional medicines
  - over-the-counter medicines
  - recreational drugs, including alcohol, tobacco, and drugs obtained by other means, such as sildenafil purchased on the internet.

Anaphylaxis

Symptoms and signs of anaphylaxis 26
Treatment of anaphylaxis 28
Prevention of anaphylaxis 31

Symptoms and signs of anaphylaxis

Anaphylaxis is defined as an immediate systems hypersensitivity event produced by IgE-mediated release of chemicals from mast cells and basophils. Theoretically, prior exposure to the agent is required and the reaction is not dose- or route-related, but in practice anaphylaxis to injected antigen is more frequent, severe, and rapid in onset than following exposure to oral or topical antigen.

Agents which commonly cause anaphylaxis include:
- drugs—e.g. penicillins, aspirin
- insect stings—e.g. wasp and bee venoms
- food—e.g. nuts.

Urticaria and angioedema are the most common symptoms (Table 3.1) and absence of these suggests that the reaction may not be anaphylaxis.

Airways oedema, bronchospasm, and shock are life-threatening and immediate emergency treatment is usually required.

The onset of symptoms following parenteral antigen (including stings) is usually within 5–30min. With oral antigen, there is often a delay. Symptoms usually occur within 2h, but may be immediate and life-threatening. A late-phase reaction may also occur with recrudescence of symptoms after apparent resolution. Recurrence is a fairly frequent phenomenon and healthcare workers should be aware of this. Patients should not be discharged too quickly as they may require further treatment.

End-of-needle reactions

Some patients may experience an anaphylactic-like reaction during rapid intravenous (IV) drug administration. This is known as an end-of-needle reaction. Initial symptoms may suggest anaphylaxis, but in fact this is a vasopressor effect and can be distinguished from anaphylaxis as bradycardia occurs which is rare in anaphylaxis. Skin symptoms are also rare in end-of-needle reactions. Stopping or slowing down the infusion or injection usually leads to resolution of symptoms, and administration at a slower rate usually avoids a repeat event.

Table 3.1 Signs and symptoms of anaphylaxis

F	Urticaria
R	Angioedema
E	Dyspnoea, wheeze
Q	Nausea, vomiting, diarrhoea, cramping abdominal pain
U	Flush
E	Upper airway oedema
N	
T	
R	Headache
A	Rhinitis
R	Substernal pain
E	Itch with no rash
	Seizure

Treatment of anaphylaxis

Anaphylaxis is a life-threatening condition; therefore rapid recognition and treatment is essential. The first response is to secure the airway and lay the patient flat to reduce hypotension. If the patient cannot tolerate a supine position (because this can worsen breathing difficulties), a semi-recumbent position is preferable.

In hospital and some community settings (e.g. home IV antibacterial therapy), it might be appropriate to keep an 'anaphylaxis box' for emergency use, which contains the following essential drugs:
- adrenaline (epinephrine)
- an antihistamine (usually chlorphenamine injection)
- a steroid (usually hydrocortisone injection).

Adrenaline

In adults, 500micrograms of adrenaline (1:1000 solution) should be administered intramuscularly if the patient is showing clinical signs of shock, airway swelling, or breathing difficulty (stridor, wheezing and cyanosis). The sub-cutaneous route is not used because absorption is too slow. IV adrenaline is hazardous and should only be administered in the hospital setting. The IV route is preferred if there are concerns about intramuscular (IM) absorption; however, time should not be wasted looking for IV access in the event of vascular compromise. For IV administration, use a dilution of at least 1:10 000 and administer the injection over several minutes. The 1:1000 solution is never used intravenously. In the community, patients and carers can be taught to administer adrenaline using a pre-loaded device, such as an EpiPen® (ALK-Abello) or AnaPen® (Lincoln Medical). Note that both types of pen contain a residual volume after use and patients should be warned about this (Table 3.2). Trainer pens can be purchased from the manufacturers. Adrenaline minijets are no longer recommended for self-administration. See Table 3.3 for doses of adrenaline for adults and children.

Emergency administration of adrenaline without a prescription

Adrenaline (1:1000 solution) is exempt from prescription-only control if it is used for the purpose of saving a life in an emergency. The Royal Pharmaceutical Society (RPS) considers that a pharmacist is justified in supplying and administering adrenaline without a prescription in a life-threatening situation.

Chlorphenamine

In adults, a dose of 10–20mg chlorphenamine should be given after adrenaline and continued as needed for 24–48h to prevent relapse. It should be administered intramuscularly or by slow IV injection to ↓ the risk of exacerbating hypotension.

Hydrocortisone sodium succinate

In adults, a dose of 100–300mg hydrocortisone is administered by IM or slow IV injection after severe attacks to help prevent relapse. The onset of action is delayed for several hours. Asthmatics who have previously received a steroid are at special risk of delayed symptoms.

Additional treatment

Symptomatic and supportive care as needed: salbutamol or terbutaline unit dose vials or IV aminophylline can be used to treat bronchospasm, with oxygen (O_2) or other respiratory support given as needed. Crystalloid infusion (e.g. sodium chloride 0.9%) might be needed to treat severe hypotension.

All patients treated initially in the community should be transferred to hospital for further treatment and observation.

Algorithms for the treatment of anaphylaxis in adults and children in hospital and community settings are available from the Resuscitation Council (UK) website.[1]

Late sequelae

Patients should be warned of the possibility of symptom recurrence, and if necessary kept under observation for up to 24h. This is especially applicable in the following circumstances.

- Past history of a recurrence (biphasic reaction).
- Severe reaction, with slow onset.
- Possibility that allergen could still be absorbed (e.g. oral administration).
- Past history of asthma or a severe asthmatic component to the reaction.

Table 3.2 Adrenaline for self-administration (IM only)

EpiPen®/AnaPen®: for children and adults >30kg body weight, adrenaline 300micrograms
Junior EpiPen®/Junior AnaPen®: children 15–30kg body weight adrenaline 150micrograms
EpiPen®/Junior EpiPen®: 1.7mL remains in the pen after use (initial volume, 2mL)
AnaPen®/Junior AnaPen®: 0.75mL remains in the pen after use (initial volume, 1.05mL)

1 The Resuscitation Council (UK). ✆ http://www.resus.org.uk/pages/glalgos.htm

Table 3.3 Dose of IM adrenaline for anaphylaxis (dose can be repeated at 5min intervals, as needed)

Age	Dose	Volume of adrenaline in 1:1000 solution (1mg/mL)
<6yrs	150micrograms	0.15mL
6–12yrs	300micrograms	0.3mL
>12yrs*/adults	500micrograms	0.5mL
*If child small or prepubertal	300micrograms	0.3mL

Doses of IV adrenaline injection for anaphylaxis

Age	Dose	Volume of adrenaline in 1:10 000 solution (100micrograms/mL)
Children	10micrograms/kg body weight	0.1mL/kg body weight
Adults	500micrograms	5mL (1mL/min; stop when response obtained)

Prevention of anaphylaxis

The risk of an anaphylactic reaction can be reduced by good drug history-taking and antigen avoidance:

- Check the patient's drug history for reports of allergy. If necessary, clarify the details of the reaction with the patient or a relative. A previous history of a mild penicillin-associated rash in infancy might not be a contraindication to future use, but bronchospasm would be.
- Be aware of cross-sensitivity between drug classes.
  - Up to 7% of people allergic to penicillin are also allergic to cephalosporins.
  - Patients allergic to aspirin are frequently also allergic to other prostaglandin inhibitors.
- Advise patients with severe allergies to carry some form of warning information (e.g. MedicAlert® bracelet).
- Some drugs (e.g. NSAIDs and ACE inhibitors) can exacerbate or ↑ the risk of a reaction. Avoid concomitant use of these drugs in situations where the patient could be exposed to the allergen (e.g. desensitization programmes).
- Remember that patients with peanut allergies should avoid pharmaceutical products containing arachis oil.

Clinical pharmacy skills

Ward etiquette 34
Patient etiquette 36
Dealing with medical staff 38
Understanding medical notes 40
Guidelines for prescription endorsement of hospital or
    institutional drug charts by pharmacists 50
Prescription screening and monitoring 54
Drug history (DHx) taking 58
Writing on drug (medicine) charts 60
Writing in medical notes 61
Medication review 62
Intervention monitoring 66
Drug use evaluation (DUE) 70
Dealing with mistakes 72
Dealing with aggressive or violent patients 74
Dealing with distressed patients 76
Dealing with dying patients 78
What if your patient is dead in the bed? 81
Ethical dilemmas 82
Financial reports and budget statements 84
Hospital budget statements 85
Writing reports 86
Managing meetings 91
Assertiveness 92
Communication skills 94
Oral presentation skills 98
Prioritizing 99
Project planning 100
Time management 102
Using Medicines Information services 104

Ward etiquette

Starting work on a new ward

- If possible, speak to the pharmacist who previously covered that ward.
- Introduce yourself to the ward manager, key medical staff, nursing staff, and other relevant staff (e.g. the ward clerk).
- Check how the ward functions.
- Find out the best time for your visit.
- Establish if there are any handover meetings or ward rounds that would be useful for you to attend.
- Check whether the ward has a pharmacy book in which nursing staff write down their supply requests or whether there is another system in place (e.g. it is the responsibility of the pharmacist or medicines management technician to check supply needs).
- Find out the ward system that the multidisciplinary team use to know which patients are in which beds.
- Explain how much time you can spend on the ward and the degree of pharmaceutical care that you can provide.
- Establish what sort of pharmaceutical care service the ward is expecting from you.
- Be aware of local policies/guidelines that pertain to your ward work.
- Comply with any rules regarding handwashing and wearing an apron, gloves, and mask.

Each ward visit

- Introduce yourself to the nursing coordinator.
- Check whether there are specific pharmaceutical care issues they would like you to follow up that day.
- Check which patients are new admissions and which ones are not, to prioritize work if necessary.
- Check which patients are being discharged that day so that take-home medication is dispensed on time, especially for patients requiring ambulance or similar transport.
- If the curtains are around a patient with whom you need to consult, check why.
- If patients in side rooms have their doors shut, knock before entering.
- Make the nursing staff aware when you leave the ward.

Patient etiquette

When delivering pharmaceutical care to patients, it is essential that pharmacists follow an appropriate code of conduct:

- Introduce yourself to the patient, stating your name and job title or role.
- Ask if it is convenient for you to speak to the patient about their medication.
- Check the patient's identity against the drug chart/notes.
  - In accordance with guidance from the national patient safety agency, before taking a history from any patient, the patient should always be asked to confirm their name, date of birth, and allergy status. This should correspond to what is written on their wrist band. If they have any form of allergy the patient should have a red wrist band confirming what they are allergic to. The wrist band will also have a hospital number. The name, date of birth, hospital number, and allergy status should then be cross-checked with the details on the drug chart and the patient notes. If any of these details are inaccurate or missing you should not proceed until either you or the nursing staff have made the necessary amendments. Additionally, patients admitted through Accident & Emergency (A&E) will often be admitted under an A&E attendance number. However, as soon as the patient's Medical Records Number (MRN) and/or NHS number is known the drug chart and wrist band should be amended accordingly. If the patient has multiple MRN numbers these should be merged into one clinical record by the clinical records team. A large number of clinical incidents and patient deaths have been directly attributed to this check not being properly carried out (e.g. two patients with similar names on the ward have medication for one patient prescribed on the other patient's drug chart, patients are administered penicillin-based antibiotics when they are penicillin allergic because they did not have a wristband or had the wrong coloured wrist band).
- Ask the patient how they would like to be addressed—e.g. by first name or Mrs/Mr.
- Explain what you will be doing—e.g. checking the medicine chart, checking the patient's own drugs (PODs), taking a medicines history, counselling patients on their new medicine. Use the term 'medicine' rather than 'drug' when talking to patients.
- Check whether the patient has any questions at the end of the consultation.
- If you are sorting out any problems with the medication, ensure that the patient is kept fully informed.
- Avoid consultations while patients are having their meals. If it is essential to speak to the patient at that time, check that it is acceptable with the patient to interrupt their meal.
- If patients have visitors present, check with the patient if it is all right to interrupt. If so, check with the patient whether they are happy for the visitors to be present during the consultation. If the patient does not want the visitors present, ask the visitors to return after a set period of time.

- If the curtains are around the patient's bed, check with the ward staff as to the reason. If necessary, speak to the patient from outside the curtain to check whether it is all right for them to see you or whether you should return later.
- If the patient becomes distressed, or is too unwell, try to sort out the task with the help of the notes/ward staff/relative or return later when the patient can be involved with the consultation.
- Be polite at all times.
- Respect the patient's privacy.

Dealing with medical staff

Medical hierarchy

In the UK, doctors must complete a five-year medical degree (or 6 years including an intercalated BSc/BMedSci degree) which leads to provisional registration with the General Medical Council. They then undertake a two-year period of foundation training. During the foundation training, doctors will be known as 'foundation house officer 1' (F1) in year 1 and 'foundation house officer 2' (F2) in year 2. The important distinction within the two-year foundation programme is that FY1 doctors are working under direct supervision, whereas FY2 doctors can work without direct supervision. This is important because a number of NHS Trusts now require FY1 doctors to pass a prescribing examination or may have restrictions imposed as to what drugs they can or cannot prescribed, whereas FY2 doctors will not.

Foundation training is almost universally followed by a period of 2–3 years of core training (the CT1 and CT2 grades) followed by a period of run-through training (starting at ST3 and extending up to ST8 depending on speciality) which leads to a CCT (Certificate of Completion of Training) at which point the doctor is able to apply for consultant posts. Junior doctors are often *not* training to work in the consultant's speciality, but rotate into that speciality for a 3–6-month post as part of their training programme. GP trainees will rotate through hospital medical specialities as part of their Vocational Training Scheme (VTS) training programme.

A consultant leads a team of junior doctors who are rotating through or training to work in the consultant's specialty. Other doctors who work in the team include clinical assistants, clinical fellows, and staff grade doctors. The specialist registrars often rotate between teams of the same speciality to ↑ their experience.

Dealing with medical staff

- Deal with the correct team of doctors. Ideally, talk directly to the prescriber if a change in the prescription is required.
- Be aware of the medical hierarchy, and deal with the appropriate grade of doctor.
- Be assertive.
- Be confident with your knowledge of the subject. If necessary, do some background reading.
- Try to anticipate questions and have answers ready.
- Explain succinctly.
- Repeat, if necessary.
- Understand and explore their viewpoint.
- Be prepared with alternative suggestions.
- Come to a mutual agreement.
- Do not be bullied.
- Be honest.
- Acknowledge if you 'don't know', and be prepared to follow up.
- If necessary, walk away from a difficult situation and seek the support of a more experienced colleague.
- Occasionally, you might need a discussion with a more senior grade of doctor if you are unhappy with the response from the junior doctor. This should be approached with tact and diplomacy.

Understanding medical notes

When a patient is first admitted to hospital, a fairly standard series of questions, investigations, and results relating to their physical examination is recorded in the notes. This is known as 'medical clerking' and is essentially the story (history) of the patient's illness to date. After interpretation of the initial clerking is mastered, it is usually fairly easy to understand subsequent entries in the notes because these are mostly brief updates. Notes written by GPs follow a similar format but are generally less detailed.

Medical clerking

Clerking usually uses the following format, although not every history includes every step.

- General information about the patient—name, age, gender, marital status and occupation.
- 'Complaining of ' (C/O) or 'presenting complaint' (PC)—a statement of what symptoms or problems have lead to the patient's admission or attendance, ideally using the patient's own words.
- 'History of presenting complaint' (HPC)—more detail about the symptoms (e.g. timing, whether they have occurred previously, whether anything improves or worsens them, severity and character).
- 'Past medical history' (PMH)—does the patient have a past history of any medical complaint, including the following:
  - previous hospital admission
  - surgery
  - chronic disease (e.g. diabetes mellitus or asthma).
- 'Drug history' (DHx)—the patient's current drugs and any drugs stopped recently are listed. Ideally, this should include any frequently used over-the-counter and herbal medicines. ADRs and allergies are also recorded here.
- 'Social history' (SH) and 'family history' (FH)—relevant details of the patient's occupation, home circumstances, and alcohol and tobacco consumption are recorded. Significant information about the medical history of close family members is noted.
  - Whether parents and siblings are alive and well (A&W).
  - Does anyone in the family have a medical problem related to the presenting complaint?
  - If close family members have died, at what age and what was the cause of death?

All the information in this section is found by asking the patient questions before the doctor examines the patient. This is known as 'systems review' (S/R). Negative findings are recorded, in addition to positive findings.

- On examination (O/E)—this is a general comment about what the patient looks like (e.g. pale, sweaty, or short of breath (SOB)).
- The doctor examines each body system in turn, recording what they have found by looking, listening, and feeling. They concentrate on any systems that are most relevant to the symptoms described by the patient (e.g. if the patient has complained of chest pain, the cardiovascular system (CVS) and respiratory system (Resp) are most relevant). The following body systems are usually covered:
  - CVS
  - Resp
  - gastrointestinal system (GI, GIT or abdo)
  - central nervous system (CNS)
  - peripheral nervous system (PNS)
  - bones and joints (ortho).

Much of the information is recorded using abbreviations and medical 'shorthand' (Table 4.1).

- 'Investigations' (Ix)—the results of any investigations, such as chest X-rays (CXRs), are recorded.
- 'Diagnosis' (Dx or Δ)—the doctor now draws a conclusion from the history and examination and records the diagnosis. If it is not clear what the diagnosis is, they might record several possibilities. These are known as 'differential diagnoses' (DDx or ΔΔ).
- The doctor now writes a plan for treatment, care, and further Ix.
- Finally, the doctor signs the report and writes down their bleep number or other contact details.

Other clinical information

Remember that the complete clinical record is much more than the medical notes. To obtain a complete picture of the patient's history and progress you might need to use other information.

- Admission form (includes the patient's address, next of kin, and GP details).
- GP's referral letter.
- Nursing notes.
- Observation charts—e.g. temperature, BP, blood glucose levels, and fluid balance.
- Laboratory data—may be paper copies in notes or on computer.
- Results of investigations, e.g. X-ray, MRI, ECG—may be paper copies in notes or on computer.
- Notes from previous admissions or out-patient attendances (including discharge summaries and clinic letters).
- Old drug charts.
- The current drug chart.

Table 4.1 Abbreviations commonly found in medical notes

+	increased, enlarged, or present (more +s indicates increased severity)
↑	increase
↓	decrease
→	normal
⬡	represents the thoracic and abdominal areas
↔	normal
♀	female
♂	male
#	fracture
O	normal or none
†	dead or died
ABG	arterial blood gases
ACTH	adrenocorticotrophic hormone
ADH	antidiuretic hormone
AF	atrial fibrillation
AFB	acid-fast bacilli
Ag	antigen
AIDS	acquired immunodeficiency syndrome
ALL	acute lymphoblastic leukaemia
AML	acute myeloid leukaemia
ANF	antinuclear factor
APTT	activated partial thromboplastin time
ARDS	acute respiratory distress syndrome
ASD	atrial septal defect
AST	aspartate transaminase
A&W	alive and well
AXR	abdominal X-ray
Ba	barium
BBB	bundle branch block
BMT	bone marrow transplant

Table 4.1 (*Contd.*)

BP	blood pressure
BS	breath sounds or bowel sounds
C/O	complaining of
Ca	carcinoma or cancer
CABG	coronary artery bypass graft
CAPD	continuous ambulatory peritoneal dialysis
CCF	congestive cardiac failure
CHD	congenital heart disease
CHF	chronic heart failure
CLL	chronic lymphoblastic leukaemia
CML	chronic myeloid leukaemia
CMV	cytomegalovirus
CNS	central nervous system
COPD	chronic obstructive pulmonary disease
CPAP	continuous positive airways pressure
creps	crepitations
CSF	cerebrospinal fluid
CSU	catheter specimen of urine
CT	computed tomography
CVA	cerebrovascular accident
CVP	central venous pressure
CVS	cardiovascular system
CXR	chest X-ray
D&C	dilatation and curettage
D&V	diarrhoea and vomiting
DDx, ΔΔ	differential diagnoses (used if there is more than one possible diagnosis)
DHx	drug history
DIC	disseminated intravascular coagulation
DM	diabetes mellitus
DNA	did not attend or deoxyribose nucleic acid

(continued)

Table 4.1 (*Contd.*)

DVT	deep vein thrombosis
D/W	discussed or discussion with
Dx, Δ	diagnosis
DXT	deep X-ray therapy, i.e. radiotherapy
EBV	Epstein–Barr virus
ECF	extracellular fluid
ECG	electrocardiogram
EEG	electroencephalogram
ELISA	enzyme-linked immunosorbent assay
EMU	early morning urine
ENT	ear, nose, and throat
ERCP	endoscopic retrograde cholangiopancreatography
ESR	erythrocyte sedimentation rate
EUA	examination under anaesthesia
FBC	full blood count
FEV_1	forced expiratory volume in 1 second
FFP	fresh frozen plasma
FHx	family history
FSH	follicle-stimulating hormone
FSHx	family and social history
FVC	forced vital capacity
G6PD	glucose 6-phosphate dehydrogenase
GA	general anaesthesia
GABA	γ-aminobutyric acid
GFR	glomerular filtration rate
GGT	γ-glutamyl transpeptidase
GH	growth hormone
GI	gastrointestinal
GU	gastric ulcer or genitourinary
GVHD	graft versus host disease
Hb	haemoglobulin

Table 4.1 (*Contd.*)

HBV	hepatitis B virus
HCV	hepatitis C virus
HIV	human immunodeficiency virus
HLA	human leucocyte antigen
HPC	history of presenting complaint
HRT	hormone replacement therapy
HSV	herpes simplex virus
IBD	inflammatory bowel disease
ICP	intracranial pressure
IDDM	insulin-dependent diabetes mellitus
Ig	immunoglobulin
IHD	ischaemic heart disease
IM	intramuscular
INR	international normalized ratio
ISQ	*idem status quo* (i.e. unchanged)
IT	intrathecal
ITP	idiopathic thrombocytopenic purpura
IUD	intra-uterine device
IV	intravenous
IVC	inferior vena cava
Ix	investigations
JVP	jugular venous pressure
KCCT	kaolin cephalin clotting time
LBBB	left bundle branch block
LFT	liver function tests
LH	luteinizing hormone
L°K°S°	liver, kidneys, spleen (° = normal)
LP	lumbar puncture
LVF	left ventricular failure
MC&S	microscopy, culture, and sensitivities

(continued)

Table 4.1 (*Contd.*)

MCHC	mean corpuscular haemoglobin concentration
MCV	mean corpuscular volume
MI	myocardial infarction
MND	motor neuron disease
MSU	midstream urine
N&V	nausea and vomiting
NAD	nothing abnormal detected
NG	nasogastric
NIDDM	non-insulin-dependent diabetes mellitus
NKDA	no known drug allergies
O/E	on examination
OA	osteoarthritis or on admission
OC&P	ova, cysts, and parasites
OGTT	oral glucose tolerance test
PC	presenting complaint
PCP	*Pneumocystis jirovecii* (previously *carinii*) pneumonia
PCV	packed cell volume
PDA	patent ductus arteriosus
PE	pulmonary embolism
PEEP	positive end-expiratory pressure
PEFR	peak expiratory flow rate
PERLA	pupils equal reactive to light and accomodation
PID	pelvic inflammatory disease
PM	post-mortem
PMH	past medical history
PR	per rectum or pulse rate
PT	prothrombin time
PTH	parathyroid hormone
PTT	partial thromboplastin time
PUO	pyrexia of unknown origin
PV	per vaginum

Table 4.1 (Contd.)

RA	rheumatoid arthritis
RAST	radio-allergosorbent test
RBBB	right bundle branch block
RBC	red blood cell
RF	renal function
RIP	rest in peace (i.e. dead or died)
Rh	Rhesus
ROS	rest of systems
RS/RES	respiratory system
RTA	road traffic accident
RTI	respiratory tract infection
RVF	right ventricular failure
$S_1 S_2$	heart sounds (first and second)
SCD/SCA	sickle cell disease/anaemia
SIADH	syndrome of inappropriate diuretic hormone
SLE	systemic lupus erythematosus
SOA	swelling of ankles
SOB	shortness of breath
SOBOE	short of breath on exercise/exertion
ST	sinus tachycardia
SVC	superior vena cava
SVT	supraventricular tachycardia
TB	tuberculosis
TBG	thyroxine-binding globulin
TFT	thyroid function tests
THR	total hip replacement
TIA	transient ischaemic attack
TIBC	total iron-binding capacity
TLC	tender loving care
TOE	transoesophageal echocardiogram
TOP	termination of pregnancy

(continued)

Table 4.1 (*Contd.*)

TPN	total parenteral nutrition
TRH	thyrotrophin-releasing hormone
TSH	thyroid-stimulating hormone
TURP	transurethral resection of the prostate
U&E	urea and electrolytes
UC	ulcerative colitis
URTI	upper respiratory tract infection
UTI	urinary tract infection
VDRL	Venereal Diseases Research Lab (used to refer to the test for syphilis)
VF	ventricular fibrillation
VSD	ventricular septal defect
VT	ventricular tachycardia
W/R	ward round
WBC	white blood count
WCC	white cell count

Guidelines for prescription endorsement of hospital or institutional drug charts by pharmacists

Administration/prescription chart review

- Pharmacists should initial and date all sections of drug charts where drugs have been prescribed when reviewing charts on the ward—this constitutes the 'clinical check' and assumes that all patient parameters are available to the pharmacist (i.e. drug history, medical notes, urea and electrolyte (U&E) levels, patient's own drugs, etc).
- If the pharmacist clinically checks the drug chart in the dispensary, the following applies.
  - All drug entries should be clinically checked using the resources available in the dispensary (i.e. no access to patient's notes, limited access to U&E levels).
  - All entries should be initialled and dated by the pharmacist, ideally in a different coloured ink to the rest of the prescription (e.g. green ink). Any items supplied should be endorsed with the quantity, strength, and form supplied.
  - The ward pharmacist should then treat the drug chart as for a new patient (i.e. check drug history, patient's own drugs (PODs), notes, and U&E levels, as appropriate.
- Ideally, a drug history should be taken from the patient by the pharmacist or pharmacy technician. This should be indicated by DHx, date and initial, and should be documented according to local policy.
- All endorsements by pharmacists are ideally made in a different coloured ink to the rest of the prescription (e.g. green ink, to distinguish pharmaceutical input from the prescribing process), although this is not a legal requirement. Ensure that the coloured ink used can be reproduced if photocopied, in line with local policy.
- Pharmacists should check and write any identified drug allergies, sensitivities, intolerances, or ADRs, in addition to the reaction, in the appropriate space section on the drug chart.
- If the patient's name, consultant, ward name, or hospital number is missing, illegible, or incorrect, this should be added or corrected by the pharmacist. If appropriate and if it is missing from the chart, the patient's weight and/or surface area should be added by the pharmacist.
- All sections of the drug chart should be checked, including 'once-only' drugs, 'fluids', and 'patient-controlled analgesia' sections.

Drug name section

- All drugs should be endorsed by the pharmacist with their non-proprietary approved names, unless they are combination products with no approved names.
- Brand names should be added for ciclosporin, theophylline, mesalazine, interferon, and lithium as the different brands are not interchangeable. Brand names should also be added for modified release (M/R) nifedipine, diltiazem, and verapamil. They are also desirable for carbamazepine, phenytoin, oral contraceptives, hormone replacement therapy (HRT), multiple-ingredient skin products, and inhalers.
- If M/R or enteric-coated (E/C) formulations are intended but not prescribed, drug names should be endorsed M/R or E/C.
- When liquid formulations are intended but not prescribed, drug names should be endorsed as liquid. The concentration should be specified. The dose in millilitres should be calculated and specified, if possible.
- When a dose is prescribed that requires a combination of strengths, the usual combination should be clarified—e.g. digoxin 187.5micrograms, 3× 62.5micrograms or 62.5micrograms + 125micrograms tablets.
- All changes agreed with the prescriber should be endorsed 'confirmed with Dr [name]', dated, and initialled. Do not use the abbreviation 'pc'.
- Non-formulary, clinical trial, or 'named patient' items should be endorsed as such.

Advice for insulins

The source of insulin should be specified (i.e. human, bovine, or porcine). The device used should also be endorsed (i.e. vial, 1.5mL or 3mL penfill, or disposable pen). Lastly, the mixture of insulin should be specified, if appropriate (e.g. 50/50).

Advice for inhalers

The strength of inhaler and the device (e.g. metered-dose inhaler (MDI), Easi-Breathe®, Accuhaler®, etc) and whether used via a spacer should be specified.

Dose section

Doses should be endorsed as whole units when not so prescribed (e.g. 500mg not 0.5g).

Abbreviations should not be used: doses prescribed as 'micrograms' or 'µg' should be endorsed as 'micrograms', doses prescribed as 'ng' should be endorsed as 'nanograms', and similarly 'IU' or 'U' should be endorsed as 'units'.

Dose times should be amended, as appropriate.

- To suit meal times—Calcichew®).
- To avoid drug interactions related to absorption—e.g. ciprofloxacin and antacids.
- Dose interval—antibiotics.
- At night (nocte)—statins (not atorvastatin).
- In the morning (mane)—fluoxetine/paroxetine.
- At 8am and 2pm to avoid nitrate tolerance—isosorbide mononitrate.

Note: changes to dose time usually do not need to be referred to the prescriber, dependent on local policy.

The dose and/or route should be clarified where ambiguous, e.g. 'propranolol 1 tablet' or (sublingual) 'GTN po'. These details should be confirmed with the patient or their notes, and do not usually have to be referred to the prescriber, dependent on local policy. Endorse that the details were confirmed with patient/GP/notes etc.

- Endorsement of drugs administered weekly (e.g. methotrexate and alendronate) must be clear, specifying the day of the week the drug is usually taken.
- As required, drugs specifying multiple routes are not encouraged, but if prescribed are endorsed with the appropriate dose for each route— e.g. prochlorperazine buccal/po/im 3mg/5mg/12.5mg, respectively.
- As required, drugs should be endorsed with their maximum frequency or dose (e.g. analgesics) and/or instructions for use (e.g. anti-diarrhoeals).
- Prescriptions for IV drugs should be endorsed with injection or infusion rates or special requirements for boluses (e.g. furosemide). High-dependency areas could be exceptions from this requirement.
- The rates of currently running drug-containing infusions should be checked, initialled, and dated (as described in the 'Pharmacy annotation section', p.52) in the pharmacy box.
- Eye drops and ointments should have left/right/both eye(s) specified.

Pharmacy annotation section

All drugs should be initialled and dated by a pharmacist, constituting the 'clinical check'. Supply endorsements should then be made by the pharmacist:

- stock items (S).
- one-stop supply (28 days).
- controlled drugs (CDs).
- patient's own drugs (PODs), including details of quantity and strength brought in and highlighting the date supplies were checked.

Symbols, such as triangle, circle, and slash, are used to distinguish entries from people's initials.

- Although self-administration should be encouraged, such systems must be supported by specific protocols that have been agreed by your institution.
- 'Non-formulary', 'clinical trial', or 'named patient' should be written in full in the drug name box.
- Prescriptions should be endorsed with the date that a supply is made.
- Prescriptions should be endorsed with the quantity supplied each time a supply is made and the appropriate strength of the product supplied.
- When a chart is rewritten, the ward pharmacist should check each entry against the previous chart, initialling and dating each entry if it is correct. The pharmacist should add the appropriate endorsing information with the date of the last supply (for information).

Further information

- Drugs stored in the refrigerator should be endorsed 'Fridge'.
- Endorse prescriptions with guidance on unusual or complex administration (e.g. disodium etidronate or alendronate).
- Clarify bioavailability differences if relevant (e.g. phenytoin capsules and suspension).
- Alert the prescriber to clinically significant drug interactions that are identified. Communicate other potential interactions to the relevant doctor either by telephone or by documentation in the patient's notes.

Prescription screening and monitoring

In an ideal world, pharmacists would review prescriptions with all relevant patient information to hand and individualize drug therapy accordingly. In reality, time and circumstances do not allow this, and pharmacists must be able to identify problems with only limited information. Time rarely allows for a full examination of all patient data, even if it is available, so pharmacists must learn to determine whether or not this is necessary.

The choice of information sources available could range from just the prescription, the patient or their representative, or, possibly, prescription-medication records (PMRs) in the community pharmacy to full laboratory data and medical and nursing notes in the hospital setting. The following discussion assumes that all information is available but it can be adapted to situations in which there are more limited data.

First impressions

Look at the prescription and patient (if present). This might seem an obvious first step, but these simple observations can tell you a great deal.

- What does the prescription or chart tell you about the patient?
  - Age—think about special considerations in children (see 🕮 p.206) and the elderly (see 🕮 p.218).
  - Weight—is the patient significantly overweight/underweight? Will you need to check doses according to weight?
  - Ward name or consultant—may tell you the presenting illness (if this is not already obvious).
  - Other charts can also provide important information—e.g. diet sheets, blood glucose monitoring, BP, and temperature.
  - What does observation of the patient tell you?
  - Old frail patients probably need dose adjustments because of low weight or poor renal function.
  - Take extra care checking children's doses; also check that the formulation is appropriate and consider licensing issues (see 🕮 p.210).
  - Unconscious patients cannot take drugs by mouth. Will you need to provide formulations that can be administered through a nasogastric or gastrostomy tube?
  - Do they have IV fluids running? Consider fluid balance if other IV fluids will be used to administer drugs (notably antimicrobials).
  - If the patient's weight is not recorded on the prescription, do they look significantly overweight/underweight. If you have concerns, ask the patient if they know their weight or weigh them.
  - Is the patient pregnant or breastfeeding?
  - Could the patient's racial origin affect drug handling—e.g. there is a higher incidence of glucose 6-phosphate dehydrogenase (G6PD) deficiency in people of African origin (see 🕮 p.200).

At this point, you might already have decided on points that need to be checked or monitored. Make a note of these as you think of them. In many hospitals a ward patient list is produced each day, which gives patient names, diagnosis, and basic clinical details. This is a useful source of readily available patient information, and you can make notes and pharmaceutical care points on your copy. Remember that the information on the list is confidential and you should be careful how you handle it. Do not leave it lying around for others to see and dispose of it by shredding or in a confidential waste bin.

Review prescribed drugs

Check each drug on the prescription carefully. Newly prescribed drugs are the highest priority, but it is important to periodically review old drugs.

- Are the dose, frequency and route appropriate for this patient, their weight and their renal function?
- What is the indication for the drug?
  - Is it appropriate for this patient?
  - Does it comply with local or national guidelines or formularies?
  - Could the drug be treating a side effect of another drug—if so, could the first drug be stopped or changed?
- Are there any potential drug interactions (see 📖 p.20)?
  - Are they clinically significant?
  - Do you need to get the interacting drug stopped or changed, or just monitor for side effects?
- Is therapeutic drug monitoring (TDM) required?
  - Do you need to check levels or advise on dose adjustment?
  - Are levels being taken at the right time?
- Is the drug working?
  - Think about the signs and symptoms (including laboratory data and nursing observations) you should be monitoring to check that the drug is having the desired effect. Are any symptoms due to lack of effect? Talk to the patient!
- Are any signs and symptoms due to side effects?
  - Do you need to advise dose adjustment, a change in therapy, or symptomatic treatment of side effects? Remember that it is sometimes appropriate to prescribe symptomatic therapy in anticipation of side effects (e.g. antiemetics and laxatives for patients on opioids).
- Check that the patient is not allergic to or intolerant of any of the prescribed drugs. This is usually recorded on the front of hospital prescription charts or you might need to check the medical notes or talk to the patient. Community pharmacy PMRs often record drug allergies or intolerance.

Ensure that you have looked at all prescribed drugs. Hospital prescription charts usually have different sections for 'as required' and 'once-only' ('stat') drugs and IV infusions. Many patients might have more than one prescription chart, and some might have different charts for certain types of drug (e.g. chemotherapy).

By now, you will probably have added to your list of points to follow up and have some idea of which patients you should focus on.

Check the patient's drug history

When patients are admitted to hospital, it is important that the drugs they normally take at home are continued, unless there is a good reason to omit them. Check that the drugs the patient usually takes are prescribed in the right dose, frequency and form.

- Ideally, use a source of information that is different from the admission history (in case the admitting doctor has made any errors):
  - GP's referral letter or computer printout
  - copy of community prescription
  - POD supplies.
  - phone GP's surgery
  - talk to the patient/relative/carer.
- Talking to the patient often reveals drugs that might otherwise be overlooked (e.g. oral contraceptive pill, regular over-the-counter medicines or herbal medicines).
- If there are any discrepancies between what has been prescribed and what the patient normally takes that you cannot account for, ensure that the doctors are aware of this. Depending on your local practice, it might be appropriate to record discrepancies on the prescription chart or in the medical notes.
- Many patients may not remember the names and doses of medication they are taking, but they will often bring in their current tablets which can be a vital source of information. It is also important to check that they are taking their medications as directed (e.g. with or without food or at the correct time of day) rather than assuming that they are following the instructions given. Additionally, it is now best practice to ask the patient's GP to fax through a list of current medications for all in-patients as an independent cross-check.

Talk to the patient

Patients are an important source of information about their drugs, disease, and symptoms. Talk to them! You might find out important information that is not recorded in the medical notes or prescription chart. If you are reviewing charts at the bedside, always introduce yourself and explain your role and what you are doing. It is a good idea to ask the patient if they have any problems with or questions about their medicines. If the patient is on many drugs or complex therapy, check their adherence by asking if they are managing to take all their medicines at home.

Care plan

You will now have notes of various problems, questions, and monitoring that you need to do. Resolve any problems and form a plan to continue monitoring the patient. Learn to prioritize. An elderly patient with renal impairment who is taking multiple drugs is at higher risk of drug-related problems than a young fit patient who is only taking one or two drugs. If you are short of time, concentrate on the high-risk patients. Check your notes, decide what jobs are essential, and deal with these first.

In some hospitals, a formal pharmaceutical care plan is written for each patient. This can be quite time consuming, but it is good practice if you can do it (for high-risk patients if not for all).

Screening discharge prescriptions

- Are all regular drugs from all prescription charts prescribed? If not, can you account for any that are omitted?
- Are timings correct and complete (e.g. diuretics to be taken in the morning)?
- Are any 'as required' drugs used frequently and therefore needed on discharge?
- Are all the prescribed drugs actually needed on discharge (e.g. hypnotics)?
- Does the patient actually need a supply? They might have enough of their own supply on the ward or at home.
- Will the GP need to adjust any doses or drugs after discharge? If so, is this clear on the prescription or discharge letter?
- Is there any information that you need to pass on to the patient, carer, or GP (e.g. changes to therapy or monitoring requirements)?
- Does the patient understand how to take the drugs, especially any new ones or those with special instructions—e.g. warfarin (see 🕮 p.362)?
- Are adherence aids needed (see 🕮 p.6)?
- When is the patient being discharged? It is important to identify which patients are being discharged that day.
- If any changes are required to the discharge prescription, the junior doctor needs to be contacted.

Drug history (DHx) taking

Before taking a DHx from a patient ensure that relevant information is obtained from the medical and nursing notes that might aid the process. Consider whether it is beneficial to have the patient's carer present, particularly for very young or old patients, for those who have difficulty communicating, or if the carer administers the medication. It is preferable if the DHx taking is carried out in an area where interruptions from visitors or other healthcare professionals are minimized.

When taking the DHx, remember to obtain details of the following.
- Drug name.
- Dose.
- Frequency.
- Formulation.
- Duration of treatment.
- Indication.
- Any problems with medication, such as with administration (e.g. inhaler), ADRs, or allergies.
- Is the patient taking their medication according to the prescribed instructions?

It is essential that details of all types of medication are obtained for a DHx, including the following.
- Medicines prescribed by the GP.
- Medicines prescribed by the hospital.
- Over-the-counter medicines.
- Alternative (e.g. herbal or homeopathic) medicines.
- Recreational drugs—discuss with patient before documenting, as many patients may not want this documented.
- All forms of medicine (e.g. tablets, liquids, suppositories, injections, eye drops/ointments, ear drops, inhalers, nasal sprays, creams, and ointments).
- If a compliance aid (e.g. dosette box) is used, who fills it?

DHxs sometimes have to be verified if patients cannot remember the details of their medication and have not brought their medication with them. DHxs can be verified by the following means.
- Checking against the POD supply.
- Checking against GP letters.
- Checking records of prescriptions used in the community (FP10 prescriptions in UK).
- Telephoning the GP's practice, and requesting a faxed copy of the patient's current medication.

During the DHx-taking process, it is also useful to establish whether the patient has any drug allergies, including symptoms.

The following information recorded from the DHx taking should be entered in the medical notes or other record according to local procedure.

- Date and time.
- DHx, including the details already discussed.
- Allergies.
- Pharmacist recommendations.
- Information provided to the patient as a result of this process.
- Signature.
- Name, profession, and contact information.

Writing on drug (medicine) charts

All pharmacists should provide information to medical and nursing staff by writing on the drug chart (see 📖 section on guidelines on prescription endorsement, p.50). Information provided on the drug chart will vary according to local practice but should ideally include the following.

- Ensure patient details (e.g. name and ward) are complete and correct.
- Document DHx information on an appropriate page of the prescription chart. (If current drug chart doesn't have a dedicated area on chart, agree local practice).
- DHx—a list of drugs, with specific details, should be recorded. Initial and date.
- ADRs/drug and food allergies.
- Additional instructions on administration:
  - IV administration
  - information about appropriate oral administration (e.g. with or after food)
  - maximum daily dose
  - 'not with' (e.g. regular prescription).
- Brand name/form—if different version affects bioavailability (e.g. Sandimmun®/Neoral®, long-acting/M/R).
- Local formulary restrictions, as appropriate.
- Clarify dose if it is not clear or could cause confusion:
  - change 0.5g to 500mg
  - liquid—annotate the concentration and volume required
  - ensure clarity for unusual frequencies (e.g. weekly or alternate days).
- Clinical information:
  - drug interactions (e.g. drugs affecting warfarin levels).
- Monitoring requests or information:
  - potassium (K^+) levels for drugs affecting/affected by potassium
  - creatinine levels for drugs affecting/affected by creatinine
  - drug levels.
- Requests to doctors to review a prescription plan:
  - length of course of antibiotics.

All information should be set out as follows.
- Written in coloured ink according to local practice (e.g. green ink).
  - Clear, legible, and in indelible ink (if handwriting is poor, please print capitals).
  - Initialled and dated, including bleep number, as appropriate.
  - Use only well-recognized abbreviations.

Writing in medical notes

Pharmacists should write in the medical notes to communicate information relating to the pharmaceutical care of the patient to the medical staff if immediate action is not required; the information should significantly influence the care of the patient,or to ensure that information is available to all members of the medical and nursing teams. The notes are a legal document, and if the pharmacist has contributed to, or attempted to contribute to, the patient's care, this should be documented.

The following is appropriate information to write in the medical notes.
- Clinically significant interactions.
- Contraindications to medicine use.
- ADRs.
- Identification of a problem that could be related to medicine use.
- Amendments to DHxs.
- General medicines information about unusual medicines/conditions.
- Counselling details and outcome.

Pharmacists who are authorized (according to local practice) to make an entry in the patient's notes include the following.
- Registered pharmacists who have received suitable training.
- Junior pharmacists and locums should discuss potential entries with their seniors or clinical supervisor before making the entry.

The pharmacist should ensure that each entry into the notes is as follows.
- Directly relevant to that patient's care.
- At the appropriate point in the notes.
- Succinct and informative.
- Follows a logical sequence.
- Subjective—e.g. records relevant patient details.
- Objective—e.g. records clinical findings.
- An assessment of the situation.
- Recommendations are clearly expressed.
- The entry should follow a standard format:
  27/11/10 Pharmacist
  Amiodarone will ↑ plasma concentration of digoxin. As *BNF* states— halve dose of digoxin.
  Tom Smith (sign) bleep 1178

Entries in the patient's notes should be as follows.
- Clear, legible, and in indelible ink (many hospital pharmacists use green ink, provided that the ink quality can be photocopied).
- Signed, with printed name, and dated.
- Include a contact number (bleep or extension).
- Use only well-recognized abbreviations.
- Include any discussion of the issue with medical or nursing staff.
- Not be informal.
- Not directly criticize medical/nursing care.

Medication review

Definition of medication review

A structured critical examination of a patient's medicines by a healthcare professional:
- reaching an agreement with the patient about treatment
- optimizing the use of medicines
- minimizing the number of medication-related problems
- avoiding wastage.

Regular medication review maximizes the therapeutic benefit and minimizes the potential harm of drugs. It ensures the safe and effective use of medicines by patients. Medication review provides an opportunity for patients to discuss their medicines with a healthcare professional. Medication review is the cornerstone of medicines management.

What does medication review involve?

- A structured critical examination of a patient's medicines (prescription and other medicines, including alternatives) by a healthcare professional.
- Identification, management, and prevention of ADRs or drug interactions.
- Minimizing the number of medication-related problems.
- Optimizing the use of medicines.
- Simplification of regimen.
- Ensuring all drugs are appropriate and needed.
- Avoiding wastage.
- Medication counselling.
- Adherence counselling—to encourage patients to adhere to their drug regimens.
- Assessment of ability to self-medicate.
- Education of patient or carer—to help them understand their drugs better.
- Education of the patient on safe and effective medication use.
- Forum for suggesting effective treatment alternatives.
- Recommendation of compliance aids.

Principles of medication review

- Patients must be informed that their medication is being reviewed.
- Patients should have the opportunity to ask questions and highlight any problems with their medicines.
- Medication review should improve the impact of treatment for an individual patient.
- A competent person (e.g. pharmacist) should undertake the review in a systematic way.
- Any changes resulting from the review are agreed with the patient.
- The review is documented according to local policy (e.g. in the patient's notes).
- The impact of any change is monitored.

Levels of medicine review

- Level 3 (clinical medication review)—face-to-face review of medication with the patient and their notes, specifically undertaken by a doctor, nurse, or pharmacist. Provides an opportunity to discuss what medication the patient is actually taking and how medicine-taking fits in with the patient's daily life.
- Level 2 (treatment review)—review of medicines, with reference to the patient's full notes, in the absence of the patient and under the direction of a doctor, nurse, or pharmacist.
- Level 1 (prescription review)—technical review of a list of the patient's medicines in the absence of the patient and under the direction of a doctor, nurse, or pharmacist.
- Level 0 (ad hoc review)—unstructured, opportunistic review of medication.

Who to target

- Patients on multiple medications or complicated drug regimens.
- Patients experiencing ADRs.
- Patients with chronic conditions.
- Elderly patients.
- Non-adherent patients.

Potential benefits of medication review

- Identification, management, and prevention of ADRs.
- Ensuring patients have maximum benefit from their medicines.
- ↓ risk of drug-related problems.
- ↑ appropriate use of medicines.
- Improved clinical outcomes.
- Cost-effectiveness.
- ↑ quality of life.
- Optimizing therapy.
- ↓ waste of medicines.
- Enables patients to maintain their independence.
- ↓ admissions to hospital.
- ↓ in drug-related deaths.

Problems identified during a medication review

- Potential ADRs.
- Potential interactions (drug–drug or drug–food).
- Suboptimal monitoring.
- Adherence/lack of concordance issues.
- Misunderstanding of dose directions.
- Impractical directions.
- Incorrect/inappropriate dosages.
- Drugs no longer needed (e.g. one medication used to treat the side effects of another).
- Difficulties with using certain dose forms (e.g. inhaler or eye drops).

Recording medication reviews

- There is no universally agreed way of documenting medication reviews.
- Local guidance for recording medication reviews needs to be followed.
- The minimum information that should be recorded is as follows:
  - current medication history
  - problems identified
  - advice given
  - suggested time-frame for the next medication review
  - date, signature, name, position, and contact details.

Further reading

Room for Review—A Guide to Medication Review: The Agenda for Patients, Practitioners and Managers. (2002). ℘ http://www.npc.nhs.uk/review_medicines/intro/resources/room_for_review_briefing.pdf

A Guide to Medication Review. (2008). ℘ http://www.npc.nhs.uk/review_medicines/intro/resources/agtmr_web1.pdf

Intervention monitoring

Clinical pharmacists can audit their impact on patient care by intervention monitoring. Some hospitals undertake these audits at regular intervals and present the results internally or to the multidisciplinary team.

Data collection forms or electronic hand-held systems are used to collect the relevant data on a pharmacist's interventions to improve patient care. Examples of data collected for this purpose include the following.

• Patient details and demographics.
• Area of work/specialization.
• Written details of the intervention.
• Date of intervention.
• Other healthcare professionals contacted.
• Evidence used to support the intervention.
• Who initiated the intervention—e.g. pharmacist, doctor, nurse, or patient.
• Possible effect the intervention would have on patient care.
• Outcome of the intervention.
• Actual outcome on patient care that the intervention had.
• Significance of intervention (Table 4.2 shows an example of one of the ways for deciding significance of the intervention).
• Category of intervention (examples are given in the section that follows).

Examples of the categories of pharmacist interventions in drug therapy

• ADRs
• Allergy
• Additional drug therapy required
• Medication error
• Medication without indication
• Untreated condition or undertreated condition
• Minimal or no therapeutic effectiveness
• Therapeutic duplication
• Patient adherence, compliance, or drug administration issue
• Patient education
• Communication with prescriber
• Incorrect medication prescribed
• Inappropriate or suboptimal dose, schedule, or route
• Optimization of drug therapy, including improving cost-effectiveness
• Dose advice
• Advice on drug choice
• Drug–drug, drug–food, or drug–disease interaction
• Side effect/toxicity
• Therapeutic monitoring for toxicity or effectiveness
• Formulation
• Compatibility
• Formulary or protocol adherence

An example of an intervention monitoring form is shown in Table 4.3.

Table 4.2 Example of significance definitions of pharmacist interventions[1,2]

Significance of intervention	Definition
Minor	Unlikely to have effect on patient outcome
Moderate	Potentially undesirable for patient outcome
Severe	Potentially detrimental for patient outcome (e.g. potentially serious prescribing error)

[1] Dean B, Barber N, Schater M. (2000) What is a prescribing error? *Quality and Safety in Health Care* **9**: 232–7.

Dodd C (2003). Assessing pharmacy Interventions at Salisbury Health Care NHS Trust. *Hospital Pharmacist* **10**: 451–6.

Further reading

Becker C, Bjornson DC, Kuhle JW (2004). Pharmacist care plans and documentation of follow-up before the Iowa Pharmaceutical Case Management program. *Journal of the American Pharmacists Association* **44**: 350–7.

McDonough RP, Doucette WR (2003). Drug therapy management: an empirical report of drug therapy problems, pharmacists' interventions, and results of pharmacists' actions. *Journal of the American Pharmacists Association* **43**: 511–18.

Hoth AB, Carter BL, Ness J, et al. (2007). Development and reliability testing of clinical pharmacist recommendation taxonomy. *Pharmaco-therapy* **27**: 639–46.

Table 4.3 Example of an intervention monitoring form

	In-patient		TTO	Out-patient
Date				
Hospital	Ward/area			
Contact source:				
Doctor	Consultant	Specialist registrar	F2	F1	GP
Nurse	Sister	Staff nurse	Auxiliary		
Other (specify)				
Category of intervention:				
Incorrect dose				
Dose advice				
Drug choice				
Drug interaction				
Side effect/toxicity/ADR				
TDM				
Drug–disease interaction				
Formulation				

Compatibility

Patient adherence/education

Formulary/protocol adherence

Cost

Other (specify)

Solution

Prescriber contacted

Nurse contacted

Documentation in notes

Other

Outcome

Advice ignored

Advice acted upon

Acknowledged no action

Information only

Patient risk:

| Low | 1 | 2 | 3 | 4 | 5 | High |

Time taken:

| <5min | 5–15min | 15–30min | 30min |

Details of intervention:

Answer/outcome on patient care:

Drug use evaluation (DUE)

DUE is a quality assurance tool which monitors and evaluates drug use against agreed criteria/standards and, if necessary, advises on a change of practice to improve the quality, safety, and cost-effectiveness of pre-scribing. It focuses on evaluating and improving the use of medication to optimize patient outcomes. The process can be carried out retrospectively, prospectively, or concurrently. It can be performed on a medication or therapeutic class, disease state, or condition. DUE is usually used as a tool in areas where prescribing practice is not consistent with agreed standards or where a new drug becomes available.

Steps to undertake a DUE cycle include the following.
- Select a drug or therapeutic area for a DUE.
- Determine objective measurable criteria and standards of use for the target area, if these are not set already.
- Design a sample data collection sheet and pilot.
- Collect the prescribing data to evaluate current practice against the standards.
- Analyse the data.
- Evaluate the practice against the standards.
- Decide what intervention needs to be introduced to improve or encourage prescribers' compliance with the agreed criteria and action plan.
- Educate staff and introduce practice to correct any inappropriate prescribing.
- Evaluate the impact of the DUE.
- Communicate the results.

To ensure an effective DUE programme, a multidisciplinary approach should be taken. Doctors and pharmacists should agree the criteria, and accurate prescribing data should be collected. There should be critical evaluation of the data and an acceptable means of correcting any deficien-cies in prescribing.

Suitable drugs or areas for a DUE study are as follows.
- Commonly used drugs to ensure cost-effective prescribing.
- Drugs for which there is a high cost or volume of usage.
- New drugs or drug classes.
- High potential for toxicity or ADRs or interaction with other medication, food, or diagnostic procedures that would result in a potential significant health risk.
- Narrow therapeutic index.
- Under consideration for formulary addition, retention, or deletion.
- Used in patient population at high risk of ADRs.
- Already included in a therapeutic policy (e.g. antimicrobial policy).
- Drugs that could improve the quality of life or patient care.
- Areas where prescribing practice is not following the standards.
- To justify the use of resources.
- The drug is most effective when used in a specific manner.

Benefits of DUE

- Confirms appropriate quality of prescribing, with respect to safety, efficacy, and cost to an organization.
- Financial benefits with the ↓ of inappropriate drug use. However, costs may increase if a more expensive drug with a better therapeutic effect is recommended as a result of the DUE.
- Improved quality of clinical pharmacy service, with respect to targeting clinical pharmacy activity and educational benefits.
- Essential component of clinical audit.
- Improves credibility of reports on drug expenditure.
- Support of the development, implementation, and monitoring of drug formularies.

Pharmacist's role in DUE

- Develop a plan for DUE programmes and processes consistent with the organization's overall goals and resource capabilities.
- Work collaboratively with prescribers and others to develop criteria for specific medications and to design effective medication use processes.
- Review individual drug charts compared with DUE criteria.
- Manage DUE programs and processes.
- Collect, analyse, and evaluate patient-specific data to identify, resolve, and prevent medication-related problems.
- Interpret and report DUE findings and recommend changes in medication use processes.
- Provide information and education based on DUE findings.

Dealing with mistakes

Medication errors are '*patient safety incidents involving medicines in which there has been an error in the process of prescribing, dispensing, preparing, administering, monitoring, or providing medicine advice, regardless of whether any harm occurred*'.[1] Medication errors are associated with significant unexpected drug-related morbidity and mortality.

Medicines management policies and procedures should be in place to minimize the risk of medication errors occurring during the medication process (i.e. for prescribing, dispensing and administration). Pharmacists can play a prominent role in optimizing safe medication use and preventing errors in all steps of the medication process:

Prescribing

- Adequate knowledge of the patient and their clinical condition.
- Clear multi-professional treatment plans.
- Complex calculations checked by two members of staff.
- Review drug treatments regularly.
- Implement electronic care records and prescribing systems.
- Legible prescriptions.
- Avoiding abbreviations.

Dispensing

- Training and competency assessment for checking prescriptions and dispensing.
- Checking medication with a patient when it is being issued and allowing patients the opportunity to ask questions about their medication.
- Formal dispensary procedures and checking systems.

Administration

Risk management must be built into the previous steps to ensure that medication is administered safely.

- Training of staff administering medication.
- Procedures for drug administration.
- High-risk areas of administration to have a double check by a second member of staff (e.g. for IV infusions or complex calculations).
- Involving patients or their carers in the administration process if appropriate.
- Storage of medication appropriately to minimize errors. Controlling the availability of high-risk drugs (e.g. potassium chloride ampoules).
- Using information technology to support prescribing, dispensing, and administration of medication.

Create a culture where staff can learn from their mistakes. Do not have a blame culture.

- Explore why a mistake has happened.
- Remain calm.
- Find out the facts.
- Focus on the processes that allowed the mistake to happen.
- Provide support.
- Assume that the person wants to learn from their mistakes.

- See mistakes as part of a learning process.

Harness the power of mistakes.
- Create mechanisms to provide support when mistakes occur.
- Learn to question and challenge without antagonism.
- Create personal learning contracts to promote self-managed learning.
- Acquire a habit of active reflection.

Reporting mistakes.
- Use the appropriate reporting mechanism within your hospital or institution.
- Inform a more senior member of staff of the mistake.
- Inform the multidisciplinary team of the mistake.
- Document the mistake and the steps leading up to the mistake.

Dealing with mistakes.
- Dealing with your own feelings, if you are the person who made the mistake—remember that we are all human and can make mistakes. You will probably feel remorse that you have made the mistake. Reflect on how the mistake was made, and plan how you will learn from the mistake to ensure that it isn't repeated.
- Dealing with people who don't acknowledge their own mistakes or who make repeated mistakes—the person's manager should be involved in dealing with the person who does not acknowledge their mistakes. Evidence must be used to discuss the mistakes, and performance management strategies put in place to ensure that the mistakes are acknowledged and learnt from.
- Dealing with a more senior member of staff who has made a mistake—it is difficult for a junior member of staff to deal with mistakes made by a more senior member of staff. Whenever possible, it is best to speak directly to the member of staff who has made the mistake, informing them of the outcome and any action you have taken. If necessary, involve another senior member of staff or your manager in the discussion.

Remember

Mistakes can be fatal. Ensure that you are aware of local policies and procedures to minimize the risk of mistakes occurring.

Further reading

National Prescribing Centre. Reducing Medication Errors. ℘ http://www.npc.nhs.uk/improving_safety/improving_safety/resources/Medication_Error/Reducing_5mg.pdf

Smith J (2004). *Building a Safer NHS for Patients: Improving Medication Safety*. London: Department of Health.

Williams DJP (2007). Medication errors. *Journal of the Royal College of Physicians of Edinburgh* **37**: 343–6.

Dealing with aggressive or violent patients

Most pharmacy staff experience some form of threatening behaviour from patients at some stage during their working lives. This can range from a patient becoming verbally abusive because of a long wait for medicines to be dispensed to an armed robbery of a community pharmacy. Aggressive behaviour may also be via the telephone or written communication. Even if there is no physical injury, the psychological effect of a violent or aggressive encounter can be significant and could affect the victim's attitude to work, co-workers and patients. The emotional distress can be ↑ in a healthcare setting because staff might feel unprepared for this type of behaviour from a patient or customer they are trying to help. There could be feelings of guilt, embarrassment, shame, fear of blame, or denial. Incidents should not be accepted as 'part of the job' and should be reported so that appropriate action can be taken to both protect and support the victim and other members of staff. If healthcare teams have strategies to review and discuss incidents of threatening behaviour, staff find this useful for coping and learning.

Facing an aggressive or violent patient can be a frightening and shocking experience, and often the response is a 'fight or flight' reaction. Being prepared for this type of incident, and knowing strategies to deal with or defuse such a situation, is of great value.

The safety of staff and other patients/customers is of paramount importance.

- Be aware of and develop systems to avoid vulnerable times and situations—e.g. pharmacy opening and closing times, a lone pharmacist, or dealing with patients with mental health problems.
- Don't attempt any heroics—your personal safety is far more important than the contents of the shop till. Hand over any money or goods demanded, because insurance cover can replace loss but not lives.
- Be aware of 'escape routes' and try not to let the patient get between you and the door.
- Ensure that you are aware of any safety procedures—e.g. panic buttons and how to activate them.
- Aim to avoid situations where you are on your own with a potentially difficult patient. If you have to go into a room alone with them, leave the door open and make sure a colleague is close by to give you back-up if necessary.
- When dealing with an aggressive or verbally abusive patient, good handling of the incident can help defuse the situation, or at least prevent it from escalating.

Don't

- Take the threatening behaviour personally.
- Be defensive or aggressive in return.
- Attempt to appease the patient by giving in to their demands, although be prepared to compromise if appropriate.
- Ignore or tolerate the behaviour.
- Be over-apologetic.
- Argue with the patient.
- Be overly sympathetic and take the patient's side.
- Use defensive or aggressive body language.

Do

- Remain calm and state your case clearly and concisely.
- Be assertive, without being aggressive.
- Maintain eye contact.
- Speak in a manner that is calm, clear, simple, slow, and non-confrontational.
- Listen to the patient and give them a chance to voice their complaints.
- Apologize if there clearly is some justification for the patient's complaint, without being overly apologetic or apportioning blame.
- Explain to the patient how to make a written complaint if they wish (frequently the patient will back down at this point).
- Call a more senior colleague if you feel out of your depth.

Limit setting

In some situations it might not be possible to avoid continued contact with a patient who has been aggressive or violent towards staff. This might be an in-patient who needs further medical care or someone attending for further out-patient appointments or repeat prescriptions (e.g. injecting drug users on opioid replacement therapy). In these cases, it might be possible to avoid further threatening incidents by setting limits.

An effective system is to draw up a contract detailing what is expected of the patient and what behaviour is considered unacceptable, and, in return, what the patient can expect from the healthcare team. The contract should state what will happen if the patient breaks the limits—usually a single warning, followed by withdrawal of services if the limits are broken again. These contracts can be very helpful in controlling patient behaviour, but it must be a two way process—healthcare staff must also stick to their side of the contract both in terms of providing care and being prepared to carry out the threat of withdrawing care if the limits are broken.

Further reading

'We don't have to take this' NHS Zero Tolerance Resource Pack. http://www.dh.gov.uk/en/Publicationsandstatistics/Publications/PublicationsPolicyAndGuidance/DH_4007545.

Dealing with distressed patients

Occasionally pharmacists might have to deal with patients who are distressed or agitated for one of the following reasons:
• their diagnosis
• difficulty in tolerating side effects
• witnessing an upsetting event with another patient
• the behaviour of visitors, other staff, or other patients.

If faced with this situation, even the busiest pharmacist should try to spend some time comforting or supporting the patient as best they can. Spending even a little time with the patient can bring considerable relief from distress:
• Do not ignore the patient, even if you are busy or unsure how to deal with the situation. If you feel you cannot deal with the situation yourself, acknowledge the patient's distress and ask if they would like you to call another member of staff.
• Ask the patient if they would like to talk to you about what it is that is upsetting them.
• Listen and don't interrupt.
• Never say 'I know how you feel'. Even if you have had to deal with the same situation yourself, it is presumptuous to state that you know how another person feels.
• If any misunderstandings or misconceptions are contributing to the patient's distress, try to correct these. If necessary, ask the medical team to talk to the patient.
• Answer any questions the patient has as honestly and openly as you can.
• Provide reassurance about symptoms that might be causing anxiety—e.g. pain can be controlled, morphine won't make them an 'addict', and side effects can be managed.
• If the patient's distress is caused by another colleague's behaviour, do not offer any comment or judgement. Listen and make a non-committal comment, such as 'I'm sorry that's how you feel'. As appropriate, suggest that they might like to speak to a senior member of staff—e.g. ward sister or senior doctor.
• Remember that silence is often as helpful as conversation. Just sitting with a patient for a few minutes while they get their emotions under control can be very helpful.
• As appropriate, physical contact, such as holding the patient's hand or touching their arm, can be a source of comfort.
• Offer practical comfort—e.g. tissues, glass of water, a chair, or privacy.
• Don't avoid the patient or the incident next time you see them, but be careful not to become too emotionally involved. A simple question like 'How are you today?' acknowledges the patient's previous distress and allows them to talk further if they wish.

Dealing with dying patients

Death is an almost daily occurrence on most wards. Although in general, patients spend most of their final year of life at home, 90% of patients spend some time in hospital and 55% die there.

As a pharmacist, you might not be as closely involved in the care of a dying patient as the nursing or medical staff, but it is still a situation that affects most pharmacists at some stage. Some pharmacists, such as those working in palliative care, oncology, or intensive care units, may be quite involved in the care of both the dying patient and their family. Learning how to deal with your own feelings, in addition to those of the patient and their family, is important.

The patient

On being told that they are dying, a patient (or their relatives) usually go through the following stages (although not all people go through every stage):

- shock/numbness
- denial
- anger
- grief
- acceptance.

It is important to let these processes happen, while supporting the patient and family sensitively.

Providing information about the illness enables the patient and family to make informed decisions about medical care and personal and social issues, and this is where you can help. Patients and relatives may perceive doctors as being too busy to answer their questions or be embarrassed to ask. A pharmacist might be perceived as having more medical knowledge (and being less busy!) than the nursing staff, but being more approachable than the medical staff.

When talking to dying patients and answering their questions, bear the following points in mind.

- Be honest—don't give the patient false hope. Answer questions as honestly and openly as possible. If the patient asks you directly whether they are dying, it is probably not appropriate for a pharmacist to confirm this. An appropriate response might be to ask why they are asking you this or to enquire what they have been already told and then formulate an appropriate response.
- Be sensitive—some patients might want lots of information about their diagnosis and care, but others might not be interested. Respect the patient's need for privacy at a difficult time but do not be afraid of talking to a dying patient—sometimes patients can feel lonely and isolated, and even a discussion lasting a few minutes can be of real benefit. Remember that different cultures have different responses to death. Whatever your own views, respect patients' religious or secular beliefs.
- Be careful—patients might not wish family or friends to know the diagnosis or that they are dying, so be especially careful what you say if other people are present.

Patients often have questions about treatment.
- Will current treatment be continued or stopped?
- Can pain or other symptoms be controlled?
- Will they become 'addicted' to morphine?
- What happens if they can no longer take medication orally?

Answer these questions as fully as you can, without overloading the patient with information. Be practical with your information and remember that some cautions become irrelevant at this stage—e.g. do not insist on NSAIDs being taken with food if the patient is not eating. If you don't feel that it is appropriate for you to answer a question, tactfully tell the patient that it would be better to ask someone more appropriate—e.g. the doctors. However, you could help the patient to formulate the question so that they feel better able to ask the doctors.

The information you provide will depend on the situation and your level of expertise. If you feel out of your depth, ask a senior colleague for advice.

Carers and relatives

Carers' and relatives' needs and questions will often be the same as the patient's, and you might need to go over some issues more than once. If the patient is going to be cared for at home, there can be many practical questions and information needs that you can answer.
- A simpler (layman's) explanation of the diagnosis and symptom management (often carers, relatives, and patients find it difficult to ask doctors for a simplified explanation).
- Coping with (potentially complex) medication regimens.
- Side effects and what to do about them.
- What to do if the patient vomits soon after taking a dose.
- Medicine storage.
- Obtaining further supplies.
- What to with unused medicines when the patient dies.
- What to do if symptoms are not controlled.
- What to do if the patient becomes too unwell to take oral medicines.

Yourself

It is important to recognize your own emotional needs, especially if your job means that you are frequently involved in the care of dying patients or if a death is especially 'close to home'. The patient or the circumstances of their illness/death might remind you of the death of a close relative or friend. This can 'open up old wounds', which you must come to terms with.

When a patient dies, you might experience various emotions.
- Sadness—a natural response to any death, but accept that it is a 'hazard' of working in healthcare.
- Relief—a prolonged or distressing illness is over.
- Grief or loss—you might have become quite attached to the patient and/or their family.
- Guilt/inadequacy—if symptoms weren't controlled or the patient's death was unexpected.

It is important to find ways to cope with this. Talking to a colleague, hospital chaplain, or close friend might help, but bear in mind that you must maintain confidentiality.

If the patient is well known to the ward/community pharmacy staff, the family might invite them to the funeral or memorial service. Attending the funeral can benefit healthcare workers, in addition to giving the family support. Consider whether your attendance could breach confidentiality. Avoid wearing a uniform, remove identification badges and bleeps, and consider whether wearing a symbol, such as a red or pink ribbon, would be inappropriate. If you are unsure whether it would be appropriate to attend, discuss it with a senior member of staff—e.g. the ward sister or your manager.

Euthanasia

It is extremely unlikely that a patient would directly ask a pharmacist to assist them to die. However, you might be aware that a patient has expressed this desire to other staff. Whatever your personal view on the morality of euthanasia, you should treat the patient the same as any other.

Euthanasia is still illegal in most countries. However, it is generally considered acceptable to give treatment that is adequate to control symptoms, even if this could shorten the duration of life, provided that the primary intent is symptom control. If you have any concerns about the appropriateness of therapy/doses in this situation, you should discuss this with the prescriber and/or a senior colleague.

What if your patient is dead in the bed?

Although not a common occurrence, clinical pharmacists can be the first to realize that a patient has died, often quietly in their bed or a chair. Here are some things to bear in mind should this happen on your round.

- Do not panic, but remain calm.
- Withdraw yourself from that patient's area and close the bed curtains, if open.
- Speak to the member of the nursing team responsible for that patient to check that they are aware of the situation.
- Consider what you feel about the incident.
- If necessary, speak to a member of the multidisciplinary team.
- Take a break to recover.
- Speak to a colleague for support.
- Continue with the day's work.
- If a relative is with the patient, they might call the pharmacist to the bed if they are concerned that the patient has died. Inform the relative that you will get a nurse to attend. Find a nurse or a member of the medical team immediately to deal with the patient, as appropriate.

It might be useful, as part of the pharmacist induction, to visit the mortuary, because dealing with death requires professional support.

Ethical dilemmas

Medical ethics deals with situations where there is no clear course of action. This might be because of a lack of scientific evidence, but it is more frequently where moral, religious, or other values have a significant influence on decision-making. Thus, medical ethics differs from research ethics; the latter is concerned with evaluating whether clinical trials are appropriate, safe, and in the best interests of the participants and/or the wider population. Many hospitals have a medical ethics committees in addition to a research ethics committee.

The issues debated by medical ethics committees are many and varied. They might produce guidelines to cover certain issues, but frequently a committee does not give a definite answer and simply provides a forum for debate. Issues debated by medical ethics committees include the following.

- Consent to or refusal of treatment, especially with respect to those unable to make decisions themselves—i.e. children or incapacitated adults.
- End-of-life issues, such as 'do not resuscitate' orders, living wills, and withdrawal of treatment.
- Organ donation and transplantation.
- Contraception and abortion.

Like most other healthcare professionals, pharmacists are expected to conduct their professional (and to a certain extent their personal) lives according to ethical principles. In the UK, the General Pharmaceutical Council (GPhC) gives advice in a code of ethics which covers many areas of pharmacy practice. However, there are occasions where pharmacists are faced with dilemmas for which there is no clear course of action.

- The pharmacist's religious beliefs or moral values are in conflict with what is expected of them—e.g. over-the-counter sale of emergency hormonal contraception.
- There is no clear scientific or evidence-based treatment available— e.g. use of unlicensed or experimental treatments.
- Business or economic issues clash with patient or public interests.

Ethical decision-making attempts to deal with these dilemmas using the following considerations.

- The values or beliefs that lie behind the dilemmas.
- The reasons people give for making a moral choice.
- Duty of care—to the patient, to their family, and to other healthcare professionals or yourself.
- Medical law.

In many instances, there is not a right or wrong answer and different people might make different—but equally justifiable—decisions based on the same set of circumstances.

It is best not to attempt to deal with ethical dilemmas alone. Depending on the situation, it is advisable to discuss the situation with the following people:
- a colleague
- the multidisciplinary team
- other interested parties, such as management, patient advocates, religious leaders or legal advisers.

Consider the following points:
- What are the patient's wishes? It is good to ask yourself 'Do I know what the patient really wants?'
- What do the patient's relatives or representatives think? Are they adequately informed to make a decision? Do they have the patient's best interests at heart? (Remember that you need to have the patient's permission to discuss the situation with their family.)
- Would you be willing for a member of your own family to be subject to the same decision-making process?
- Could the decision made in this situation adversely affect the treatment of other patients?
- Do issues of public health or interest outweigh the patient's rights?
- Is the decision or course of action legally defensible?
- Is the decision just and fair—e.g. are scarce resources being used appropriately?

It is also important to remember the following points:
- 'Do no harm' is a good basic principle, but sometimes some 'harm' must be done to achieve a greater individual or public good.
- Ensuring patient health should include mental and spiritual health in addition to physical health.
- Acting with compassion is not necessarily the same as acting ethically.
- Slavishly following scientific or evidence-based decision-making could lead to a morally inappropriate action (or lack of action).

Financial reports and budget statements

On the basis of data provided from pharmacy computer systems, pharmacists often take responsibility for providing financial information to their clinical area. Reports are generally monthly or quarterly. At the end of the financial year, an annual finance report is usually produced. Reports are usually sent to the finance manager, clinical director, and manager of a clinical area.

The objectives of a financial report are as follows.
- Relevant and timely information.
- Easy to understand and concise information.
- Verifiable and complete numbers.
- Format enables comparison.
- Reporting is consistent in form and content.
- Reports are adequate for the audience.
- Reports are periodic.
- Data ar inclusive, analytical, and comparative.
- Assumptions are attached.

Financial reports should include the following elements:
- statistical data
- financial data
- current month
- actual versus budgeted.

The type of financial information that a pharmacist supplies is as follows:
- Overall drug expenditure for a financial year by month or quarter.
- Actual drug expenditure to date.
- Projected expenditure for the current financial year and the next financial year.
- Comparison of expenditure with that of the previous financial year (e.g. by month, quarter or year).
- Analysis of expenditure by clinical areas, in-patient/out-patient/take-home medication.
- The top 20–50 high-expenditure drugs by month, quarter, or year.
- High-expenditure therapeutic areas for a specified period of time (e.g. month, quarter, or year).
- Explanation of any areas of unexpected high expenditure.
- Interpretation of financial information, detailing areas where cost savings can be made.
- Detail where cost savings have already been achieved.
- Interpretation of changes in expenditure or drug use.
- Exceptions to previous trends.

This information can be portrayed in tabular or graphical form but should be presented in ways that are easy to interpret and include a commentary. It is helpful to determine what the recipient actually wants in the report before providing financial reports.

Hospital budget statements

- The finance department often produces budget statements, which it is useful for pharmacists to understand.
- The financial year in the UK National Health Service (NHS) runs from April 1 to March 31.
- The budget statement reflects the budget that is available and the financial position at a point in a financial year.
- These budget statements include salary (pay), non-salary (non-pay), and income budgets for a department or group of departments.
- Drug budgets are included in the non-salary budget.
- The drug budget expenditure is based on the cost of drugs issued by pharmacy.
- Budget statements usually include the following information for each of the budgets:
  - the total annual budget
  - the budget available for the year to date
  - the actual budget spent for the year to date
  - the difference between the available budget and the actual budget spent (variance)
  - the percentage of budget spent to date
  - the forecast spend for the financial year
  - total financial position.
- If a budget is overspent, it is usually represented as a positive number.
- If a budget is underspent, it is usually represented as a negative number.
- Finance department budget statements should be linked to financial reports prepared by pharmacy staff (see 📖 p.84).
- Pharmacists might be asked for a breakdown of drug expenditure information.

Writing reports

Pharmacists can be required to write reports on a variety of subjects, such as the following.
- drug expenditure analysis
- evaluation of a new drug
- proposal for a new project.

A well-written and well-presented report is more likely to be read and acted on than something that is messy and incoherent. Much of the guidance given here also applies to writing business letters, e-mails, and memos (Table 4.4).

Define the aim
- What is the purpose of the report and what are you trying to achieve? Is it simply to inform the reader or is some course of action expected as a result of the report?
- Use a title that describes the aim or the content. As appropriate, write aims and objectives.
  - Aims describe what you intend to do.
  - Objectives describe how you intend to achieve the aims.

Content
The content should all be relevant to the title/aims. Look through your notes and delete any unnecessary material.
- Ensure that the content is appropriate to the readership.
  - Who are the readers?
  - What do they already know about the subject?
  - How much time will they have to read the report?
  - Might they have certain expectations of the report or preconceptions about the subject?
  - Why are you submitting this report to them?
- What type of information will you be including and how is this best presented.
  - Drug expenditure report—graphs and tables.
  - Review of papers—predominantly text.
- Review the information and classify it under headings or sections, following the suggested structure and the rules:
  - Headings should follow a logical sequence:
    — problem/cause/solution
    — chronological order
    — priority—by urgency or need
    — drug review—follow *BNF* headings, i.e. drug, indications, contraindications, and cautions.
  - Headings should clearly tell the reader what that section is about.
  - Ideally, the maximum number of items in a section is seven; otherwise there is too much information for the reader to take in at once. If necessary, subdivide sections.
  - Ensure that the content of each section is relevant to the heading.
  - Try not to repeat information in different sections.

Table 4.4 Report structure

The following is a suggested structure. Depending on the type of report, the structure can vary.

Title

Identification

Your name, department and contact details, and the date

Distribution

It might be helpful to list the following.

Those who need to take action.

Those for whom the report is for information only.

Contents

Aims and objectives

Summary or abstract

Introduction

Provides the background and context of the report

Explains why the report was written

Gives the terms of reference

Method/procedure

There should be sufficient information for the reader to understand what you did, without giving every detail

Results/findings

Discussion

The main body of the report; use section headings here

Conclusions

A re-statement of the main findings

Includes recommendations or proposals for future work

References

Use a standard system, such as the Harvard style—i.e. author, date in brackets, title of the article, journal title, volume and page numbers

Appendices

These should include information that informs the reader but is not essential on the first reading

Glossary

Explain any unusual or scientific terms or unavoidable jargon

Footnotes

Author name, date of preparation, review date, and page numbers

Layout

Even a well-written report with good content can be overlooked if it is difficult to read. A large amount of type crowded on to a page is difficult to read and the eye soon becomes tired.

- Leave wide margins at both sides and ample space at the top and bottom of each page. This also gives the reader space to write notes and ensures that print on the left-hand side doesn't disappear into the binding.
- Avoid left and right justification. Left justifying creates spaces in the text, which is easier on the eye.
- Use 1.5 or double spacing.

Bullet points and numbering

Putting information into lists using bullet points or numbering has the following benefits:

- makes it easier to read.
- has more impact.
- cuts the number of words (and waffle).

Most word processing programs offer a selection of bullet points. Keep things simple and only use one or two different types of bullet in your report.

- Use a straightforward numbering system (e.g. 1, 1.1, 1.2, 1.2.1) and avoid over-numbering (e.g. 1.2.1.1.1!).

Font

Use a font that is clear and easy to read. Use fonts without serifs ('**sans serif** '; e.g. Arial) and use a 12-point font size for the majority of the text e.g.

('**good writing**') (Gill Sans MT, 12 point)

is easier to read than

('good writing') (Times New Roman, 12 point)

or

('**good writing**') (Gill Sans MT, 10 point).

Avoid using capitals or underlining to highlight text: **bold** is easier to read than CAPITALS or underlining. People with poor literacy skills find upper-case text especially difficult to read.

For a lesson in how font style and layout affects ease of reading, compare the *Sun* newspaper with *The Times*!

Paragraphs

A paragraph should cover only one point or argument. As a rule, it should be about seven or eight lines long, and certainly no longer than 10 lines. The most important information should be in the first or last sentence of the paragraph.

Charts and tables

These should be used to convey information, usually of numerical origin, which might be too complex to describe in words. However, overuse or inappropriate use can divert the reader from the main message, making your work confusing. When deciding whether to use a chart or table consider the following points.

• Will it save words?
• Will it clarify things for the reader?
• Is the information to be presented quantifiable in some way?
• Will it help the reader to make comparisons?
• Will it help to illustrate a specific point?

In general, bar charts are the simplest charts to produce and suit most data. They are easier to interpret and less prone to be misleading than pie charts, graphs or pictograms. When using charts, consider the following points.

• Give the chart a title.
• Make sure that bars or axes start at zero.
• If comparing two charts, the axes should have the same scale.
• Label axes and bars.
• Show actual amounts on bars and pie chart slices.
• Use only two-dimensional versions—three-dimensional bars and slices can distort the relative proportions.
• Avoid overuse of colour or hatching, which might not reproduce clearly.
• Keep it simple!

Language

• Keep language simple and to the point.
• Avoid long sentences.
• Avoid foreign language phrases—e.g. *ad hoc* and *pro rata*.
• Use active rather than passive sentences—'Use paracetamol regularly for pain' is preferable to 'Paracetamol is to be used regularly for pain'.
• Avoid double negatives as these can cause confusion—'Paracetamol is not incompatible with breastfeeding' could easily be misinterpreted as 'Paracetamol is not compatible with breastfeeding'.
• Only use common abbreviations, such as 'e.g.', without explanation. Where you wish to use an abbreviation, write in full the first time, followed by the abbreviation—e.g. Royal Pharmaceutical Society (RPS). Thereafter, the abbreviation can be used.
• Avoid jargon and clichés.

Revision and editing

As much as 50% of the time spent writing a report should be devoted to revision and editing (Table 4.5).

• Print the report and check for spelling mistakes and other obvious errors (do not just rely on computer spelling and grammar checks).
• Check punctuation.
• Work through the report using the editing checklist and revise as necessary.
• Ask a colleague to read the report and make comments. Check that they interpret the information as you intended.

Table 4.5 Editing checklist

Aim

Is the aim clear?

Is the content at the right level for the reader?

If action is required as a result of the report, is this clear?

Content

Is the structure logical?

Do the conclusions follow the argument?

Are numerical data accurate and clearly presented?

Do graphs and tables achieve their aim?

Have you quoted references and sources appropriately?

Language

Are paragraphs the right length?

Have unnecessary words, double negatives, clichés, and jargon been avoided?

Are spelling and punctuation correct?

Presentation

Are abbreviations and symbols explained and used consistently throughout?

Do page breaks fall at natural breaks in the text?

Are page numbers and footers etc. included, as needed?

Does any of the text get lost on printing?

Does the whole report look tidy and professional?

Managing meetings

To manage meetings efficiently, get the best results, and use time effectively, follow the tips:

- Ensure that the agenda is understood in advance. Circulate a written agenda at least a week before the meeting, including the following points for each item to be discussed:
  - topic
  - duration
  - responsibility.
- Circulate any necessary or pertinent materials to be read before the meeting.
- The meeting should have a chairperson who must ensure that it runs smoothly and to time, allowing all participants to be involved.
- Be clear with the participants why the meeting is being held and what it will achieve.
- Ensure that at least two-thirds of the participants have a role in every topic on the agenda. Consider rearranging the agenda so that people do not waste time listening to a topic in which they have no active interest.
- Be clear what preparation is required in advance of the meeting.
- Always start and finish on time.
- Discourage deviations from the agenda and tangential topic discussions.
- Discourage AOB (any other business).
- Consider using a flip chart and record actions on it for all to see.
- Try to ensure that individuals record their actions in their diaries before leaving, and do not wait for the arrival of the 'minutes'.
- Minute-taking depends on the culture of the organization. The material to be recorded, how and by whom it is recorded, may vary between meetings and institutions.
- Minutes should be circulated as soon as possible after the meeting, ideally delaying no longer than 2wks.
- Do not hold meetings that are only for information. Minimize the use of meetings just to distribute information that could be circulated electronically.

Assertiveness

Assertiveness is an essential skill that can be learnt, developed, and practised. Applying assertive strategies enables you to stand up for yourself and express yourself appropriately and constructively.

Definition of assertiveness

- Expressing thoughts, feelings, and beliefs in a direct, honest, and appropriate way.
- Having respect for yourself and others.
- Relating well to people.
- Expressing your needs freely.
- Taking responsibility for your feelings.
- Standing up for yourself if necessary.
- Working towards a 'win–win' solution to problems.
- Ensuring that both parties have their needs met as much as possible.

Assertive people effectively influence, listen, and negotiate so that others choose to cooperate willingly. Assertiveness promotes self-confidence, self-control, and feelings of positive self-worth, and it is the most effective means for solving interpersonal problems.

Assertive behaviour

- When you differ in opinion with someone you respect, you can speak up and share your own viewpoint.
- You stand up for your rights or those of others no matter what the circumstances.
- You have the ability to correct the situation when your rights or those of others are violated.
- You can refuse unreasonable requests made by friends or co-workers.
- You can accept positive criticism and suggestion.
- You ask for assistance when you need it.
- You have confidence in your own judgement.
- If someone else has a better solution, you accept it easily.
- You express your thoughts, feelings, and beliefs in a direct and honest way.
- You try to work for a solution that, as much as possible, benefits all parties.
- You interact in a mature manner with those who are offensive, defensive, aggressive, hostile, blaming, attacking, or otherwise unreceptive.

Non-assertive behaviour

- Aggressive behaviour involves a person trying to impose their views inappropriately on others. It can be accompanied by threatening language and an angry glaring expression, and communicates an impression of disrespect.
- Submissive behaviour is the opposite of aggressive behaviour. The person plays down their own needs and is willing to fit in with the wishes of others to keep the peace. It shows a lack of respect for the person's own needs and communicates a message of inferiority. It can be accompanied by passivity, nervousness, and lack of eye contact.

- Manipulative behaviour occurs when a person seeks to ingratiate themselves with another through flattery and other forms of deceit. It can be accompanied by over-attention and a simpering smarmy voice.

Strategies for behaving more assertively

- Identify your personal rights, wants, and needs.
- Use 'I' messages to give people complete information to address a problem. 'I' messages are assertions about the feelings, beliefs, and values of the person speaking, and the sentences used begin with 'I'. The 'I' messages should include three parts.
  - Behaviour—what it is that the other person has done or is doing?
  - Effect—what is happening because of their behaviour?
  - Feelings—what effect does their behaviour have on your feelings?
- Be direct and express your request succinctly.
- Choose assertive words.
- Use factual descriptions.
- Avoid exaggerations.
- Express thoughts, feelings, and opinions reflecting ownership.
- Convey a positive assertive attitude using the following communication techniques.
  - Maintain good eye contact.
  - Maintain a firm, factual, but pleasant, voice.
  - Pay attention to your posture and gestures.
    — Stand or sit erect, possibly leaning forwards slightly, at a normal conversational distance.
    — Use relaxed conversational gestures.
  - Listen, to let people know that you have heard what they said.
  - Ask questions for clarification.
  - Look for a win–win approach to problem-solving.
  - Ask for feedback.
- Evaluate your expectations and be willing to compromise.

Examples of assertive language

- I am . . .
- I think we should . . .
- I feel bad when . . .
- That seems unfair to me.
- Can you help me with this?
- I appreciate your help.

Communication skills

Communication is a key skill for pharmacists. Every day pharmacists communicate with a variety of different groups:
- patients/customers
- other healthcare professionals
- drug company representatives
- managerial staff.

Depending on the audience and circumstances, a different approach might be required, but the core skills are the same (Tables 4.6 and 4.7).

Planning and preparation

Before any encounter, a certain amount of planning and preparation is required, even if it is just a few words with a counter assistant to establish a customer's requirements.
- Establish the most appropriate means of communication—this might be written, in the form of a letter, memo, leaflet, or verbal, such as a conversation, seminar or oral presentation, or both.
- Know the subject—if necessary, do some background reading or research. Even if it means keeping a customer waiting, a quick look in the *BNF* could mean that ultimately your message is accepted more readily because it is well informed.
- Know the audience—understanding their background, knowledge base, and requirements aids effective communication. Communicating with one person requires different strategies compared with communicating with a small or large group.
- Prepare the message—a simple straightforward piece of information, such as dosage instructions, requires little, if any, preparation.
  However, a more complex message, such as the answer to a medicines information enquiry, might require some preparation.
  - Be clear in your own mind about what message or messages you want to get across.
  - Break the message down into a series of points.
  - Structure the message so that ideas are presented in order of importance.
  - Provide a one- or two-sentence summary/conclusion at the end.
- Think ahead—try to anticipate any questions that might arise and be prepared with the information needed to answer them.

Delivering the message

Whether communicating in writing or verbally, the same rules apply.
- Use language appropriate to the audience—avoid jargon and complex terms, and use simple direct words.
- Avoid vague terms, e.g. 'occasionally' or 'frequently', because these might mean different things to different people.
- Check understanding by asking for feedback or questions.

Remember that verbal communication is made up of three aspects:
- 55% body language
- 38% tone of voice
- 7% words that make up the communication.

Listening skills (Table 4.8)

An essential part of communication is listening. Not only does this ensure your own understanding, but it shows interest and concern and empowers the respondent by enabling them to participate fully in the communication process. The traditional active/passive roles of healthcare professional talking and patient listening, respectively, are not conducive to good communication. Good listening (by both parties) ensures that the encounter has the mutual participation of healthcare professional and patient. This should lead to the information elicited being of more value; any message is more likely to be remembered and acted upon.

- Reflecting back—clarify your understanding by repeating back ('mirroring') information, but in paraphrase.
- Summarizing—'What I think I hear you saying is. . . .'
- Body language.
  - Use facial expressions and postures to show empathy.
  - Mirror facial expression.
  - Nod encouragingly.
  - Adopt a listening posture—as appropriate, lean towards the speaker while being careful to avoid invading their personal space.
  - Maintain eye contact.
  - Avoid signs of impatience or being in a hurry.
- Ask open-ended questions—e.g. how and why.
- Use closed questions, as appropriate–i.e. those with a 'yes' or 'no' response.
- Use silences appropriately.
  - Allow the speaker to finish what they want to say and avoid the temptation to jump in.
  - Do not interrupt or finish the speaker's sentences.
  - If necessary, allow a short period of silence to elapse, especially if the speaker is slow or hesitant in their speech.
  - Silences can be helpful in giving thinking time.
- Use verbal or non-verbal signals to show that you are listening and encourage the speaker—e.g. nodding and saying 'yes' or 'mm'.
- If necessary, note down key points while the other person is speaking, but avoid scribbling throughout. Warn the speaker that you will be doing this so that they don't find it off-putting.
- In responding, avoid the following.
  - Exclamations of surprise, intolerance, or disgust.
  - Expression of over-concern.
  - Moralistic judgements, criticism, or impatience.
  - Being defensive and getting caught up in arguments.
  - Making false promises, flattery, or undue praise.
  - Personal references to your own difficulties.
  - Changing the subject or interrupting unnecessarily.
  - Speaking too soon, too often, or for too long.

Questioning

Questioning is also an important skill for communicating effectively. As pharmacists, this often involves direct questioning of a colleague regarding a course of action or prescribing decision. However, when dealing with patients, a broader approach might be required to obtain all the information required.

- Use open questions to enable the respondent to elaborate and give new information—e.g. 'How are you getting on with your medications'?
- Phrasing questions in different ways often elicits different information—e.g. asking 'Do you have any problems with your medicines?' can elicit more information than asking 'Do you have any side effects?'.
- Avoid leading questions, e.g. 'You're not getting any side effects are you?', because usually the respondent will give the answer that they think the questioner wants (in this case, 'No').
- Closed questions can be used to establish specific information—e.g. 'Are you taking this medicine with food?'
- Be specific because the respondent might interpret certain terms differently to you—e.g. 'Are you taking these medicines regularly?' could mean the respondent is taking them once daily, once weekly, or once monthly!
- Avoid questions that the respondent might interpret as being judgemental or critical.
- As appropriate, ensure that you understand the answer by paraphrasing it back to the respondent—e.g. 'Just to be clear, I think you are saying . . .'.

Table 4.6 Barriers to good communication

Physical barriers

- Speech problems
- Hearing impairment
- Communicating in a language that is not the audience's first language or through a translator
- Visual impairment
- Learning difficulties
- Noisy or distracting environment

Emotional barriers

- Preconceptions and prejudice
- Fear
- Aggression

Table 4.7 Checklist of essential interpersonal skills to improve communication

- Body language:
  - be aware of body language when interacting with people
  - mirror body language
  - ensure that body language, tone, and words are sending out the same messages
- Rapport with people
- Social poise, self-assurance, and confidence
- Tact and diplomacy
- Consideration of others
- Assertiveness and self-control
- High standards
- Ability to analyse facts and solve problems
- Tolerance and patience
- Ability to make good decisions
- Honesty and objectivity
- Organizational skills
- Good listening habits
- Enthusiasm
- Persuasiveness
- Ability to communicate with different types of people

Table 4.8 Ten ways to become a better listener

- Schedule a time and place to listen
- Create comfort
- Avoid distractions
- State the reasons for the conversation
- Use non-verbal signals
- Use reflection, paraphrasing, and summarizing
- Listen for the message behind the emotions
- Be patient
- Write down any commitments
- Follow up

Oral presentation skills

Pharmacists often make presentations to a variety of audiences. These can be both formal and informal. Some suggestions on how to prepare and effectively deliver an oral presentation:

- Know the expected duration of the presentation.
- Know the composition of the audience.
- Know the format—e.g. workshop or formal presentation.
- Know about the facilities—e.g. availability of audiovisual aids.
- Prepare approximately one slide per 1–2min of presentation.
- Find out whether you are expected to supply handouts to the audience, how many, and what level they should be aimed at.
- Check whether you are expected to send the presentation slides in advance, and, if so, the timelines for this.
- Plan and prepare your presentation.
- A presentation usually consists of three parts.
  - Tell the audience what you are going to talk about.
  - Talk about it.
  - Tell the audience what you told them.
- Always take a back-up option for the presentation—have the presentation saved on more than one USB stick and take a paper copy to refer to if the technology fails.
- Arrive at the presentation in plenty of time to ensure that the equipment can be tested or your presentation can be downloaded.
- Familiarize yourself with the venue and the equipment available— e.g. pointer or computer equipment.
- Ensure that you are not blocking the audience's view of your slides from where you are standing.
- Check that your slides are in focus.
- Look at the audience and NOT the screen!
- Make sure you look at ALL of the audience, so that they all feel included.
- Minimize how much you move around.
- Ensure that the audience can hear you.
- Introduce yourself, why you are presenting, and your background experience to the subject.
- Use a pointer to highlight points of data; avoid overuse and excessive circling.
- Involve the audience by asking questions or for input, as appropriate.
- Ask if the audience have any questions. Depending on the time and format, invite questions during the presentation and/or at the end.
- When responding to questions, consider repeating the question asked so that all audience members can hear the question and response, and to ensure that the question was understood.

Prioritizing

Pharmacists can be called upon to undertake a variety of tasks. Work often has to be prioritized to use time effectively and to complete tasks in a timely manner. The ability to understand the priorities of others and to prioritize your own work is a very important skill to learn. Some tips on prioritizing:

- When deciding the priority of a particular task, consider both its importance (is it worth doing?) and its urgency (does it need to be done right now?):
- Figure 4.1 shows a useful tool for prioritizing your work—write tasks in the boxes according to whether they fit the labels.
  - Urgent and important tasks take first priority.
  - Important tasks that are not urgent take second priority.
  - Unimportant tasks that are also not urgent take lowest priority.
- When deciding whether to do a particular task, consider the number of people it affects and the cost of undertaking the task.
- Numbered daily checklists are often helpful.
- To understand the priorities of others requires excellent communication skills, especially the ability to ask good-quality questions, listen to the answers, and notice body language.
- Knowing where your plan fits into the plans of others is useful in predicting problems, solving problems, and influencing solutions.
- Knowing where your plan fits in your own organization's priorities ensures access to and release of resources.

Fig. 4.1 Tool for prioritizing work—write tasks in the boxes according to where they fit the labels.

Project planning

The purpose of a project plan is to determine and facilitate the achievement of a set of objectives, i.e. achievement of milestone objectives en route to achievement of goal objectives. Planning is done in the context of the stated mission of the organization and the vision of the organization. Planning is about the following:

• Ensuring that every individual involved knows what to do, when, how, where, and why.
• Communicating the plans to those who need to be confident that the ambitions will be delivered to the specification required, on time, and within budget.
• Forecasting what might occur in order that action can be taken to achieve the desired goal and avoid undesirable outcomes.
• Making decisions about actions that will be taken prior to and during anticipated situations.

A project plan needs to be broken down into tasks that need to be done, and then sequencing the tasks in a logical order. Tasks are actions. Accurate identification of the tasks is essential as they are the basis of:

• developing schedules
• identifying milestones
• implementing change plans
• planning communication
• resource planning: manpower, materials, and machinery
• monitoring
• maintaining records
• managing risk
• measuring progress
• forecasting remaining work.

It can be useful to complete a one-page summary of each task that contains all the information needed to delegate the responsibility for completion of the task to one person, as each task is effectively a 'mini-project'.

The quickest and most effective way to produce outline plans is to do it in five phases.

1. Describe the scope of the project.
2. Identify the tasks.
3. Schedule the tasks into a sensible order that will achieve the outcome of the plan.
4. Identify milestones. Milestones are the significant objectives that are to be achieved on the way to completing the project, and serve as visible indications of progress. They enable people to know that the plan is being implemented without having to know the details.
5. Implement the plan.

When scoping the project, the questions to be considered are as follows.
- Obtain a simple description.
- Why it is being considered?
- Where does it fit with other projects?
- What are the benefits to the organization?
- What are the downsides or penalties of not doing it?
- What are the major issues?
- What are the risks?
- What are the measures of success?
- What is the return on investment? Obtain a summary for this.
- What are the names of key stakeholders and stakeholder groups?
- Get an indication of whether to invest resources in a project plan.

Software is available to help with project planning and the production of time flowcharts (Gantt charts).

Time management

Quick techniques for managing time include the following.
- The four Rs of paperwork:
  - recycle (bin)
  - refer (out-tray and delegation)
  - respond
  - record (file).
- Invest time, don't spend it.
- De-clutter.
- Use a system for time management:
  - Use a list system to write down ideas, thoughts, and tasks as you think of them.
  - Use a diary system.
  - Use a name and address system.
  - Bracket tasks, appointments, and travel time.
  - Set time limits, with interruptions.
  - Use 'scrap time' wisely.
  - Take frequent quick breaks to ↑ productivity.
  - Do the most important tasks first.
  - Or, do the fastest and easiest tasks first.
  - Demand completed work from your staff.
  - Communicate upwards when you have problems:
    — description of problem
    — list of possible solutions
    — recommended solution
    — list of necessary resources
    — implementation of the solution.

Using Medicines Information services

The Medicines Information (UKMI) service is a countrywide network comprising two national (Wales and Northern Ireland),14 regional, and 220 local MI centres. Local services range from one pharmacist, providing information part-time, to a large centre, with pharmacists, technicians, and administrative staff. Most MI centres provide an information service to hospital-based and community-based enquirers, including members of the public, but some only answer enquiries from within their NHS trust. For both community pharmacists and hospital pharmacists, it is a good idea to check who provides the MI service for your area.

Some centres provide a specialist information service (Table 4.9) but it is usually advisable to contact your local service first. Remember to contact local specialists as well, because advice from another centre might not reflect local practice.

Before contacting your MI centre with an enquiry, do some basic research. Most MI centres expect pharmacist colleagues to have checked basic sources before contacting them—e.g. BNF, Summary of Product Characteristics, and Martindale. Before contacting the MI centre, try to anticipate what background information they might require and have this ready. Depending on the type of enquiry, this might include the following:

• Drug details, including dose, route, formulation, brand, and indication.
• Patient details, including underlying condition, relevant laboratory results, age, weight, and past medical history.
• The identity of the original enquirer.
• Urgency.
• Contact details.
• Whether a written or verbal response is required.
• Any sources already checked for information and what was found.
• ADRs—nature of reaction, timing of the event, other drugs, any de-challenge/re-challenge and the outcome.
• Pregnancy—number of weeks gestation, whether or not the drug has already been taken by the mother, and indication.
• Breastfeeding—age, weight, medical status of infant, and whether the treatment is short or long term.
• Drug interactions—which drugs/drug classes are involved and the nature of the event, if a suspected interaction has already occurred.

After the enquiry is complete, it is really helpful if you feed back the outcome to your MI centre. It is rare that they hear what happened as a result of the answer given, and it is useful information to add to their enquiry records. Remember to fill in a yellow card for any significant ADRs (see 📖 p.18).

Further reading

www.ukmi.nhs.uk
www.nelm.nhs.uk

Table 4.9 UKMI specialist information centres

Specialist topic	Centre
Drugs in pregnancy	Wolfson Unit Regional Drugs and Therapeutics Centre (Newcastle)
Drugs in lactation	Trent and West Midlands MIC
Complementary medicine	Welsh MIC
Drugs in cardiothoracics	Royal Brompton and Harefield NHS Foundation Trust MIC
Drugs in dentistry	North West MIC
Medicines in children	Alder Hey Royal Liverpool Children's Trust MIC
Drugs in liver impairment	Leeds MIC
Drugs in renal impairment	South West MIC
Drugs in porphyria	Welsh MIC
Drugs in psychiatry	Pharmacy Department, Maudsley Hospital
Ophthalmic drugs	Moorfields Hospital MIC
HIV/AIDS	Chelsea and Westminster Hospital MIC
Toxicology and poisoning (not emergency enquiries)	Wolfson Unit Regional Drugs and Therapeutics Centre (Newcastle)/Regional Medicines and Poisons Information Centre, Northern Ireland

Contact details are on the UKMI website: www.ukmi.nhs.uk

Clinical trials

Clinical trial regulations 108
Licensing of a clinical trial 109
Clinical trial development phases 110
Trial design, randomization, and blinding 111
European Clinical Trials Directive 112
Clinical trials: hospital pharmacy guidance 114
Ethical committees 116

Clinical trial regulations

Clinical trials form a fundamental part in the research, development, and licensing of new medicines. Research of how the drug interacts in humans is essential to ensure safe and effective medicines are licensed as new treatments. It is an exciting and varied role at the cutting edge of modern research with trials ranging across all therapeutic specialities. Clinical Trial pharmacists are therefore required to have a broad clinical knowledge and a specialist knowledge of the regulations that clinical trials have to follow.

New regulations were introduced in 2004 to help regulate the field of clinical trials in human subjects. The European Clinical Trials Directive (2001/20/EC) was implemented across the European Union (EU) in 2004 and transposed into local law (Statutory Instrument (SI)1031 in the UK). Its primary aim is to ensure that patient safety is paramount in all clinical trials. Its secondary aim is to ensure the integrity of the data that is collected so that the decisions that are made from the outcomes of the trial are representative of true effects of the medicine and not due to bias in the trial.

All clinical trials involving investigational medicinal products (unlicensed drugs in a clinical trial) have to follow the principles outlined as good clinical practice (GCP). This is a defined quality standard devised by the International Conference on Harmonisation (ICH) which provides guidelines on how clinical trials should be conducted and defines the roles and responsibilities of clinical trial sponsors, clinical research investigators, and monitors.

GCP aims to ensure that the safety of the patient and the integrity of the data collected are paramount at all times. The guidelines include protection of the human rights of subjects in a clinical trial and provide assurance of the safety and efficacy of the newly developed compounds. Everyone involved in running a clinical trial (clinicians, nursing staff, pharmacists, radiologists, etc.) must have GCP training to ensure that they complete their role to the required standard.

Licensing of a clinical trial

Before a clinical trial starts, the following authorizations/approvals must be obtained:

- Clinical trial authorization from a competent authority—in the UK this is the Medicines and Healthcare Products Regulatory Agency (MHRA).
  - The competent authority must consider the application within 60 days (maximum). This application can run in parallel with the ethics opinion.
  - This application outlines the design and outcomes of the trial so that the competent authority can assess whether the trial safe to conduct.
  - The competent authority must notify the sponsor within 35 days if there are grounds for refusal.
- A favourable opinion from one ethics committee, if the trial is deemed ethical to complete.
- Permission from the NHS trust for the trial to take place within that trust (R&D approval) for each site. This now also includes an opinion on the suitability of the local investigator and facilities (used to be obtained from the local research ethics committee).
- A EudraCT number must be obtained from the EudraCT database. The EudraCT number is a unique number allocated to each trial by the competent authority (MHRA). The EudraCT database registers details of all trials approved in the EU.
- The MHRA enforces these standards in the UK by performing inspections of GCP and good manufacturing practice (GMP). The MHRA is also responsible for ensuring that suitable safety monitoring occurs in all clinical trials.
- There is no distinction between commercial and non-commercial trials, and there are no exemptions for any trials using a drug that is prescribed outside of its licence.
- All clinical trials will follow a protocol which will contain detailed information about the design of the trial and the drugs involved. All processes and requirements outlined in the trial must be followed as the protocol will have been written in compliance with GCP to ensure the study follows the required regulations.

Clinical trial development phases

The development of new drugs has four phases of clinical trials in humans. These trials can only occur following extensive modelling of the effects of drugs and testing in animals.

Phase I trials

- First time that the drug is given to humans.
- Provide data on the tolerability of a range of doses and assess Maximum tolerated dose (MTD) and toxicity of a drug used for the first time in humans.
- Provide data on pharmacokinetics and pharmacodynamics of the drug.
- Often designed to start at a single low dose, which is gradually increased depending on the side effects until the MTD is reached.
- Usually only involve small numbers of participants, and are usually undertaken in healthy volunteers unless it is unethical (e.g. cytotoxic drugs must be tested in cancer patients).

Phase II trials

- Usually the first time that the drug is given to a patient with the disease state it is thought to treat (with the exception of anti-cancer drugs). Often called proof of concept studies.
- Assess efficacy and define therapeutic dose range and dosing regimen for a specific indication, with minimum side effects.
- Provide further information on safety, pharmacokinetics, and pharmacodynamics in the presence of the disease process.
- Provide information on the doses that should be tested in phase III studies.
- Relatively small numbers of patients are studied under close supervision, usually by specialized investigators.

Phase III trials

- Assess treatment outcomes in a variety of patients approximating to the population of patients who will receive the drug once it is launched.
- Often compare new treatments with existing treatments.
- Aim to demonstrate long-term safety and tolerance.
- Undertaken in large numbers of patients, often in multiple centres across the globe.

Phase IV trials

- Performed after a product licence is obtained.
- Aim to investigate the incidence of relatively rare ADRs or to compare drugs with comparative treatments, often to extend the range of approved indications.

Trial design, randomization, and blinding

- The most robust trials include blinding and randomization.
- Controlled clinical trials compare a test treatment with another treatment or placebo agent. These can be designed as parallel or crossover studies.
  - Parallel studies assign patients to receive one study treatment only. They do not receive the other agent during the trial, i.e. the two groups of patients continue in the study 'in parallel'.
  - Crossover studies assign patients to receive one study treatment for a set period of time and, following a washout period, the same patients receive the second treatment.
- Randomized trials assign treatments to successive patients in a predetermined random way.
  - Randomized trials aim to show that one treatment is superior to another, and they avoid investigator bias.
  - Patients are randomly allocated to the new drug, or an existing recognized treatment, or a placebo agent, which provides comparisions for treatment outcomes.
- These trials are often blinded.
  - Open-label studies—no one is blinded and everyone is aware of which treatment has been administered.
  - Single-blind study—the investigator or assessor does not know which treatment has been administered but the patient is aware.
  - Double-blind study—neither the subject nor the investigator knows which treatment has been given. This is the preferred type of study. Often the pharmacist is the only person who is aware of which subject is receiving which treatment. ▶ Care must be taken to ensure that participants in the trial are not inadvertently unblinded as this can introduce bias to the outcomes of the study and invalidate the trial.

Controlled randomized double-blind parallel-group studies are the reference standard for comparing treatments.
- There can be problems with blinding in a clinical trial.
  - If the drugs have obvious differences—e.g. IV versus oral forms, different looking or tasting tablets/capsules.
  - When ADRs are associated with only one arm of the trial.
  - Ethical issues of withholding information from patients on the exact treatment they are receiving.
- When trials are blinded, mechanisms must be in place (ideally accessible 24 hours a day) to ensure that individuals can be unblinded in the case of emergencies.
- If an attending clinician needs information about a patient participating and needs information about treatment options, the worst-case scenario is usually to treat as if the patient is on active treatment.
  - Many clinical trials now have web pages containing information on the treatments involved and contact information for emergencies. There is usually a study identifier (a shortened name of the title) which can be researched on Google to provide additional information.

European Clinical Trials Directive

The Clinical Trials Directive provides regulations that need to be followed for all clinical trials to ensure patient safety. The Clinical Trials Directive was first implemented in 2004 and there have been three subsequent amendments to ensure that it covers current requirements and has been expanded to include blood products used in a clinical trial. The latest amendment was completed in 2008 and was transposed in the UK in SI 2008/941.

There are some specific requirements within the Directive that are particularly relevant to pharmacy or are in areas where pharmacists can help ensure compliance:

- Trials have to be under the control of a named sponsor. The sponsor is the person legally responsible for the conduct of a clinical trial. This is usually the chief executive of the body registered as the sponsor (this can be a pharmaceutical company or a clinician in a hospital trust or university department). This person is responsible for ensuring that the required systems are in place and that all the regulations are complied with.
- All staff involved in clinical trials must have evidence of suitable training in their CPD log.
- All sites who manufacture, label, or assemble clinical trial materials must hold an Investigational Medicinal Product Manufacturing Authorization (MIA(IMP)).
- Hospitals or healthcare centres with patients who are participating in a clinical trial fall under the Section 37 exemption within SI 1030. This allows a pharmacist (or a person under their authorization) to reconstitute, assemble, or label a clinical trial material without this license. This does not allow pharmacies to manufacture a drug. Definitions of what constitutes manufacture and what is reconstitution are available from the MHRA.
- An individual in the pharmacy department will be named as the responsible pharmacist for clinical trials within that hospital or trust. This pharmacist must liaise with the trust's research and development department to ensure that the trials are valid and acceptable. They are also the contact person for any pharmaceutical company or investigator who wish to run a clinical trial within that hospital.
- Clinical trial protocols must be made available to the pharmacy department in advance of consideration by an ethics committee, so that the practical details, such as doses and method of administration, packaging, labelling, and study documentation appropriate for each individual trial, can be checked. The protocol must specify the duration of and responsibility for the storage of all pharmacy records relating to the trial.
- Failure to comply with the EU clinical trials directive is a criminal offence.
- On completion of a clinical trial the sponsor must notify the competent authority within 90 days of the conclusion of the trial.

- If the trial terminates early, the sponsor must notify the competent authority within 15 days.
- The competent authority can suspend or terminate any trial if there are doubts about the safety or scientific validity.

In summary, the Clinical Trials Directive sets standards to ensure the following.

- Safety of clinical trial participants.
- Quality assurance of clinical trials and investigational medicinal products (IMPs).
- An appropriate regulatory approval system for clinical trials in the EU.
- Ethics committees were established on a statutory basis.
- Appropriate requirements for the manufacture, import, and labelling of IMPs.
- Manufacture and labelling of clinical trial drugs are compliant with GMP.
- Adequate safety monitoring of patients participating in trials.
- Procedures for reporting and recording ADRs.

Clinical trials: hospital pharmacy guidance

All investigational medicinal products (IMPs) used in a clinical trial should be received from an approved EU supplier and must be verified by a qualified person (QP) from within the EU. Any supplies manufactured outside the EU must be imported into the EU with an import licence.

Receipt of supplies

The pharmacy department is responsible for maintaining the traceability of all IMPs used in the trial.

- All clinical trial supplies should be checked on receipt to ensure that they have been received in good condition and are in accordance with the shipping paperwork.
- Receipt of supplies may need to be acknowledged. This can be done using an electronic system or by faxing the paperwork back to the company who shipped the drug. This is to ensure that the supplies reached their intended destination.

Storage and handling

- All IMPs must be handled by the pharmacy department in a hospital/trust.
- IMPs must be kept in a separate secure storage area, with sufficient segregation to ensure that there is no confusion between trial materials.
- The designated pharmacist should ensure that the formulation, presentation, and storage of clinical trial medications are appropriate.
- Records of storage conditions must be kept.
- Clinical trial medication must be dispensed against appropriate prescription forms, which have been agreed by the trial investigators and pharmacy department and which help to identify clearly that the subject is participating in a clinical trial.
- Each clinical trial drug prescription must contain the agreed title of the study and a protocol number unique to the study to enable the study to be easily identified and avoid confusion.
- The pharmacy department should be involved in the reconciliation and disposal of unused medication. Guidance is available from the regional quality assurance pharmacists' document on waste disposal.

Labelling, packaging, and stability issues

- All IMP labels must comply with labelling requirements for IMPs, as outlined in Annex 13 of the GMP guide.
- Pharmacists, and those working under their supervision, do not need to hold a manufacturing authorization to repackage or change the packaging of clinical trial materials if this is done in a hospital or health centre for patients of that establishment.

Documentation and records

- The pharmacy department must keep appropriate records of the dispensing of clinical trial drugs and detailed drug accountability.

- Clinical trial documentation should be retained in the pharmacy for the life of the trial, and must be retained for a minimum of 15 years and in the case of a paediatric trial until the subject is 21 years of age.
- All training must be documented and available for inspection. Only people who are suitably trained in the trial procedures should be involved in the running of the trial.
- Clinical trial randomization codes should be held in the pharmacy department. Arrangements for the codes to be broken outside normal pharmacy working hours must be made. Criteria for code breaking should be available and records made in the relevant trial documentation.
- Departmental standard operating procedures must be in place, which are suitably version-controlled and reviewed at regular intervals.

Charging for clinical trials
- The pharmacy department should have a standard method of charging for clinical trials, which has been agreed with the R&D department.
- Arrangements should be made for the levy of prescription charges in accordance with current guidance.
  - Prescription charges do not apply in trials where patients could receive a placebo substance.
  - A prescription charge should be levied (subject to the usual prescription charge exemption criteria) for trials comparing active substances or different doses of an active substance.

Ethical committees

The EU directive (2001/20/EC) ensures that there are national ethics committees operating within a legal framework, with firm deadlines for approval. The UK ethics review system is the National Research Ethics Service (NRES).

The composition of a research ethics committee is as follows.
- 12–18 members (lay and medical).
- Balanced age and gender distribution.
- Subcommittees encouraged.
- Lead reviewers suggested.
- Quorum of seven members stipulated and defined.
- Co-opted members allowed, as defined, to ensure the balance of the committee is maintained.

Ethics committees consider the following.
- The relevance of the clinical trial and trial design.
- Whether the evaluation of the anticipated benefits and risks are satisfactory and conclusions justified.
- The protocol.
- The suitability of the investigator and supporting staff.
- The Investigators' Brochure (document that details results of previous trials and the chemical composition of the IMP).
- The quality of the facilities.
- The consent form and patient information sheet.
- The procedure to be followed for obtaining informed consent.
- Justification for research on persons incapable of giving informed consent.
- The arrangements for the recruitment of subjects.
- Provision for indemnity or compensation in the event of injury or death.
- Insurance or indemnity to cover the liability of the investigator and sponsor.
- The arrangements for rewarding or compensating investigators and trial subjects, including the amount, and the relevant aspects of any agreement between the sponsor and the site.

Timelines for ethics committees
- Ethics committees meet monthly.
- The ethics committee has a maximum of 60 days from the date of receipt of the valid application to give its 'reasoned opinion'.
- Ethics committees must give favourable opinions within 35 days.
- There might be a single request for supplementary information.
- There is no extension to the 60-day period except for trials involving gene therapy, somatic cell therapy, or xenogenic cell therapy.

Pharmacists advising ethics committees

Pharmacists advising ethics committees should be able to use their pharmaceutical expertise to advise on issues including the following.

- Quality assurance.
- GCP issues.
- GMP issues.
- Storage.
- Issues surrounding drug administration—e.g. blinding.
- Monitoring ADRs.
- Clinical trial design and randomization.
- Licensing arrangements for the trial.
- Indemnity arrangements for the trial.
- Safety and efficacy of any drugs involved.
- Appropriateness of the proposed dosage regimens.
- Appropriateness of the formulation.
- The method of monitoring compliance with drug regimens.
- Patient education.
- Continuing supply of medications for 2 years following the trial.
- Availability of a QP (if required).

Further reading

Medicines Healthcare Regulatory Agency: www.mhra.gov.uk.
Clinical Trials Toolkit: www.ct-toolkit.ac.uk.
NRES website: www.nres.npsa.nhs.uk.
Royal Pharmaceutical Society: www.rpharms.com.
European Clinical Trials Directive (2001/20/EC).
The Medicines for Human Use (Clinical Trials) Regulations 2004 – SI 2004/1031.
The Medicines for Human Use (Clinical Trials) Amendment Regulations 2006–SI 2006/1928..
The Medicines for Human Use (Clinical Trials) Amendment (No. 2) Regulations 2006–SI 2006/2984.
The Medicines for Human Use (Clinical Trials) and Blood Safety and Quality (Amendment) Regulations 2008 – SI 2008/941.
Day S (2007). *Dictionary for Clinical Trials*. John Wiley.
Raven A (1997). *Consider it Pure Joy, Introduction to Clinical Trials* (3rd edn). Cambridge Healthcare Research.

Controlled drugs

Suspected loss of controlled drugs within hospitals *120*
Patients' own controlled drugs in a hospital setting *122*

Suspected loss of controlled drugs within hospitals

Ward or clinic level

On discovering a discrepancy in a stock balance two nurses, midwives, or operating department practitioners (ODPs) must immediately check the following.

- All requisitions received have been entered on the correct page of the record book(s).
- Administered controlled drugs prescribed for in-patients have been entered into the Controlled Drug Record Book (or Patients' Own Controlled Drug Record Book).
- No item has been accidentally put in the wrong place or cupboard.
- All calculations of previous balance checks are correct.

If the error or omission is traced, the two nurses, midwives, or ODPs must make an entry in the Controlled Drug Record Book (or the Patients' Own Controlled Drug Record Book), clearly stating the reasons for the entry and the correct balance, and sign the entry.

If no reason for the error or omission is found it must be reported to the ward pharmacist (if available—resident pharmacist out of hours) without delay, and an incident form and suspected loss of controlled drug form completed.

If the pharmacist confirms the discrepancy, the Accountable Officer must be informed immediately by the pharmacist.

The Health Act 2006 created a new role of Accountable Officer for controlled drugs who is charged with the responsibility for the safe, appropriate, and effective management and use of controlled drugs within their organization.

It is the responsibility of the Accountable Officer or Chief Pharmacist to inform the police if criminal activity is reasonably suspected. The police should NOT be contacted by ward staff unless instructed to do so.

If theft by a member of staff involving controlled drugs is witnessed or there is strong suspicion that a member of staff has diverted a controlled drug for their own purposes, the senior nurse, midwife, or ODP in charge of the shift should deal with the issue as for any other witnessed or suspicion of theft situation as this falls under a performance and conduct issue. They must also inform the pharmacist (if available—resident pharmacist out of hours) without delay who will immediately inform the senior pharmacist on call who will in turn inform security, the Accountable Officer, and the Chief Pharmacist. The police should not be involved without prior permission from the Accountable Officer and the Chief Pharmacist.

The record of suspected losses should be reported to the clinical governance committee, or a similar body, that has responsibility for the administration of medicines.

Notes for the investigating pharmacist

On investigating identified discrepancies, it is good practice to check the following initially.

- Arithmetic details in the register.
- Identify the time interval when the suspected drug balance was correct.
- Enquire about the probable number of staff who could have had access to the keys for controlled drug storage during the investigated period.
- Check whether the senior nurse has organized all administrations for the drug to be checked against the patient's drug chart during the time period being investigated.
- Ensure that regular checks of controlled drug stocks have been performed.
- Check when nurse and pharmacist stock accountability was last undertaken.

Note that small discrepancies involving liquid preparations are not uncommon, but could need to be monitored in case a pattern emerges.

If an arithmetical error explains the loss, it is not usually considered necessary to complete an incident form or report the incident to senior managers.

Hospital pharmacy department

Suspicion of loss must be reported immediately to the appropriate manager—e.g. the dispensary manager or stores manager. The manager must undertake an inventory check and decide if staff are following the department's standing operating procedures for receipt and supply of controlled drugs. It is GCP to check the following.

- Arithmetic details in the register.
- Identify the time interval when the suspected drug balance was correct.
- Department's standard operating procedures have been complied with—e.g. only designated staff have access to operate in controlled drug preparation area, including out-of-hours staff, and that all such staff have received appropriate training.
- Receipt and invoice procedures are in place.
- Access to the department by visitors is enforced and visitors have no access to controlled drug preparation areas.
- All supply requisitions are checked.

If a discrepancy exists, the loss should be submitted in writing to the Chief Pharmacist and Accountable Officer, who should review the standard operating procedures. The incident should be reported to the clinical governance committee, or a similar body, that has responsibility for medicine management.

The decision to involve an external investigator must be undertaken with the involvement of the Chief Pharmacist and the Accountable Officer.

Patients' own controlled drugs in a hospital setting

Patients admitted into hospital

Patients' own controlled drugs refer to those drugs brought in by patients when admitted to hospital and those that may be supplied as part of discharge medication (TTO).

Whenever a patient is admitted with his/her own controlled drug(s) they should be encouraged to return these home via an identified adult. Responsibility for security is given to the adult, and therefore it is essential that this is recorded in the patient notes/care plan. They do not need to be entered in the Patients Own Controlled Drug Record Book unless considered as an added documented precaution.

If a patient is admitted with his/her own controlled drugs and it has been decided to retain the patient on the ward, two registered nurses should check these into the ward's Patients' Own Controlled Drugs Register.

The drug and its form, strength, and quantity should be checked, and the drug(s) should then placed in a controlled drugs cupboard, with the details entered in a separate Patients' Own Controlled Drugs Record Book.

The patients name must be written on the label. If unlabelled strips of medicine are brought in, these should not be administered to the patient and the supplies should be highlighted to a pharmacist, who should organize their destruction or return to the patient, or their relative, on discharge.

Use of patients' own controlled drugs

Ideally, the use of the patients own supplies for in-patients should be restricted to the following.
- Non-formulary drugs or drugs which are otherwise unavailable.
- While awaiting supplies from the pharmacy.
- Administration records should be completed on the relevant page of the Patients' Own Controlled Drugs Record Book.

Nurses should be encouraged to order supplies from their pharmacy as soon as feasible.

Return of patients' own controlled drugs

When the patient goes home, their medicines must be signed out of the Patients' Own Controlled Drug Record Book by the patient's nurse/ midwife, which should be checked by a second nurse/midwife and handed directly to the patient, assuming that the nurse has previously checked that the patient's drug and labelled dose schedule hasn't changed during the in-patient stay.

A patient's own controlled drug should never be used to treat other patients but must be returned to the patient before their discharge if there is no change to the prescription. If they have been issued with a new and revised prescription for controlled drugs, those brought in with them must be returned to pharmacy as soon as is practical after the patient has been discharged.

Disposal and destruction of controlled drugs including patients own medicines

A controlled drug ceases to be classified as a controlled drug once it has been rendered irretrievable, i.e. all controlled drugs, once disposed of, should be unrecognizable as controlled drugs and non-usable as a controlled drug.

Only small amounts of controlled drugs can be destroyed on wards—e.g. the surplus when a dose smaller than the total ampoule or vial is drawn up, when a dose is drawn up but not used, broken ampoules of controlled drugs, or left-over syringe/opiate infusion residue.

For all other controlled drugs (e.g. expired stocks, PODs, and excess stock) the pharmacist responsible for the ward or department MUST be notified. these controlled drugs MUST NOT be destroyed on the ward.

Wards and departments who do not receive a routine pharmacy visit, must either arrange for a pharmacist to come to the ward or agree a mutually convenient time for the nurse, midwife, or ODP to take their controlled drugs and the Controlled Drug Record Book to the Pharmacy, where a pharmacist will sign for their return.

The process for destruction of controlled drugs in pharmacy should be found in your Local Standard Operating Procedure

Records of destruction

All destruction must be documented in the appropriate section of the Controlled Drug Record Book or the Patients' Own Controlled Drug Record Book. It must be witnessed by a second person who may be another nurse, midwife, ODP, doctor, or pharmacist.

Evidence-based medicine

Evidence-based medicine (EBM) and clinical pharmacy 126
Statistical versus clinical significance 128
Odds ratios and relative risk 130
Binary and continuous data 132
L'Abbé plots 133
Mean difference and standardized mean difference 134
Assessing the quality of randomized studies 136
Critical appraisal of systematic reviews 138
Critical assessment of papers 140
Guidelines 143
Number needed to treat (NNT) 144
Confidence intervals 147

Evidence-based medicine (EBM) and clinical pharmacy

EBM has become standard practice during recent years, although it is probably more widely practised in primary care in the UK. The following definition of EBM can be adapted for clinical pharmacy.

Definition of EBM

> EBM is the conscientious, explicit and judicious use of current best evidence in making decisions about the care of individual patients.[1]

The authors of the definition go on to state that the practice of EBM requires the integration of individual clinical expertise with the best available external clinical evidence from systematic research.

The second definition comes from the McMaster University website:

> EBM is an approach to healthcare that promotes the collection, interpretation and integration of valid, important and applicable patient-reported, clinician-observed and research-derived evidence. The best available evidence, moderated by patient circumstances and preferences, is applied to improve the quality of clinical judgements.[2]

Evidence-based clinical pharmacy

Borrowing the Sackett definition, a definition might be as follows: *Evidence-based clinical pharmacy is the conscientious, explicit and judicious use of current best evidence in making decisions about the care of individual patients.*

This entirely fits with the concept of pharmaceutical care (see 📖 p.244) and challenges clinical pharmacists not only to keep abreast of developments in their chosen specialty, but also to apply clinical developments to patient circumstances and preferences.

One of Bandolier's maxims is that EBM is essentially 'tools not rules'.[3] Pharmacists need to remember this when applying current best evidence to patient care.

Strengths of evidence

A hierarchy of evidence (Table 7.1) is helpful in avoiding types of studies that are inherently biased. A number of grading systems are currently available which are useful in terms of identifying the level of evidence available and as a tool for categorizing recommendations made in clinical guidelines, for example. For updated information on this topic, see the GRADE website.[4]

Some evidence tables regard large randomized trials as level I evidence. Evidence from levels IV and V should not be overlooked if it is all that is available. Conversely, recommendations should not be made on level V evidence if level I or II evidence is available.

1 Sackett DL *et al.* (1996). *British medical Journal* **312**: 71–2.
2 McMaster University. http://hiru.mcmaster.ca.
3 www.ebandolier.com.
4 www.gradeworkinggroup.org.

Table 7.1 Type and strength of efficacy evidence

I	Strong evidence from at least one systematic review of multiple well-designed randomized controlled trials
II	Strong evidence from at least one properly designed randomized controlled trial of appropriate size
III	Evidence from well-designed trials without randomization, single group, cohort, time series, or matched case-controlled studies
IV	Evidence from well-designed non-experimental studies from more than one centre or research group
V	Opinions of respected authorities, based on clinical evidence, descriptive studies, or reports of expert committees

Further reading

Useful resource for pharmacy is available on the Bandolier website www.medicine.ox.ac.uk/bandolier/booth/booths/pharmacy.html.

Statistical versus clinical significance

Simply because a study finding is statistically significant, does not mean that the finding is important. Large trials or large meta-analyses have the potential to find very small statistically significant differences between groups. An important consideration when interpreting significant findings is assessment of how clinically significant the finding is.

'*Clinical significance*' refers to a value judgement people must make when determining the meaningfulness of the magnitude of an intervention effect.

For example, if an expensive medication was found to significantly ↓ systolic blood pressure (SBP) by an average of 2mmHg, it would be important to consider the clinical merit of the intervention. Would there be any important health benefits to a patient of a ↓ in SBP of just 2mmHg? Would it be worth investing in an expensive intervention if it delivered such a meagre ↓ in SBP? Are there any cheaper medications available that produce greater ↓ in BP?

Well-conducted rigorous randomized controlled trials should recruit enough participants to detect a difference between groups which is determined as clinically significant before the study.

Odds ratios and relative risk

What is an odds ratio?

The number needed to treat (NNT) is a very useful way of describing the benefits (or harms) of treatments, both in individual trials and in systematic reviews. Few papers report results using this easily interpretable measure. However, NNT calculations come second to working out whether an effect of treatment in one group of patients is different from that found in the control groups. Many studies, particularly systematic reviews, report their results as odds ratios or as a ↓ in odds ratios, and some trials do the same. Odds ratios are also commonly used in epidemiological studies to describe the probable harm an exposure might cause.

Calculating the odds

The odds of an event occurring are calculated as the number of events divided by the number of non-events. For example, 24 pharmacists are on call in a major city. Six pharmacists are called. The odds of being called are 6 divided by 18 (the number who were not called) or 0.33. An odds ratio is calculated by dividing the odds in the treated or exposed group by the odds in the control group. In general, epidemiological studies try to identify factors that cause harm—those with odds ratios >1. For example, if we look at case–control studies investigating the potential harm of giving high doses of calcium-channel blockers to treat hypertension. Clinical trials typically look for treatments that ↓ event rates, and that have odds ratios <1. In these cases, a percentage ↓ in the odds ratio is often quoted instead of the odds ratio. For example, the ISIS-4 trial reported a 7% ↓ in the odds of mortality with captopril treatment, rather than reporting an odds ratio of 0.93.

Relative risks

Few people have a natural ability to interpret event rates that are reported in terms of odds ratios. Understanding risks and relative risks seems to be easier to grasp.

The risk (or probability) of being called in the example already described in 'Calculating the odds' is 6 divided by 24 (the total number on call) or 0.25 (25%). The relative risk is also known as the 'risk ratio', and if reporting positive outcomes, such as improvement, it can be called 'relative benefit'.

Risks and odds

In many situations in medicine, we can get a long way in interpreting odds ratios by pretending that they are relative risks. When events are rare, risks and odds are very similar. For example, in the ISIS-4 study 2231 out of 29 022 patients in the control group died within 35 days: a risk of 0.077 (2231/29 022) or an odds of 0.083 (2231/(29 022−2231)). This is an absolute difference of 6 in 1000 or a relative error of ~7%. This close approximation holds true when we talk about odds ratios and relative risks, provided that the events are rare.

Why use an odds ratio rather than relative risk?

If odds ratios are difficult to interpret, why don't we always use relative risks instead? There are several reasons for continuing with odds ratios, most of which relate to the superior mathematical properties of odds ratios. Odds ratios can always take values between zero and infinity, which is not the case for relative risks.

The range that relative risk can take depends on the baseline event rate. This could obviously cause problems if we were performing a meta-analysis of relative risks in trials with greatly different event rates. Odds ratios also possess a symmetrical property: if you reverse the outcomes in the analysis and look at good outcomes rather than bad outcomes, the relationships have reciprocal odds ratios. Again, this is not true for relative risks.

Odds ratios are always used in case–control studies where disease prevalence is not known: the apparent prevalence depends solely on the ratio of sampling cases to controls, which is totally artificial. To use an effect measure that is altered by prevalence in these circumstances would obviously be wrong, so odds ratios are the ideal choice. This, in fact, provides the historical link with their use in meta-analyses: the statistical methods that are routinely used are based on methods first published in the 1950s for the analysis of stratified case–control studies. Meta-analytical methods that combine relative risks and absolute risk reductions are now available, but more caution is required in their application, especially when there are large variations in baseline event rates.

A fourth point of convenience occurs if it is necessary to make adjustments for confounding factors using multiple regression. When measuring event rates, the correct approach is to use logistic regression models that work in terms of odds and report effects as odds ratios. All of which makes odds ratios likely to be in use for some time—so it is important to understand how to use them. Of course, it is also important to consider the statistical significance of an effect in addition to its size: as with relative risks, it is easy to spot statistically significant odds ratios by noting whether their 95% confidence intervals do not include 1, which is analogous to a <1 in 20 chance (or a probability of <0.05 or gambling odds of better than 19:1) that the reported effect is solely due to chance.

Formula to calculate an odds ratio

$$\text{Odds ratio} = \frac{\text{odds on treatment}}{\text{odds on control}}$$

Where odds ratio = 1, this implies no difference in effect

Formula to calculate a relative risk

$$\text{Risk ratio} = \frac{\text{risk on treatment}}{\text{risk on control}}$$

Where risk ratio = 1, this implies no difference in effect

Binary and continuous data

Broadly, statistical tests can be grouped into those used to compare *binary* (also called 'dichotomous') outcome data and those used to compare *continuous* outcome data. Binary outcomes are those that can only take two possible values, such as dead or alive, pain or no pain, and smoker or non-smoker. Statistical tests on binary data, such as relative risks, compare the rate of an event between the groups; it also makes the calculation of NNT possible. Continuous outcomes are derived from data that can take any value on a scale. Some examples of continuous data include height, BP, time, or the score in a test. Statistical tests on continuous data (e.g. *t* tests) compare the difference between means of each group (see 📖 p.134).

L'Abbé plots

L'Abbé plots are named after a paper by Kristen L'Abbé and colleagues and are an extremely valuable contribution to understanding systematic reviews. The authors suggest a simple graphical representation of the information from trials. Each point on a L'Abbé scatter plot represents one trial in the review. They are a simple and effective way to present a series of results, without complex statistics. The proportion of patients achieving the outcome with the experimental intervention is plotted against the event rate in the control group. Even if a review does not show the data in this way, it is relatively simple to determine this if the information is available.

For treatment, trials in which the experimental intervention was better than the control are in the upper-left section of the plot, between the y-axis and the line of equality. If the experimental intervention was no better than the control, the point falls on the line of equality, and if the control was better than the experimental intervention, the point is in the lower-right section of the plot, between the x-axis and the line of equality (Fig. 7.1).

For prophylaxis, this pattern is reversed. Because prophylaxis ↓ the number of bad events (e.g. death after myocardial infarction following the use of aspirin), we expect a smaller proportion of patients harmed by treatment than in the control group. So if the experimental intervention is better than the control, the trial results should be between the x-axis and the line of equality.

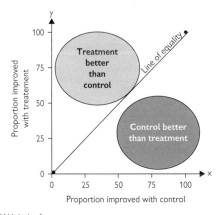

Fig. 7.1 L'Abbé plot for treatment.

Mean difference and standardized mean difference

Analyses of continuous data often show the difference between the means of the groups being compared. In a meta-analysis, this can involve either comparing the mean difference of trials in two groups directly if the unit of measurement of the outcome is the same (e.g. if height is the outcome of interest and all trials measure height in centimetres) or standardizing the outcome measure and comparing the difference between the standardized means if different assessment scales are used to measure subjective conditions, such as mood, depression, or pain.

In a meta-analysis of continuous data, if an experimental intervention has an identical effect as a control (or comparison), the mean difference or standardized mean difference is zero. Therefore if the lower limit of a confidence interval around a mean difference or standardized mean difference is >0, the mean of the experimental intervention group is significantly greater than that of the control group. Similarly, if the upper limit of the confidence interval is <0, the mean of the experimental intervention is significantly lower than that of the control. However, if the confidence interval incorporates the value 0, there is no significant difference between the means of the groups being compared.

Consider the output from a Cochrane review which compared the effect of very low calorie diets (VLCDs) with other interventions for weight loss in patients with type 2 diabetes mellitus (Fig. 7.2). In this case, weight loss is measured in kilograms so there is no need for standardization. As can be seen, the meta-analysis of the two trials indicated that the mean difference in weight with the management with a VLCD and other interventions is −2.95kg. This suggests that patients with type 2 diabetes mellitus on a VLCD are, on average, 2.95kg lighter than patients with type 2 diabetes mellitus on the comparison interventions. However, the range of the 95% confidence intervals includes 0, which indicates that the difference in weight loss between the two groups is not statistically significant.

Review: Long-term non-pharmacological weight loss interventions for adults with type 2 diabetes mellitus
Comparison: 01 VLCD vs different intervention (1–10: fixed models. 11–20: random models, rho = 0.75)
Outcome: 01 weight loss (kg)

Study	Treatment		Control		Weighted mean difference (fixed) 95% CI	Weight (%)	Weighted mean difference (fixed) 95% CI
	N	Mean (SD)	N	Mean (SD)			
Wing, 1991a	17	−8.60 (9.20)	16	−6.80 (6.90)		39.5	−1.80 [−7.33, 3.73]
Wing, 1994	48	−14.20 (10.30)	45	−10.50 (11.60)		60.5	−3.70 [−8.17, 0.77]
Total (95% CI)	65		61			100.0	−2.95 [−6.42, 0.53]

Test for heterogeneity chi-square = 0.27 df = 1 p = 0.60 I^2 = 0.0%
Test for overall effect z = 1.66 p = 0.1

−10.0 −5.0 0 5.0 10.0
Favours treatment   Favours control

Fig. 7.2 Meta-analysis of a VLCD versus other interventions for weight loss in patients with type 2 diabetes mellitus.

Assessing the quality of randomized studies

Assessment tools for randomized studies are widely available and all have problems because they do not cover all the issues that could be considered to be important. This simple method picks up on the main issues of randomization, blinding, and patient withdrawal from studies (Table 7.2). The maximum quality score is 5 if all the criteria are fulfilled.

In addition, a more general appraisal tool is presented (Table 7.3). It picks up details from the scoring system described in Table 7.2.

Table 7.2 Simple assessment tool for a randomized trial[1]

Is the study randomized?	Score
Yes	1
Is the randomization appropriate?	
Yes—e.g. random number tables	1
No—e.g. alternate patients, date of birth, or hospital number	−1
Was the study double blind?	
Yes	1
Was blinding correctly carried out?	
Yes—e.g. double dummy	1
No—e.g. treatments did not look identical	−1
Were withdrawals and drop-outs described?	
Yes	1

[1] Jadad A et al. (1996). Assessing the quality of reports of randomized clinical trials: is blinding necessary? Controlled Clinical Trials. **17**: 1–12.

Table 7.3 General appraisal tool for a randomized trial

Was the method of randomization appropriate (e.g. computer generated)?
Was the study described as 'double-blind'? And was the method of blinding adequate (e.g. double dummy, or identical tablets)?
Was the trial sensitive, i.e. able to detect a difference between treatment groups (e.g. use of a placebo, or additional active groups)?
Were baseline values for each treatment group adequate for trialists to measure a change following treatment?
Were the groups similar at the start of the trial?
Similar patients?
Diagnostic criteria clearly stated?
Similar baseline measures?
Was the size of the trial adequate?
How many patients were there in each group?
Were outcomes clearly defined and measured appropriately?
Were they clinically meaningful?
Were they primary/surrogate outcomes?
Were the outcome data presented clearly?
If multiple tests were conducted, were single positive results inappropriately presented?
Quality score[1]

Randomization	Double-blinding	Withdrawals/ drop-outs	Total score

Critical appraisal of systematic reviews

Systematic reviews are considered to be the best level of evidence if they are well conducted and evaluate a number of randomized trials. They can be particularly useful when seeking to answer clinical questions. However, they are only reliable if the process of the review has followed rigorous scientific principles. Authors should explicitly state the topic being reviewed and have made a reasonable attempt to identify all the relevant studies. The 10 questions listed in Table 7.4 help in that assessment. If the paper fails either of the first two questions, it is not worth proceeding further.

Table 7.4 Ten questions to make sense of a review[1]

For each question answer : Yes, No, or Don't Know

A. Are the results of the review valid?

1. Did the review address a clearly focused issue (e.g. the population, intervention, and/or outcomes)?

2. Did the authors look for the appropriate sort of papers?

   Check that the authors looked for randomized controlled trials or had clear reasons for including other types of studies.

Is it worth continuing?

3. Do you think the relevant important studies were included?

   Look for search methods, use reference list, unpublished studies and non-English language articles.

4. Did the authors do enough to assess the quality of the studies included?

   This would routinely be in the form of an assessment tool for randomized controlled trials.

5. If the results of studies were combined, was it reasonable to do so?

B. What are the results?

6. What is the overall result of the review?

   Is there a clear numerical expression?

7. How precise are the results?

   What were the confidence intervals?

C. Will the results help my local situation?

8. Can the results be applied locally?

9. Were all important outcomes considered?

10. Are the benefits worth the harms and costs?

[1] Oxman AD et al. (1994). Users guide to the medical literature. VI: How to use an overview. *Journal of the American Medical Association* **272**: 1367–71.

Critical assessment of papers

When reading a clinical trial paper, it is too easy to read the abstract quickly and skim through the main text. Taking the time to critically evaluate the paper might seem daunting and too time-consuming. In many situations a quick read through is all that is needed. However, if the information gleaned from the paper is going to be used to decide on treatment options or might be used to support a formulary application, a more thoughtful approach is required. The information in this section specifically relates to critically evaluating a clinical trial paper, but the same process, adapted to the content, can be used for other types of clinical paper.

It is not necessary to be a statistician or an expert in trial design to critically evaluate a paper. Much of the evaluation is common sense. A full critical evaluation should take all the following points into account, but even simply bearing them in mind will help you get more out of any paper you read.

- Title—does this accurately reflect the content of the paper? Ideally, the title should state the question under investigation, rather than potentially biasing readers by declaring the results. Cryptic titles are a popular way of attracting readers' attention, but if it is too obscure, could it be because that the authors don't really know what they are writing about? Before progressing, consider how useful this trial is in the clinical setting. If it is too esoteric, it might not be worth reading any further!
- Authors—should be from professions/institutions appropriate to the subject studied. Be cautious with papers authored by pharmaceutical industry employees, but don't dismiss these out of hand. Too many authors might mean that the work is scrappy. Multicentre studies should list the key authors and acknowledge other participants at the end of the paper. Is a statistician listed as an author or acknowledged? This should provide reassurance that the statistics are correct.
- Journal—don't assume that because a paper is published in a mainstream journal it is a good paper. However, be more cautious about papers from obscure journals.
- The introduction—should give relevant background information, building logically to the study topic. If the introduction is waffly or irrelevant, ask yourself if the authors really know what they are writing about.
- Method—a well-written method should give sufficient information for another person to reproduce the study. The information given should include the following.
  - Type of study (e.g. randomized controlled trial, cohort, or case study).
  - Numbers involved, ideally including details of powering.
  - Patient selection and randomization—details of patient demo-graphics should be given and the baseline characteristics of each group should be roughly the same (and should be acknowledged if not).
  - Inclusion/exclusion criteria—consider whether these are appropriate. If there are too many exclusion criteria, the study might not be relevant to the clinical setting.

- Outcome measurements—by now, the question that the authors are trying to answer should be clear. The factors used to measure the outcome should be appropriate and, if possible, directly related to the question. Be cautious of surrogate markers. In many clinical settings, it might be unethical, too invasive, or take too long to use the target outcome. However, check that the surrogate marker closely reflects the target outcome as a whole and not just one aspect of it.
- An appropriate comparator drug should be used at its standard dose. Any new drug should be tested against standard therapy. If a drug is compared with placebo or an outdated or rarely used drug, ask yourself why. With the exception of the study treatment, all other interventions should be the same.
- A randomized controlled trial should ideally be double-blinded (i.e. neither the study participants nor the investigators know which subjects are receiving the study drug and which subjects are receiving the comparator). Sometimes this is not feasible or ethical, but there might be bias if the trial is open-label (both subjects and investigator know who is receiving which treatment) or single-blind (the investigator but not the participants know who is receiving each treatment).
- Be cautious with crossover trials—if the disease studied could improve with time without treatment (especially if it is self-limiting or seasonal), a crossover trial is inappropriate. An adequate 'washout' period between treatments is essential.
- The details of statistical tests should be given—the tests should be appropriate to the type of data presented. Beware of trials that use numerous statistical tests. Why are so many tests needed? Is it that there is nothing to prove? Further discussion of statistical tests is beyond the scope of this topic. Consult relevant textbooks for further information.
- Results—should answer the question originally asked and be easy to comprehend.
  - Graphs and tables should be relevant and clear. Too many graphs and tables suggest that the authors are having difficulty proving their point! Watch labelling of axes on graphs. Sometimes labelling is skewed (e.g. does not start at zero) to give more impressive results.
  - If means are quoted, the variance and/or median should also be quoted. This helps determine whether the mean is a true 'average' or whether extreme values have skewed the results.
  - The results might be statistically significant, but are they clinically significant? Results presented as odds ratios, relative risks, or NNT are generally easier to apply to a clinical setting.
- The discussion—should logically build from the results to answer the original question, one way or another. If the authors make statements such as 'further study is required . . .', ask yourself why. Is this because the original study design was unsuitable? Any doubts or inconsistencies should be dealt with satisfactorily, not just explained away.

- The conclusion—should be appropriate to the data presented and give a definite final answer. If the conclusion is woolly, was there any point in the study in the first place or were the authors just 'paper chasing'?
- The bibliography—should be up to date and relevant. Beware of too many references from obscure journals. You should be able to satisfactorily follow up statements made in the rest of the paper by reference to the original papers quoted.
- Acknowledgements—look for any specialists not in the author list, which might provide reassurance if you had any doubts about the authors' expertise in any angle of the study. Watch out for funding or sponsorship from parties with a vested interest in the outcome of the study (notably the pharmaceutical industry!). However, don't dismiss studies sponsored by the pharmaceutical industry out of hand. Much good work is supported by the pharmaceutical industry.

Further reading

Sackett DL et al. (2005). *Evidence-based Medicine*. Churchill Livingstone.
Jones C (2002). Evidence-based medicine. 1: Research methods. *Pharmaceutical Journal* **268**: 875–7.
www.clinicalevidence.com

Guidelines

Guideline development is a common way of either seeking to introduce new practices or attempting to stop some current practices. Guidelines can be time consuming and costly to develop. There is evidence that they can be effective if carefully prepared and peer reviewed. Shekelle et al.[1] proposed the following key steps that need to be followed.

- Identify and refine the subject area.
- Create a guideline development group.
- Based on systematic reviews:
  - assess the evidence about the clinical question or condition
  - translate the evidence into a recommendation within the guideline.
- Ensure that the guideline is externally reviewed.

A useful checklist for guidelines is provided by Shaneyfelt et al.[2] This review of some 270 guidelines lists some 25 points to consider when preparing a guideline. These include stating the purpose of the guideline, using an expiry date, and grading the recommendations according to the strength of the evidence.

1 Shekelle PG et al. (1999). Developing clinical guidelines. *Western Journal of Medicine* **170**: 348–51.
2 Shaneyfelt TM et al (1999). Are guidelines following guidelines? *Journal of the Amereican Medical Association* **281**: 1900–5.

Number needed to treat (NNT)

The NNT is a measure of clinical significance and changes view from 'Does a treatment work?' to 'How well does a treatment work?'. This concept is widely used and useful not only in its own right, but also to enable direct comparisons of treatments. The league table of treatments from the Oxford Pain Research Unit (Fig. 7.3) illustrates the value of such an approach. Ideally, we would want an NNT of 1. Although there are treatments that meet this criterion (e.g. anaesthetic agents) in practice NNTs are >1 for the reasons discussed here.

The NNT is defined as follows: the number of people who must be treated for one patient to benefit. The NNT is expressed in terms of a specific clinical outcome and should be shown with confidence intervals.

Calculating the NNT for active treatments

The NNT calculation is based from the understanding of risk ratios (Fig. 7.4). Although the NNT is the reciprocal of the absolute risk reduction, it is not necessary to understand this concept to calculate the NNT. A worked example is included so that the process is transparent. The equation is quite simple, and it is easy to calculate the NNT in published trials using a pocket calculator.

The NNT was initially used to describe prophylactic interventions. The NNT for prophylaxis is given by the following equation:

> 1/(proportion of patients benefiting from the control intervention minus the proportion of patients benefiting from the experimental intervention).

The NNT for active treatment is given by the following equation:

> 1/(proportion of patients benefiting from the experimental intervention minus the proportion of patients benefiting from the control intervention).

From the equation in Fig. 7.4 it should be apparent that any response in the control arm leads to NNT >1. People often ask what a good NNT is; it depends whether the NNT is for treatment (ideally in the range 2–4) or prophylaxis (the NNT is generally larger). Issues such as toxicity have an influence, including the cost. For example, a cheap and safe intervention that prevents a serious disease but has an NNT of 100 might well be acceptable.

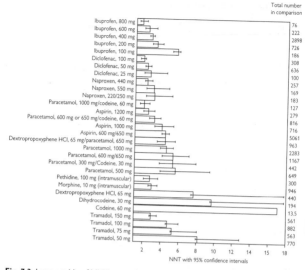

Total number in comparison

Ibuprofen, 800 mg	76
Ibuprofen, 600 mg	222
Ibuprofen, 400 mg	2898
Ibuprofen, 200 mg	726
Ibuprofen, 100 mg	186
Diclofenac, 100 mg	308
Diclofenac, 50 mg	636
Diclofenac, 25 mg	100
Naproxen, 440 mg	257
Naproxen, 550 mg	169
Naproxen, 220/250 mg	183
Paracetamol, 1000 mg/codeine, 60 mg	127
Aspirin, 1200 mg	279
Paracetamol, 600 mg or 650 mg/codeine, 60 mg	816
Aspirin, 1000 mg	716
Aspirin, 600 mg/650 mg	5061
Dextropropoxyphene HCl, 65 mg/paracetamol, 650 mg	963
Paracetamol, 1000 mg	2283
Paracetamol, 600 mg/650 mg	1167
Paracetamol, 300 mg/Codeine, 30 mg	442
Paracetamol, 500 mg	649
Pethidine, 100 mg (intramuscular)	300
Morphine, 10 mg (intramuscular)	946
Dextropropoxyphene HCl, 65 mg	440
Dihydrocodeine, 30 mg	194
Codeine, 60 mg	13.5
Tramadol, 150 mg	561
Tramadol, 100 mg	882
Tramadol, 75 mg	563
Tramadol, 50 mg	770

NNT with 95% confidence intervals

Fig. 7.3 League table of NNT to produce ≥50% pain relief for 4–6h compared with placebo in patients with pain of moderate or severe intensity.

	Controls	Active treatment
Number of patients	N_{con}	N_{act}
Improved = clinical end point	Imp_{con}	Imp_{act}

$$NNT = \cfrac{1}{\cfrac{Imp_{act}}{N_{act}} - \cfrac{Imp_{con}}{N_{con}}}$$

Fig. 7.4 Number needed to treat (NNT).

Using the NNT to express harm

The number needed to harm (NNH) can also be helpful, in addition to the NNT. The NNH is calculated using a similar formula derived from data for adverse events rather than desired effect (Fig. 7.5).

Fig. 7.5 Number needed to harm (NNH).

Confidence intervals

Most pharmacists are aware of *p* values in terms of an answer being significant (in a statistical sense) or not. However, the use of *p* is increasingly redundant, and new methods of reporting significance have emerged.

The most common method is the confidence interval, which enables us to estimate the margin of error. For example, if we measured BP in 100 adults, we could derive a mean result. If we then took a further 100 adults and repeated the experiment, we would arrive at a similar, but not identical, figure. The confidence interval, expressed as a percentage, enables calculation of the margin of error and tells us how good our mean is. Generally, the figure is set at 95%, so we can be confident that the true mean lies somewhere between the upper and lower estimates (Fig. 7.6). Expressed a different way, there is only a 5% chance of the result being outside the calculated limits.

The statistics involved are derived from a range of 1.96 standard deviations above and below the point estimated. For a 99% confidence interval, a figure of 2.58 standard deviations is used.

Calculating confidence intervals

Although the formulae are available in standard statistics works, there are a number of confidence interval calculators on the web that require the use of the calculated point estimate and the number of samples to derive the confidence interval at a given percentage.

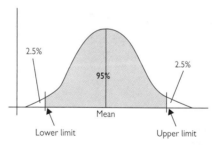

Fig. 7.6 Illustration of the data incorporated within a 95% confidence interval.

Herbal medicines

Herbal drugs *150*
General information about commonly
    used herbal medications *154*
Chinese herbal medicine *157*
Herbal interactions *158*
Perioperative considerations for herbal drugs *160*

Herbal drugs

The efficacy and safety of herbal drugs present a number of issues to pharmacists. Herbal drugs are more often complex mixtures of active constituents that vary in quality for a number of reasons, such as environmental and genetic factors. Furthermore, the constituents responsible for the claimed therapeutic effects are frequently unknown or only partly explained.

The position is further complicated by the traditional practice of using combinations of herbal drugs, and it is not uncommon to have as many as five or more herbal drugs in one product. There is potential risk from impurities/adulterations of herbal medicine mixed with toxic plant extracts because of misidentification or intentional addition of allopathic drugs.

The European pharmacopoeia includes 120 monographs on herbal drugs. Control of the starting materials is essential to ensure the reproducible quality of herbal medicinal products. Herbal drugs must be accurately identified by macroscopic and microscopic comparison with authentic material. Herbal drugs are referred to by their binomial Latin names of genus and species; only permitted synonyms should be used. Different batches of the same herbal ingredient can differ in quality because of a number of factors.

- Inter- or intra-species variation.
- Environmental factors.
- Time of harvesting.
- Plant part used—active constituents usually vary between plant parts, and it is not uncommon for a herbal drug to be adulterated with parts of the plant that are not normally used.
- Storage conditions and processing treatments can greatly affect the quality of an herbal ingredient.
- Instances of herbal remedies adulterated with other plant material and conventional medicines.
- Extraction/drying methods.

Identity tests establish the botanical identity of a herbal drug.
- Chemical (e.g. colour or precipitation) and chromatographic tests are used for identification of the ingredients.
- Assay—a herbal drug with known active principles should have an assay established to set the criterion for the minimum acceptable percentage of active substance(s).

Legislation of herbal drugs

Although herbal drugs have been used as traditional remedies for centuries and are perceived by many to be without major safety problems, the UK has a series of controls to limit general availability.

Hazardous plants, such as digitalis, rauwolfia, and nux vomica, are specifically controlled under the Medicines Act as prescription-only medicines (POMs).

Certain herbal ingredients are controlled under the Medicines (Retail Sale and Supply of Herbal Remedies) Order, 1977, SI 2130. This Order (part I) specifies 25 plants that cannot be supplied except by a pharmacy, and includes well-known toxic species such as areca, crotalaria, dryopteris and strophanthus.

Herbal remedies exempt from licensing fall under two main categories:

- Subject to the provisions of section 12 of the Medicines Act 1968, products can be compounded and supplied by a herbalist on their own recommendation.
- If no medical claims are made that are attributable to the herbal product, it can be sold as a food supplement.

Efficacy

Herbs used medicinally normally have a traditional reputation for their uses, but generally there is little scientific documentation of their active constituents, pharmacological actions, or clinical efficacy.

The current emphasis on EBM requires evidence of efficacy from rigorous randomized controlled trials. Several systematic reviews have been prepared by the Cochrane Collaboration. These reviews highlight that, in some cases, the evidence base is weak and studies are often flawed. Evidence from randomized controlled trials has confirmed the efficacy of St John's wort products versus placebo in the treatment of mild to moderate depression.

If the active constituents of a herbal drug are known, it is possible and, in most cases, desirable to standardize the extract. The aim of standardization is to obtain an optimum and consistent quality of a herbal drug preparation by adjusting it to give a defined content of a constituent or group of constituents with known therapeutic activity. Examples include senna, frangula, digitalis, belladonna, and horse chestnut.

In the case of St John's wort, early studies concentrated on the hypericin constituents, but more recent work suggests that hyperforin and, possibly, flavonoids also contribute to the antidepressant properties.

Safety and adverse effects

Information on herbal medicines is lacking in many areas including active constituents, metabolites, pharmacokinetics, pharmacology, toxicology, adverse effects, long-term effects, use by specific patient groups, and contraindications.

- Herbal drugs could present a potential risk to health from exposure to contaminants present in the herbal product and result in ADRs (Table 8.1).
- Reliance on self-administration of herbal drugs or products could delay a patient seeking qualified advice or cause a patient to abandon conventional treatment without appropriate advice.
- In some cases, herbal medicines could compromise the efficacy of conventional medicines through herb–drug interactions.

Table 8.1 Adverse reactions associated with herbal medications

Adverse reaction	Herbal medication
Cardiotoxicity	Aconite root tuber, ginger, licorice root, mahuang
Cross-sensitivity with ragweed	Arnica, calendula, dandelion, echinacea, feverfew, german chamomile, golden rod, march blazing star, milk thistle, mugwort, pyrethrum, stevia, tansy, wormwood oil, yarrow
Gastrointestinal (nausea, emesis, dyspepsia, etc.)	Echinacea, ephedra, evening primrose oil, garlic, ginger, milk thistle, soy
Hepatotoxicity	Borage, calamus, chaparral, Chinese herbs, coltsfoot, echinacea, germander, kava rhizome, kombucha, life root, mahuang, pennyroyal, sassafras, skullcap, soy, valerian
Neurotoxicity	Aconite root tuber, ginkgo seed or leaf, kava rhizome, mahuang, penny royal
Renal toxicity	Chinese yew, hawthorn, impila root, penny royal, star fruit
Sedation	Chamomile, ginger, St John's wort, valerian

General information about commonly used herbal medications (Table 8.2)

Table 8.2 General information about commonly used herbal medications

Herbal drug	Use(s)	Proposed mechanism of action	Other considerations
Black cohosh	• Treat PMS and dysmenorrhea • Reduce menopausal symptoms such as hot flushes	• Possibly has oestrogen-like activity • Suppresses lutenizing hormone secretion	• Not recommended for >6 months • May relieve vasomotor symptoms • Effect on breast cancer, osteoporosis and cardiovascular risk is not known
Chamomile	• Reduce anxiety and insomnia • Relieve GI spasms	• Contains flavonoids which are the active component • Benzo-diazepine receptor binding ligand	• Allergic reactions reported esp. if patient has ragweed allergy • Sedation is additive with other therapies
Echinacea	• Treat and prevent colds • Stimulate the immune system	• Increases phagocytosis and lymphocyte activity • Anti-inflammatory	• Not recommended for longer than 8wks • Can worsen asthma
Evening primrose oil	• Treat symptoms of PMS and menopause	• Active component probably linoleic acid	• Evidence is controversial • Side effects include headache, nausea, and diarrhoea
Feverfew	• Prevent migraines • Relieve dysmenorrhea • Improve inflammatory processes	• Inhibits prosta-glandin synthesis • Analgesic properties	• Rapid with 'post feverfew syndrome' which includes anxiety, headaches, and insomnia • Must be taken daily for migraine prevention • Not used for migraine treatment • Contraindicated in pregnancy

Table 8.2 (Contd.)

Herbal drug	Use(s)	Proposed mechanism of action	Other considerations
Garlic	• Lower cholesterol • Treat hypertension • Prevent stomach and colon cancer	• Antioxidant and antiplatelet activity • Smooth muscle relaxant and vasodilator • HMG-CoA reductase inhibitor	• Odourless preparations have less of the active component • Enteric coating ensures proper absorption
Ginger	• Decrease GI upset and nausea • Reduce post-surgical nausea	• Serotonin antagonist at 5-HT3 receptor in ileum • Anti-inflammatory	• Toxicity includes sedation and arrhythmias • Adverse effects include gas, heartburn, and bloating
Ginkgo biloba	• Enhance memory • Treat or prevent dementia	• Antioxidant • Increases blood circulation by decreasing viscosity • Regulates vascular smooth muscle	• Uncooked seeds contain ginkgo toxin which can cause seizures
Ginseng	• Stimulate the immune system • Improve blood glucose and BP control	• Increases cortisol concentrations • Stimulates natural killer cells	• Limit use to 3 months • May cause sleep disturbances • Avoid large amounts of caffeine
Hawthorn	• Treat heart failure • Improve hypertension • Treat coronary heart disease	• Anti-inflammatory properties • Lipid-lowering properties	• May decrease dyspnoea and fatigue • No mortality or morbidity data
Horse chestnut	• Improve symptoms of chronic venous insufficiency • Decrease leg oedema	• Seeds contain aescin which reduces venous capillary permeability • Anti-inflammatory • Weak diuretic activity	• May increase bleeding when in combination with warfarin • Can turn urine red • Can cause kidney or liver damage
Licorice	• Treat stomach ulcers • Relieve constipation	• Glycyrrhizin and glycyrrhetinic acid prevent the degradation of prostaglandins in the gastric mucosa • Antioxidant activity	• Can cause sodium and water retention and hypokalemia • Avoid in patients with cardiovascular or renal disorders

(continued)

Table 8.2 (Contd.)

Herbal drug	Use(s)	Proposed mechanism of action	Other considerations
Milk thistle	• Protect the liver	• Seeds contain silymarin • Antioxidant, anti-inflammatory activity • Inhibits mitochondrial damage	• GI side effects are common including nausea, diarrhoea, and fullness • Cross-sensitivity to ragweed allergy
Pepper-mint	• Reduce nausea and indigestion • Treat headaches • Improve irritable bowel syndrome	• Direct relaxing on GI smooth muscle • Inhibits potassium depolarization in intestine	• Avoid in patients with pre-existing GI disorders • May decrease absorption of iron
Saw palmetto	• Treat benign prostatic hyperplasia	• May inhibit 5-α-reductase • Local anti-androgenic and anti-inflammatory effects on prostate	• Symptom improvement similar to that seen with finasteride • No long-term data
Soy	• Decrease cholesterol • Relieve menopausal symptoms • Improve bone mineral density	• Isoflavones bind to α and β oestrogen receptors	• Causes nausea, bloating, and constipation
St John's wort	• Treat depression and anxiety	• Active components, hypericin and hyperforin, inhibit serotonin, dopamine, and norepinephrine re-uptake	• May cause photo-sensitivity • Avoid in patients with psychiatric illness including bipolar and schizophrenia • May have withdrawal effect after chronic use
Valerian	• Treat anxiety and insomnia	• Binds with GABA receptor in CNS	• Can cause excitability with high doses • Takes weeks for effect

Chinese herbal medicine

Most of the substances used in Chinese herbal medicine originate from China. The Chinese pharmacopeia lists over 6000 different medicinal substances; there are currently over 600 different herbs in common use. Herbs are used for their abilities to treat specific Chinese diagnoses and alleviate specific complaints. For example, there are assortments of herbs that can alleviate coughing, but each one is appropriate for a cough with a different Chinese diagnosis. The variety and degree of different combinations of herbal medicines makes Chinese herbal medicine very complex.

Combination of herbal products

The one characteristic of Chinese herbal medicine that most differentiates it from other types of herbal medicine is the degree of combination undertaken. Chinese herbalists very rarely prescribe a single herb to treat a condition; instead, a mixture could contain >20 herbs. Pre-prepared formulas are available; however, these products are not usually as potent as the traditional preparation of 'decoction'.

Decoction is the traditional method of preparing herbal medicine. A decoction is a concentrated form of tea. The practitioner weighs out a day's dosage of each herb and combines them in a bag. A patient is given a bag for each day the herbal formula must be taken. The herbs are then boiled in water by the patient at home; the boiling process takes 30–60min and the resulting decoction is consumed several times during the day.

Quality issues

The quality and safety of Chinese herbs has repeatedly come into question after media coverage of concerns over heavy-metal contamination, adulteration, and use of endangered animal species. Heavy-metal contamination has been detected in several Chinese herbal products, usually as a result of poor manufacturing. Adulteration of herbal medicines with prescription drugs has been found in a few herbal products. The use of endangered animals in Chinese herbal medicine is very rare.

Herbal interactions

Information on herb–drug interactions (Table 8.3) is generally limited to case reports, although recognition is improving, with the result that clinically important interactions are increasingly being identified and prevented by healthcare professionals.

Variability of constituent ingredients and the pharmaceutical quality of unlicensed herbal products can often be the main reason for the low incidence of reported interactions.

Types of interaction

Pharmacokinetic interactions with drugs

- Absorption
- Distribution
- Metabolism
- Excretion

Pharmacodynamic interactions with drugs

- One substance affecting the response of another at its site of action.

Herb–disease interaction

Certain underlying diseases could be exacerbated by ingestion of herbal ingredients with the following properties:

- hypertensive properties.
- hyperglycaemic/hypoglycaemic activity.

Table 8.3 Some important herb–drug interactions

Herb	Drug interaction	Considerations
Black cohosh (Actaea racemosa)	Antihypertensives	May ↓ BP
Chamomile (Chamaemelum nobile)	Anticoagulants	Consider discontinuing 2wks before surgery
Echinacea purpurea	Immunosuppressants (eg corticosteroids)	Immune suppression can result from prolonged use for >14 days Loss or ↓ in therapeutic effect of some drug therapies; probably induction of CYP enzymes
Ephedra (ma huang)—active constituent is ephedrine	Will have the same interactions as ephedrine	Misuse has resulted in death
Evening primrose oil	Could interact with anti-coagulants or antiplatelet drugs Can ↓ seizure threshold	

Table 8.3 (Contd.)

Herb	Drug interaction	Considerations
Feverfew (*Tanacetum parthenium*)	Could interact with anti-coagulants or antiplatelet drugs	Consider discontinuing 2wks before surgery
Fish oil supplements (omega-3 fatty acids)	Reports of ↓ platelet aggregation	Unlikely to have clinical significance
Garlic (*Allium sativum*)	Could interact with anti-coagulants or antiplatelet drugs	Consider discontinuing 2wks before surgery Loss or ↓ in therapeutic effect of the drug therapies; probably induction of CYP enzymes
Ginger (*Zingiber officinale*)	Could interact with anti-coagulants or antiplatelet drugs	Consider discontinuing 2wks before surgery
Ginseng (*Panax ginseng*)	Could interact with anti-coagulants or antiplatelet drugs Interacts with hypoglycaemic drugs Avoid concurrent monoamine oxidase inhibitors (MAOIs)	Varying effects on BP Hypoglycaemia Could potentiate action of MAOIs Limit use to 3 months
Hops (*Humulus lupulus*)	Could have additive effect with CNS depressants	Avoid in depressive states
Horse chestnut (*Aesculus hippocastanum*)	Could interact with anti-coagulants or antiplatelet drugs	↑ risk of bleeding
Passion flower (*Passiflora incarnate*)	Additive effects with CNS depressants Avoid concurrent MAOIs	Reports of hepatic and pancreatic toxicity
Saw palmetto (*Serenoa serrulata*)	Caution with finasteride	Potential of additive effect
St John's wort (*Hypericum perforatum*)	Anticonvulsants Ciclosporin Digoxin Protease inhibitors and non-nucleoside reverse transcriptase inhibitors (NNRTIs) Oral contraceptives Theophylline Warfarin Irinotecan	Loss or ↓ in therapeutic effect of the drug therapies; probably induction of CYP enzymes by St John's wort constituents
Valerian (*Valeriana officinalis*)	Additive effects with CNS depressants	
Milk thistle (*Silybum marianus*)	CYP3A4 enzyme inducer Protease inhibitors and NNRTIs Phenytoin	↓ blood levels and hence chance of treatment failure

Please note that this is not an exhaustive list but a point of general reference. New information about herbal interactions can be obtained from ⌕ http://www.mhra.gov.uk

Perioperative considerations for herbal drugs

- Herbal medicines have the potential to pose problems in the peri-operative setting because patients often fail to communicate concurrent herbal remedies during DHx taking by healthcare professionals.
- Few data exist in the medical literature regarding the use of herbal products and the development of ADRs or interactions associated with anaesthesia.
- The most important risks associated with herbal products during the perioperative and immediate postoperative periods are cardiovascular, coagulation, and sedative effects.
  - Cardiovascular effects—ephedra, ginseng, and garlic:
    — ephedra can cause a dose-dependent ↑ in heart rate and BP.
    — ginseng ↑ BP and its use is not recommended during the surgical period in patients with cardiovascular disease.
    — garlic could ↓ BP, but its effects are normally brief and usually require high dosages.
  - Bleeding effects—garlic, ginseng, gingko, evening primrose oil, feverfew, fish oils, ginger, horse chestnut, and kava kava.
  - Sedative effects—chamomile, kava kava, valerian, hops, passion flower, and St John's wort.

Although there continues to be debate on the incidence of reactions to herbal products during the perioperative period, it might be prudent to recommend discontinuation of these agents for at least 2wks before surgery.

Medical gases

Clinical uses *162*
Cylinder identification coding *168*
Guideline for oxygen use in adult patients *170*
Domiciliary oxygen therapy *172*

Clinical uses

Air
Clinical indications
- In ventilators and incubators—to provide uncontaminated and controlled airflows.
- Replacement for contaminated atmospheric air.
- Carrier for volatile anaesthetic agents.
- Power source for pneumatic equipment.

Carbon dioxide
Clinical indications
- To rapidly ↑ depth of anaesthesia when volatile anaesthetic agents are administered.
- To facilitate blind intubation in anaesthetic practice.
- To facilitate vasodilatation, lessening the degree of metabolic acidosis during the induction of hypothermia.
- To ↑ cerebral blood flow in arteriosclerotic patients undergoing surgery.
- To stimulate respiration after a period of apnoea.
- To prevent hypocapnia during hyperventilation.
- For clinical and physiological investigations—e.g. insufflation into Fallopian tubes.
- For tissue-freezing techniques.

Entonox (50:50 mixture of nitrous oxide and oxygen (O_2))
Clinical indications
Used exclusively for the relief of pain:
- trauma
- dental work
- wound and burn analgesia
- childbirth analgesia.

Administration of Entonox
The gas is administered using a facemask or mouthpiece; gas flow is controlled by a sensitive demand valve which is activated by the patient's inspired breath. This enables pressurized gas from the cylinder to flow through a pressure regulator into the lungs at a steady rate. Longer and deeper breaths enable greater volumes of gas to be taken into the lungs, if necessary.

The gas is rapidly absorbed on inhalation, providing analgesia within minutes. The patient safely controls the dosage and, under normal conditions, there is no risk of overdose because the patient's level of consciousness governs their ability to maintain the flow of gas.

Helium

Clinical indications

Helium is used with at least 21% O_2:

- to assist O_2 flow into the alveoli of patients with severe respiratory obstruction
- to prevent atelectasis.
- for gas-transfer lung function tests.

Oxygen

Clinical indications

- To provide life support by restoring tissue O_2 levels—e.g. asthma, myocardial infarction (MI), and sickle cell crisis.
- Management of sudden cardiac or respiratory arrest.
- Resuscitation of the critically ill.
- Anaesthesia.

Oxygen delivery systems are listed in Table 9.1.

Typical dosing for O_2 in acute conditions

- Cardiac or respiratory conditions: 100%.
- Hypoxaemia with Pa_{CO_2} <5.3kPa: 40–60%.
- Hypoxaemia with Pa_{CO_2} >5.3kPa: 24% initially.

Long-term O_2

Used to improve mortality and morbidity in patients with chronic hypoxia caused by chronic obstructive pulmonary disease (COPD), pulmonary malignancy, heart failure, and other lung diseases such as cystic fibrosis and interstitial lung disease. Should be considered if arterial Pa_{O_2} <7.3kPa or 7.3–8kPa if the patient has polycythaemia or evidence of pulmonary hypertension.

Nitrous oxide

Clinical indications

- Nitrous oxide is used as an inhalation anaesthetic in combination with either a volatile or an IV anaesthetic agent.
- Used in combination with 50% O_2 as an analgesic agent.

Table 9.1 Oxygen delivery systems

Type	Flow rate	Inspired O_2 concentration
Low flow (Ventimask-controlled)		24%/28%/31%
Nasal prongs	1–2L	24–28%
High-flow mask	1–15L	24–60%
Non-rebreathing mask		≤90%
Anaesthetic mask or endotracheal tube		100%

Oxygen — Integral valve

Cylinder code	CD	HX	ZX	ZH[2]	DF[2]
Cylinder order code	101-CD	101-HX	101-ZX	101-ZH	101-DF
Nominal contents (litres)	460	2300	3040	2400	1360
Nominal cylinder pressure (bar)	230	230	300	300	137
Nominal outlet pressure (bar)	4	4	4	4	4
Valve outlet flow connection	6mm firtree	6mm firtree	6mm firtree	6mm firtree	6mm firtree
Valve outlet pressure connection	Oxygen Schrader (BS 5682)	Oxygen Schrader (BS 5682)	Oxygen Schrader (BS 5682)	Oxygen Schrader (BS 5682)	
Valve operation	handwheel	handwheel	handwheel	handwheel	handwheel
Flow-rate (litres/min)	Firtree: 1-15/Schrader: 40	Firtree: 1-15/Schrader: 40	Firtree: 1-15/Schrader: 40	Firtree: 2-45/Schrader: 40	2-4
Dimensions L×D (mm)	520×100	930×140	930×143	595×175	690×175
Water capacity (litres)	2.0	10.0	10.0	8.0	9.4
Nominal weight full (kg)	3.5	19.0	14.0	14.0	12.0

Cylinder code	ZA	ZB	ZC[2]	AD[1]	DD[2]
Cylinder order code	101-ZA	101-ZB	101-ZC	139-AD	109-DD
Nominal contents (litres)	300	300	300	460	460
Nominal cylinder pressure (bar)	300	300	300	230	230
Nominal outlet pressure (bar)	4	4	4	4	4
Valve outlet flow connection	6mm firtree	6mm firtree	6mm firtree	6mm firtree	6mm firtree
Valve operation	handwheel	handwheel	handwheel	handwheel	handwheel
Flow-rate (litres/min)	0.1-15	1-15	0.1-15	8	8
Dimensions L×D (mm)	366×85	390×85	390×85	480×100	520×100
Water capacity (litres)	1.0	1.0	1.0	2.0	2.0
Nominal weight full (kg)	1.55	2.7	2.7	4.0	3.5

Oxygen — Standard valve

Cylinder code	AZ	C	D	E	J[2]
Cylinder order code	298121-AZ	101-C	101-D	101-E	101-J
Nominal contents (litres)	170	170	340	680	6800
Nominal cylinder pressure (bar)	137	137	137	137	137
Valve outlet connection	Pin-index	Pin-index	Pin-index	Pin-index	Pin-index (side spindle)
Valve outlet specification	ISO 407	ISO 407	ISO 407	ISO 407	ISO 407
Valve operation	key	key	key	key	key
Dimensions L×D (mm)	290×106	430×89	535×102	865×102	1320×229
Water capacity (litres)	1.2	1.2	2.3	4.7	47.2
Nominal weight full (kg)	2.5	2.5	3.9	6.5	78.0

Cylinder code	AF[2]	F	G
Cylinder order code	101-F	101-F	101-G
Nominal contents (litres)	1360	1360	3400
Nominal cylinder pressure (bar)	137	137	137
Valve outlet connection	5/8" BSP (F)	5/8" BSP (F)	5/8" BSP (F)
Valve outlet specification	BS 341 No.3 (Bullnose)	BS 341 No.3 (Bullnose)	BS 341 No.3 (Bullnose)
Valve operation	key	key	key
Dimensions L×D (mm)	670×175	930×140	1320×178
Water capacity (litres)	9.4	9.4	23.6
Nominal weight full (kg)	12.0	17.0	39.0

Keynotes: [1] The indicated cylinders are for specialised applications and availability is restricted. [2] For domiciliary use only. (Inc. valve) † White

Fig. 9.1 Medical cylinder data. Information is current and is UK specific. Reproduced with permission from BOC Medical, part of the BOC Group PLC.
http://www.bochealthcare.co.uk/en/index.shtml

Nitrous Oxide* — Standard valve

Cylinder code	AZ	C	D	E	F	G	J
Cylinder order code	298122-AZ	141-C	141-D	141-E	141-F	141-G	141-J
Nominal contents (litres)	450	450	900	1800	3600	9000	18000
Nominal cylinder pressure (bar)	44	44	44	44	44	44	44
Valve outlet connection	Pin-index	Pin-index	Pin-index	Pin-index	11/16"×20TPI(M)	11/16"×20TPI(M)	11/16"×20TPI(M)
Valve outlet specification	ISO 407	ISO 407	ISO 407	ISO 407	BS 341 No 13	BS 341 No 13	BS 341 No 13
Valve operation	key	key	key	key	handwheel	handwheel	handwheel
Dimensions* L×D (mm)	290×106	430×89	535×102	865×102	930×140	1320×178	1520×229
Water capacity (litres)	1.20	1.20	2.32	4.68	9.43	23.60	47.20
Nominal weight full (kg)	3.0	2.0	5.0	9.0	22.0	52.0	105.0

ENTONOX† (50% O_2/50% N_2O) — Integral valve

Cylinder code	EA	ED	HX
Cylinder order code	211-EA	211-ED	211-HX
Nominal contents (litres)	350	700	2200
Nominal cylinder pressure (bar)	137	137	137
Nominal outlet pressure (bar)	4	4	4
Valve outlet connection	Entonox Schrader (BS 5682)	Entonox Schrader (BS 5682)	Entonox Schrader (BS 5682)
Valve operation	handwheel	handwheel	handwheel
Valve outlet pressure connection	Schrader-40	Schrader-40	Schrader-40
Dimensions* L×D (mm)	366×85	520×100	940×140
Water capacity (litres)	1.00	2.00	10.00
Nominal weight full (kg)	2.4	4.0	19.0

ENTONOX† (50% O_2/50% N_2O) — Standard valve

Cylinder order code	D	F	G
Cylinder order code	211-D	211-F	211-G
Nominal contents (litres)	500	2000	5000
Nominal cylinder pressure (bar)	137	137	137
Valve outlet connection	Pin-index	Pin-index (side spindle)	Pin-index
Valve outlet specification	ISO 407	ISO 407	ISO 407
Valve operation	key	key	key
Dimensions* L×D (mm)	535×102	930×140	1320×178
Water capacity (litres)	2.32	9.43	23.60
Nominal weight full (kg)	4.0	18.0	34.5

Helium‡ — Standard valve

Cylinder code	F
Cylinder order code	163-F
Nominal contents (litres)	1200
Nominal cylinder pressure (bar)	137
Valve outlet connection	5/8" BSP (F) (Bullnose)
Valve outlet specification	BS 341 No. 3
Valve operation	key
Dimensions* L×D (mm)	930×140
Water capacity (litres)	9.43
Nominal weight full (kg)	17.0

HELIOX21§ (79% He/21% O_2) — Integral valve

Cylinder code	HX
Cylinder order code	173-HX
Nominal contents (litres)	1780
Nominal cylinder pressure (bar)	200
Nominal outlet pressure (bar)	4
Valve outlet flow connection	6mm firtree
Valve outlet connection	Heliox Schrader (BS 5682)
Valve operation	handwheel
Valve outlet pressure connection	Firtree:1:15/Schrader-40
Dimensions* L×D (mm)	940×140
Water capacity (litres)	10.0
Nominal weight full (kg)	15.5

HELIOX21§ — Standard valve

Cylinder code	HL
Cylinder order code	173-HL
Nominal contents (litres)	8200
Nominal cylinder pressure (bar)	200
Nominal outlet pressure (bar)	4
Valve outlet connection	Side outlet
Valve outlet specification	ISO 5145 No. 26
Valve operation	handwheel
Dimensions* L×D (mm)	1540×230
Water capacity (litres)	50.0
Nominal weight full (kg)	85.0

* Blue, †Blue and white quarters, ‡Brown, §Brown and white quarters

Fig. 9.1 (Contd.)

Carbon Dioxide * — Standard valve

Cylinder code	C	E	VF	LF
Cylinder order code	201-C	201-E	201-VF	201-LF
Nominal contents (litres)	450	1800	3600	3600
Nominal cylinder pressure (bar)	50	50	50	50
Valve outlet connection	Pin-index	Pin-index	0.860"×14TPI(M)	0.860"×14TPI(M)
Valve outlet specification	ISO 407	ISO 407	BS 341 No.8	BS 341 No.8
Valve operation	key	key	handwheel	handwheel
Dimensions¹ L×D (mm)	430×89	865×102	930×140	930×140
Water capacity (litres)	1.20	4.68	9.43	9.43
Nominal weight full (kg)	3.0	8.5	22.0	22.0

Oxygen/Carbon Dioxide mixture† (95% O₂/5% CO₂)

Cylinder code	F	G	J
Cylinder order code	131-F	131-G	131-J
Nominal contents (litres)	1360	3400	6800
Nominal cylinder pressure (bar)	137	137	137
Valve outlet connection	5/8" BSP (F)	5/8" BSP (F)	5/8" BSP (F)
Valve outlet specification	BS 341 No.3 (Bullnose)	BS 341 No.3 (Bullnose)	BS 341 No.3 (Bullnose)
Valve operation	key	key	key
Dimensions¹ L×D (mm)	930×140	1320×178	1520×229
Water capacity (litres)	9.43	23.6	47.2
Nominal weight full (kg)	17.0	39.0	78.0

Air‡ — Standard valve

Cylinder code	AZ	E	F	G	J
Cylinder order code	298123-AZ	191-E	191-F	191-G	191-J
Nominal contents (litres)	160	640	1280	3200	6400
Nominal cylinder pressure (bar)	137	137	137	137	137
Valve outlet connection	Pin-index	Pin-index	5/8" BSP (F)	5/8" BSP (F)	5/8" BSP (F)
Valve outlet specification	ISO 407	ISO 407	BS 341 No.3 (Bullnose)	BS 341 No.3 (Bullnose)	BS 341 No.3 (Bullnose)
Valve operation	key	key	key	key	key
Dimensions¹ L×D (mm)	290×106	865×102	930×140	1320×178	1520×229
Water capacity (litres)	1.2	4.7	9.4	23.6	47.2
Nominal weight full (kg)	2.5	6.5	17.0	39.0	78.0

Lung Function mixtures Types 1-4§

Cylinder code	AV	AK
Cylinder order code	Various	Various
Nominal contents (litres)	1500	6000
Nominal cylinder pressure (bar)	150	150
Valve outlet connection	5/8" BSP (F) (L+H) (Side Outlet)	5/8" BSP (F) (L+H) (Side Outlet)
Valve outlet specification	BS 341 No.3 (Bullnose)	BS 341 No.3 (Bullnose)
Valve operation	handwheel	handwheel
Dimensions¹ L×D (mm)	680×180	1540×230
Water capacity (litres)	10.0	40.0
Nominal weight full (kg)	18.0	59.0

Carbon Dioxide/Oxygen mixtures§

	(5% CO₂/95% O₂)		(10% CO₂/90% O₂)		(20% CO₂/80% O₂)	
Cylinder code	AV	L	AV	L	AV	L
Cylinder order code	299031-AV-PC	299031-L-PC	299032-AV-PC	299031-L-PC	299954-AV-PC	299033-L-PC
Nominal contents (litres)	1440	7300	1460	7300	1530	7650
Nominal cylinder pressure (bar)	137	137	137	137	137	137
Valve outlet connection	5/8" BSP (F) (Side Outlet)	5/8" BSP (F) (Side Outlet)	5/8" BSP (F) (Side Outlet)	5/8" BSP (F) (Side Outlet)	5/8" BSP (F) (Side Outlet)	5/8" BSP (F) (Side Outlet)
Valve outlet specification	BS 341 No.3 (Bullnose)	BS 341 No.3 (Bullnose)	BS 341 No.3 (Bullnose)	BS 341 No.3 (Bullnose)	BS 341 No.3 (Bullnose)	BS 341 No.3 (Bullnose)
Valve operation	handwheel	handwheel	handwheel	handwheel	handwheel	handwheel
Dimensions¹ L×D (mm)	680×180	1540×230	680×180	1540×230	680×180	1540×230
Water capacity (litres)	10.0	50.0	10.0	50.0	10.0	50.0
Nominal weight full (kg)	19.0	85.0	19.0	86.0	19.0	87.0

* Grey; † Grey (Grey with white quarters); ‡ Black and white quarters; § Green

Fig. 9.1 (Contd.)

⊙ Carbon Dioxide/Air mixture† (5% CO₂/95% Air)

Cylinder code	AV	L
Cylinder order code	299034-AV-PC	299034-L-PC
Nominal contents (litres)	1350	6750
Nominal cylinder pressure (bar)	137	137
Valve outlet connection	5/8" BSP (F) (Side Outlet)	5/8" BSP (F) (Side Outlet)
Valve outlet specification	BS 341 No.3	BS 341 No.3
Valve operation	(Bullnose) handwheel	(Bullnose) handwheel
Dimensions* L×D (mm)	680×180	1540×230
Water capacity (litres)	10.0	50.0
Nominal weight full (kg)	18.0	82.0

†(inc valve) Green

⊙ Helium/Oxygen/Nitrogen mixture† (56% N₂/35% O₂/9% He)

Cylinder code	AV	L
Cylinder order code	299035-AV-PC	299035-L-PC
Nominal contents (litres)	1310	6580
Nominal cylinder pressure (bar)	137	137
Valve outlet connection	5/8" BSP (F) (Side Outlet)	5/8" BSP (F) (Side Outlet)
Valve outlet specification	BS 341 No.3	BS 341 No.3
Valve operation	(Bullnose) handwheel	(Bullnose) handwheel
Dimensions* L×D (mm)	680×180	1540×230
Water capacity (litres)	10.0	50.0
Nominal weight full (kg)	18.0	81.0

Cylinder types

6ft. (1.83m)

AZ ZA/ZB ZC C AD CD DD PD RD D E AF DF F LF VF AV HX G AK J L/HL

Valve types

Pin-index Side Spindle valve   Integral valve   Handwheel valve   Bullnose valve   Pin-index valve   Handwheel side outlet

Pin index types

Oxygen   Nitrous Oxide   Entonox   Air   Carbon Dioxide

BOC Medical
Customer Service Centre, Priestley Road, Worsley, Manchester
M28 2UT
Tel: 0800 111 333 Fax 0800 111 555 Email: bocmedical-uk@
boc.com
www.bocmedical.co.uk
The words BOC, BOC Medical are registered trade marks of The
Linde Group of companies in the UK.
© Copyright BOC Limited
MED130946/SAPUK/0709/SM

Fig. 9.1 (Contd.)

Cylinder identification coding

Cylinders are made from either from steel or, more recently, aluminium wrapped with Kevlar. Each cylinder is marked with a specific colour for each gas type, according to standards BS1319C and ISO 32, and fitted with outlet valves of various types. The top of the cylinder has a tapered thread into which is permanently fitted a valve. The valve can be opened by a handwheel, thumbwheel, or special key. The gas outlet from this valve is connected to a pressure-reducing regulator, pressure gauge, and other devices, depending on the application.

Four main types of cylinder outlet valves are in use: bullnose, pin index, handwheel, and valve and side spindle pin-index valves. More recently, cylinders have been introduced that carry an integrated valve/regulator. These are also known as 'star valves' or 'combi-valves'.

The most important valve in use is the pin-index valve, which has a system of non-interchangeable valves designed to ensure that the correct gas is filled into the cylinder and that the cylinder can only be connected to the correct equipment.

Medical gas flowmeters

Medical O_2 and air flowmeters normally have differently calibrated flow tubes, but the fitting of the cylinder onto the regulator is the same. The Entonox cylinder is fitted with a demand valve, because administration depends on patient demand.

The cylinder labelling includes details of the following (Fig. 9.1).
- Product name, chemical symbol, and pharmaceutical form.
- Safety phrases.
- Cylinder size code.
- Nominal cylinder contents in litres.
- Maximum cylinder pressure in bars.
- Product shelf-life and expiry date.
- Reference to the medical gas data sheet (which details clinical indications, dosage schedules, and contraindications—ensure that you are aware of location of this information in the pharmacy).
- Storage and handling precautions.

At the pressures used, some gases liquefy within the cylinder and therefore behave differently during storage and delivery.

O_2 and Entonox remain gases, whereas nitrous oxide and carbon dioxide (CO_2) liquefy. The liquids will cool considerably during expansion and this can cause problems, although this drawback is put to good use in cryosurgery where nitrous oxide evaporation and expansion are used as the energy source. Entonox should not be stored below freezing point (0°C) because the mixture (50% nitrous oxide and 50% O_2) can separate.

Guideline for oxygen use in adult patients

Oxygen has traditionally been used in hospitals in an uncontrolled manner, sometimes with inadequate monitoring. It is a treatment that should be used with discrimination and responsibility, as with any form of treatment.

Clinical indication, policy, and potential errors.

Additional inspired oxygen is used to improve oxygen delivery to the tissues, i.e. it is a treatment for hypoxaemia not breathlessness.

Each hospital should develop guidelines to ensure a requirement for oxygen to be prescribed according to a target saturation range and for those who administer oxygen therapy to monitor the patient and keep within the saturation target range.

Oxygen prescription

Oxygen should be prescribed to achieve a target saturation of 94–98% for the most acutely ill patients or 88–92% for those at risk of hyper-capnic respiratory failure.

Oxygen administration

Oxygen should be administered by staff who are trained in oxygen administration. These staff should use appropriate devices and flow rates in order to achieve the target saturation range.

Monitoring and maintenance of target saturation

Oxygen saturation and delivery system should be recorded on the patient's monitoring chart alongside the oximetry result. Oxygen delivery devices and flow rates should be adjusted to keep the oxygen saturation in the target range.

Oxygen should be signed for on the drug chart on each drug round.

Weaning and discontinuation

Oxygen should be reduced in stable patients with satisfactory oxygen saturation, assuming that corrective action has been undertaken to resolve the cause of hypoxaemia. Oxygen should be crossed off the drug chart once the decision has been taken to stop oxygen therapy.

Errors

- Patients with chronic ventilatory failure are sometimes given inappropriately high concentrations of oxygen, which results in worsening carbon dioxide retention and respiratory acidosis.
- Patients who are otherwise hypoxic, including those with acute ventilatory failure, are given unnecessarily low inspired oxygen concentrations.

Management of respiratory failure

Type 1 respiratory failure (hypoxia with normal $Paco_2$)

- Occurs in a wide variety of patients with acute or chronic cardiac or respiratory disease.
- Hypoxia can be confirmed by measurements of oxygen saturation but arterial blood gas analysis is required to exclude CO_2 retention.
- The objective of treatment is to achieve normal levels of oxygenation.

Type 2 respiratory failure (hypoxia with elevated $Paco_2$)

Acute ventilatory failure

- This occurs in most conditions resulting in acute respiratory distress— e.g. asthma, pulmonary oedema, pneumonia, etc.
- Hypoxia can be confirmed by measurements of oxygen saturation. Blood gas analysis is required to confirm acute ventilatory failure with an elevated $Paco_2$, low pH, and normal bicarbonate (acute respiratory acidosis).
- The objective of treatment is to restore normal oxygenation. High concentrations of inspired oxygen are *not* contraindicated.
- There should be urgent assessment of the need for assisted ventilation.

Chronic ventilatory failure (± acute component)

- This should be suspected in a variety of situations including patients with chronic lung disease (COPD), neuromuscular disease, and skeletal disorders.
- It is confirmed on the basis of blood gas analysis, which shows an elevated $Paco_2$, normal or reduced pH, and elevated bicarbonate.
- The objective is to achieve safe but not normal levels of oxygen. A Pao_2 of 6–8 or saturations of 80–90% are acceptable.
- Low concentrations of oxygen should be administered using a system working on the Venturi principle, which delivers precise concentrations of 24%, 28%, 31%, etc.
- If, in the chronic situation, nasal cannulae are used, oxygen saturation should be monitored to achieve saturation levels of ~85%.

Further reading

O'Driscoll BR *et al.* (2008). BTS guideline for emergency oxygen use in adult patients. *Thorax* **63** (Suppl vi): vi1–68.

Domiciliary oxygen therapy

Domiciliary oxygen therapy, of which there are three forms, is the administration of oxygen at concentrations greater than that available in room air (which is 21%). It is prescribed for the following reasons.

- To correct hypoxaemia—a deficiency of oxygen in arterial blood, leading to an arterial oxygen tension (PaO_2) ≤ 7.3kPa (normal values are 11.5–13.5kPa). Complications, if left untreated, include cor pulmonale, secondary polycythaemia, and pulmonary hypertension.
- To prevent hypoxia—a lack of oxygen in the tissues resulting in cell death.

Long-term oxygen therapy

There are several conditions which may lead to long-term oxygen therapy (LTOT) being prescribed to correct the chronic hypoxaemia which can result. Screening patients with the use of pulse oximetry is advisable for those with an underlying condition, with a referral for an LTOT assessment made if oxygen saturations fall below 92%. The LTOT assessment must include arterial blood gas analysis so that oxygen and carbon dioxide levels can be reviewed.

The assessment should take place during a period of clinical stability and therefore requires consideration in terms of timing as the treatment for the underlying condition needs to be reviewed and optimized. If an assessment is undertaken during an exacerbation of a condition, LTOT may be inappropriately indicated and subsequently prescribed.

Conditions that could result in chronic hypoxaemia include:

- COPD (the disease for which LTOT is most commonly prescribed)
- cystic fibrosis
- bronchiectasis
- interstitial lung disease
- pulmonary lung disease
- primary pulmonary hypertension
- pulmonary malignancy
- chronic heart failure.

Studies have shown improved exercise endurance in COPD patients breathing supplemental oxygen, with improved walking distance and ability to perform daily activities. Additional benefits of LTOT in COPD patients include reduction of secondary polycythaemia, improved sleep quality, and reduced sympathetic outflow, with increased sodium and water excretion, leading to improvement in renal function.[1–3]

1 Chapman S et al. (eds) (2005). Long-term oxygen therapy. Oxford Handbook of Respiratory Therapy, pp.632–5. Oxford: Oxford University Press.

2 National Clinical Guideline Centre (2010). Chronic Obstructive Pulmonary Disease: Manage of Chronic Obstructive Pulmonary Disease in Adults in Primary and Secondary Care. London: National Clinical Guideline Centre (available online at: http://guidance.nice.org.uk/CG101/ Guidance/pdf/ English I(accessed 1 June 2010).

3 Esmond G, Mikelsons C (2009). Oxygen therapy. Non-invasive Respiratory Support Techniques: Oxygen Therapy, Non-invasive Ventilation and CPAP, pp.47–88. Chichester: Wiley–Blackwell.

The term LTOT refers to the number of hours per day therapy is used rather than the number of years it is used for, although it is likely to be lifelong treatment once commenced. This form of therapy is based on two landmark trials conducted in the 1980s, in which the main outcome was improved survival in those patients receiving oxygen for at least 15h per day and an increase in 5-year survival and an overall improvement in quality of life.[4,5] For this to be achieved, the following is necessary.

- The daytime oxygen tension should be kept at or above 8kPa (the equivalent to an oxygen saturation (SpO_2) ≥92%.
- The equipment used to deliver LTOT is suitable to administer oxygen therapy for at least 15h per day.

When therapy is indicated, an oxygen concentrator is a more convenient and reliable way to supply LTOT than oxygen cylinders. This runs off the normal household electricity supply and does not require replenishing like an oxygen cylinder does. However, it requires yearly maintenance. This device draws in atmospheric/room air (consisting of approximately 78% nitrogen and 21% oxygen) and separates these gases through the use of zeolite, which captures nitrogen molecules, resulting in a continuous supply of oxygen in the home of up to a flow rate of ~5L/min. A back-up oxygen cylinder should be supplied to patients using an oxygen concentrator in case of emergencies such as mechanical breakdowns or an electricity supply failure.

Nasal cannulae, designed to deliver a typical low flow of oxygen at 1–4L/min, are more frequently used than facemasks to deliver oxygen to the patient because:

- they are less obvious and obtrusive
- communication is not hindered
- the patient is able to eat and drink while using oxygen.

NB: higher flows of oxygen (>4L/min) may cause the nasal passages to become dried out, resulting in inflammation, nosebleeds, and pain, which could affect adherence to treatment.)

Facemasks are seldom used in LTOT as they are often considered to act as a barrier to communication and need to be removed in order for the patient to eat and drink. However, there are circumstances which would warrant provision of a facemask. Such instances include the presence of a nasal defect or high flow rates not being tolerated via nasal cannulae. When a mask is used, the most appropriate is a fixed-concentration mask in the form of a Venturi mask which will deliver a more accurate concentration of oxygen. It is also advisable to provide the patient with nasal cannulae so that oxygen can continue to be delivered during periods of eating and drinking.

4 Nocturnal Oxygen Therapy Trial Group (1980). Continuous or nocturnal oxygen therapy in hypoxemic chronic obstructive pulmonary disease: a clinical trial. *Annals of Internal Medicine* **93**: 391–8.

5 Medical Research Council (1981). Long term domiciliary oxygen therapy in hypoxemic cor pulmonale complicating chronic bronchitis and emphysema. Report of the Medical Research Council Working Party. *Lancet* i: 681–6.

Ambulatory oxygen therapy

Ambulatory oxygen therapy provides oxygen during exercise and activities of daily living for patients who have chronic hypoxaemia or exercise oxygen desaturation. It enables patients to leave home for a longer period of time to fulfil activities of daily living and improve their quality of life. Several factors need to be taken into account when deciding if a prescription of ambulatory oxygen is indicated. This may involve patients having to undertake a timed walking test or a shuttle walking test during assessment.

Patients suitable for this type of therapy can be divided into two main categories:

- those with PaO_2 ≤7.3 kPa (i.e. those patients already on LTOT) who are also mobile.
- Patients with PaO_2 of 7.3–8.0kPa who desaturate on exercise or show an improvement in exercise capacity or dyspnoea with oxygen.

Different types of equipment can be used to deliver ambulatory oxygen.
- Portable oxygen cylinders, of which there are four types available.
  - DD—a lightweight cylinder containing 460L of oxygen that lasts for 3h 50min at 2L/min.
  - F size—contains 1360L of oxygen and lasts approximately 11.5h at 2L/min.
  - PD—a smaller but heavier cylinder than the DD type which contains 300L of oxygen and lasts for 2.5h at 2L/min.
  - E size—a lightweight portable cylinder containing 600L of oxygen which lasts for 5h at 2L/min.

NB: the duration of use of the chosen cylinder may be increased by adding an oxygen-conserving device into the circuit, which ensures that oxygen is only delivered on inspiration.
- Liquid oxygen.
- Portable concentrator.

Apart from E size portable oxygen cylinders and portable concentrators, ambulatory oxygen equipment is available on the NHS.

Short-burst oxygen therapy

Short-burst oxygen therapy (SBOT) lasts for 10–15min at a time and is frequently given to patients with normal oxygen levels to alleviate breathlessness due to hypoxia after exercise. Some patients are noted to use a burst of oxygen prior to exertion, such as climbing the stairs.

SBOT is an expensive treatment, best provided by using one or more oxygen cylinders (usually F size) placed strategically round the house, with little published evidence to support its use. It is considered for patients with episodes of severe breathlessness due to hypoxia which is not relieved by other means, such as the use of oral morphine or benzodiazepines. This mode of therapy may also be used for palliation—e.g. terminal stages of lung cancer, which causes distressing shortness of breath, where some patients describe a subjective benefit in their breathlessness from using short bursts of oxygen during this time.

The practicalities of domiciliary oxygen therapy

- Patients needing domiciliary oxygen therapy should have stopped smoking before commencing therapy. Studies indicate that the benefit of such therapy, LTOT in particular, is limited in continued smokers, with an increased risk of fire.[1,3]
- The specialist home oxygen assessment services should be contacted when domiciliary oxygen is indicated for a patient. This service assesses, prescribes, reviews, and follows up patients requiring domiciliary oxygen in the UK. (Previously, oxygen was prescribed by a GP following recommendation from a respiratory physician.)
- These services are funded by the primary care trust (PCT), which can give details of who should be contacted if an assessment is needed.
- Once a patient has been assessed for domiciliary oxygen, a home oxygen order form (HOOF) is completed by the specialist oxygen assessment service for the provision of the correct form of domiciliary oxygen.
- The completed HOOF is faxed to the oxygen supplier, who then contacts the patient to arrange a date for installation. (Details of oxygen suppliers can be found on the primary care contracting website www.pcc.nhs.uk)
- Follow-up reviews of patients are carried out by the specialist home oxygen assessment service to ensure compliance and ongoing requirement for domiciliary oxygen.
- Patient education in the use and maintenance of long-term, ambulatory, or short-burst oxygen therapy and maintenance of equipment is important and requires the involvement of specialist respiratory nurses.

Patient management issues

Drug use in liver disease *178*
Drug dosing in liver disease *180*
Hepatorenal syndrome (HRS) *183*
Drugs in renal impairment *184*
Drugs in pregnancy *190*
Drugs in breastfeeding *194*
Drugs and dietary considerations *198*
Glucose 6-phosphate dehydrogenase (G6PD) deficiency *200*
Drugs in porphyria *202*

Drug use in liver disease

Terminology used in liver disease is summarized in Table 10.1. The liver is the main site of drug metabolism and the principal location for CYP450 metabolism (see 🕮 p.21). In most cases, metabolism leads to inactivation of the drug, although some drugs have active metabolites (e.g. morphine) or require metabolism to be activated (e.g. cyclophosphamide). Despite this, it is frequently unnecessary to modify the dose (or choice) of drug in liver disease because the liver has a large reserve of function, even if disease seems severe. However, special consideration of drugs and doses are required in the following situations:

- **Hepatotoxic drugs**—whether the hepatotoxicity is dose-related or idiosyncratic, these drugs are more likely to cause toxicity in patients with liver disease and so should be avoided if possible.
- **Protein binding**—the liver is the main source of synthesis of plasma proteins (e.g. albumin). As liver disease progresses, plasma protein levels fall. Thus, with less protein available for binding, there is more free drug available, which can lead to ↑ effects and toxicity, especially if the therapeutic index is narrow or the drug is normally highly protein bound (e.g. phenytoin). If albumin levels are significantly ↓, serum levels measured for TDM might have to be adjusted to give a corrected level.
- **Anticoagulants/drugs that cause bleeding**—the liver is the main source of synthesis of clotting factors and there is an ↑ risk of bleeding as liver function deteriorates. Anticoagulants should be avoided (and are rarely indicated because of the ↓ in clotting factors) and drugs that ↑ the risk of bleeding (e.g. NSAIDs, selective serotonin re-uptake inhibitors (SSRIs)) should be used with caution. Avoid intramuscular injections because there is a risk of haematoma.
- **Liver failure**—patients with clinical signs of liver failure (e.g. significantly deranged liver enzymes, ascites, or profound jaundice) usually have altered drug handling (Table 10.2). In addition, drugs that could worsen the condition should be avoided:
  - Hepatic encephalopathy could be precipitated by certain drugs. Avoid all sedative drugs (including opioid analgesics), drugs causing hypokalaemia (including loop and thiazide diuretics) and drugs causing constipation.
  - Oedema and ascites could be exacerbated by drugs that cause fluid retention (e.g. NSAIDs and corticosteroids). Drugs with high sodium content (e.g. soluble/effervescent formulations, some antacids and IV antibacterials) should also be avoided.

Table 10.1 Terminology in liver disease

Hepatocellular injury	Damage to the main cells of the liver (hepatocytes)
Hepatitis	Inflammation of the liver, a type of hepatocellular injury. Could be caused by viruses, drugs, or other agents, or could be idiosyncratic.
Cirrhosis	Chronic, irreversible damage to liver cells, usually caused by alcohol or hepatitis C. If the remaining cells cannot maintain normal liver function (compensated disease), ascites, jaundice, and encephalopathy can develop (decompensated disease).
Cholestasis	Reduction in bile production or bile flow through the bile ducts.
Liver failure	Severe hepatic dysfunction where compensatory mechanisms are no longer sufficient to maintain homeostasis. Could be acute and reversible, or irreversible (e.g. endstage cirrhosis).

Drug dosing in liver disease

The effects of liver disease, and consequent impairment of drug handling, are diverse and often unpredictable. Unlike renal disease, drug clearance does not ↓ in a linear fashion as liver function worsens. In addition, whereas in renal disease measuring creatinine clearance gives a good predictor of drug clearance, in liver disease there is no good clinical factor that predicts drug clearance and thus dose adjustment.

Impaired elimination is usually only seen in advanced liver disease. The following markers indicate significant impairment:

- ↓ albumin (↑ or ↓ in acute liver disease)
- ↑ prothrombin time
- ↑↑ liver function tests (LFTs).

The following four main factors affect drug clearance:

Hepatic blood flow

Hepatic blood flow might be altered in liver disease because of cirrhosis (fibrosis inhibits blood flow), hepatic venous outflow obstruction (Budd–Chiari syndrome), or portal vein thrombosis. Even in the absence of liver disease, hepatic blood flow might be ↓ in cardiac failure or if BP is massively ↓ (e.g. in shock).

The clearance of drugs that are highly metabolized by the liver (high-extraction/high-clearance drugs) is directly related to blood flow. When these drugs are administered orally, their first-pass metabolism is significantly ↓ (if hepatic blood flow is ↓) and so bioavailability ↑. Administration by non-enteral routes, especially IV administration, avoids the effect of first-pass metabolism and therefore bioavailability is unaffected. Thus the effect of liver impairment on the clearance of these drugs is fairly predictable, being directly related to hepatic blood flow.

Drugs that are poorly metabolized (low-extraction/low-clearance drugs) are unaffected by changes in hepatic blood flow. Clearance of these drugs is affected by a variety of other factors.

In both situations doses should be titrated according to clinical response and side effects (Table 10.2).

Decreased hepatic cell mass

Extensive liver cell damage can occur in both acute and chronic liver disease. High-extraction drugs are metabolized less efficiently and therefore doses should be ↓ because peak plasma levels are ↑. Low-extraction drugs will have ↓ systemic clearance, leading to delayed elimination. Thus the dose should remain the same but the dose interval should be ↑ (Table 10.2).

Table 10.2 High- and low-extraction drugs

High-extraction drugs

Dose at 10–50% normal for oral administration
Dose at 50% normal for IV administration
↑ dose interval in portal systemic shunting

- Clomethiazole
- Glyceryl trinitrate
- Lidocaine
- Metoprolol
- Morphine
- Pethidine
- Propranolol
- Verapamil

Low-extraction drugs

Dose at 50% normal (all routes)
↑ dose interval

- Ampicillin
- Atenolol
- Chloramphenicol
- Chlordiazepoxide
- Cimetidine
- Diazepam
- Digoxin
- Furosemide
- Lorazepam
- Naproxen
- Prednisolone
- Spironolactone
- Tolbutamide
- Warfarin

Portal systemic shunting

If cirrhosis or portal hypertension is present, a collateral venous circulation, which bypasses the liver, could develop. This means that drugs absorbed by the GI tract might enter the systemic circulation directly. Thus there is minimal first-pass metabolism of high-extraction drugs and peak concentrations are ↑. The half-life of both high- and low-extraction drugs is prolonged, and so the dose interval should be ↑.

Cholestasis

In cholestasis, substances that are normally eliminated by the biliary system accumulate. This includes some drugs that are eliminated by bile salts (e.g. rifampicin and sodium fusidate). Because lipid absorption depends on bile salt production, it is theoretically possible that there is a ↓ in absorption of lipid-soluble drugs. In cholestasis, bile salts accumulate in the blood. This could ↑ bioavailability of protein-bound drugs because of competition for binding sites.

Analgesia in liver failure

The choice of analgesic drug in liver failure is problematic because both NSAIDs and opioids are contraindicated. The analgesic of choice is paracetamol because hepatotoxicity only occurs in overdose, when glutathione is saturated. In liver failure, glutathione production is maintained. It is advisable to avoid maximum daily doses of paracetamol because this can ↑ prothrombin time.

Further reading/information

Remington H et al. (1992). Drug choice in patients with liver disease. *Pharmaceutical Journal*, **248**: 845–8.
Cavell G (1993). Drug handling in liver disease. *Pharmaceutical Journal*, **250**: 352–5.
Summaries of product characteristics.
Leeds Medicines Information Centre.
General guidelines for prescribing in liver disease are given in Table 10.3.

Table 10.3 General guidelines for prescribing in liver disease

- Avoid hepatotoxic drugs (note that many herbal medicines/adulterants are potentially hepatotoxic)
- Use renally cleared drugs preferentially
- Monitor closely for side effects of hepatically cleared drugs
- Avoid drugs that ↑ the risk of bleeding
- Avoid sedating drugs if there is a risk of encephalopathy
- Avoid constipating drugs if there is a risk of encephalopathy
- In moderate or severe liver impairment consider the following options:
  - ↓ dose of highly metabolized drugs
  - ↑ dose interval for all hepatically cleared drugs
- If albumin levels are low, consider ↓ the dose of highly protein-bound drugs
- Drugs that affect electrolyte balance should be used cautiously and monitored carefully
- In preference, use older well-established drugs if there is experience of use in liver impairment
- Start with the lowest possible dose and ↑ cautiously, according to response or side effects

---

clearance can be achieved using the Cockroft and Gault equation (Table 10.5). This equation takes into account the fact that muscle mass (and therefore serum creatinine levels) vary according to gender and weight.

Calculating the rate of creatinine clearance in this way gives a better estimate than simply using serum creatinine, but it is not exact and tends to under- or overestimate the rate by up to 20%. Ideal body weight should be used in obese or fluid-overloaded patients. The equation is particularly inaccurate in pregnant women, children, and patients with marked catabolism or rapidly changing renal function. For children a more accurate creatinine clearance can be calculated (Table 10.5).

Remember that elderly patients nearly always have some degree of renal impairment because of the normal ageing process. Despite its limitations, the Cockroft and Gault equation is extremely useful for assessing renal impairment in this setting and is preferable to using serum creatinine alone. For example, a serum creatinine of 120micromol/L might be normal in a fit young man but could represent significant renal impairment in a frail elderly woman.

Table 10.5 Calculating creatinine clearance

Adults

Cockroft and Gault equation:[1]

$$\text{Creatinine clearance (mL/min)} = \frac{F(140 - \text{age}) \times \text{weight (kg)}}{\text{serum creatinine (micromol/L)}}$$

where $F = 1.04$ in females and 1.23 in males.

Use IBW in obese or fluid-overloaded patients.

Modification of Diet in Renal Disease[2] (= eGFR)

$$\text{eGFR (mL/min/1.73m}^2) = 32788 \times \text{serum creatinine (micromol/L)}^{-1.154} \times \text{age}^{-0.203} \times X \times Y$$

where $X = 1.212$ (if African American) and $Y = 0.742$ (if female)

Children[3]

$$\text{Estimated creatinine clearance (mL/min/1.73m}^2) = \frac{40 \times \text{height (cm)}}{\text{serum creatinine (micromol/L)}}$$

Neonates[4]

$$\text{Estimated creatinine clearance (mL/min/1.73m}^2) = \frac{30 \times \text{length (cm)}}{\text{serum creatinine (micromol/L)}}$$

---

[1] Cockroft DW, Gault MH (1976). "Prediction of creatinine clearance from serum creatinine". *Nephron*, **16**(1): 31–41.

[2] Levey AS et al. (1999). A more accurate method to estimate glomerular filtration rate from serum creatinine: a new prediction equation. *Annals of Internal Medicine*, **130**: 461–70.

[3] Morris MC et al. (1982). Evaluation of a height/plasma creatinine formula in the measurement of glomerular filtration rate. *Archives of Diseases in Children*, **57**: 611–15.

[4] Schwartz GJ et al. (1984). A simple estimate of glomerular filtration rate in full term infants during the first year of life. *Journal of Paediatrics*, **104**: 849–54.

Normal creatinine clearance in adults is ~80–120mL/min (for infants and children, see Table 10.6). In the UK, the following ranges of GFR are considered to represent various degrees of renal impairment:
- mild, 50–20mL/min
- moderate, 20–10mL/min
- severe, <10mL/min.

An alternative method of estimating GFR is to use the Modification of Diet in Renal Disease (MDRD) equation, which is often quoted as estimated GFR (eGFR). This equation is more reliable than the Cockroft and Gault equation for patients with unstable renal function or acute renal failure. However, it quotes the GFR for a standard body surface area (i.e. mL/min/1.73m^2) and so it is unsuitable for patients at extremes of body weight or amputees. It is also unsuitable for certain ethnic groups. Some laboratories are now quoting eGFR in addition to serum creatinine when reporting renal function. This is appropriate in terms of giving a better indication than serum creatinine of whether the patient has any degree of renal impairment. However, most drug dosing recommendations are based on GFR not eGFR, and in this respect calculating the creatinine clearance using the Cockroft and Gault equation gives a better estimate.

Dose adjustment in renal failure
The kidney is involved in the elimination of most drugs, either in their active/unchanged form or as their metabolites, although for some drugs this might be only a very small proportion of the dose. Drugs for which the kidney is a major site of elimination usually require dosage adjustment to avoid accumulation and thus toxicity. Remember that some of these drugs might also be nephrotoxic and drug accumulation can make renal impairment worse.

In patients with mild renal impairment it might only be necessary to monitor closely for side effects, with or without further deterioration in kidney function. However, in moderate or severe renal impairment an alternative drug should be used if possible. The ideal drug in renal failure would have the following attributes:
- <25% excreted unchanged in the urine.
- No active/toxic metabolites.
- Levels/activity minimally affected by fluid balance or protein-binding changes.
- Wide therapeutic margin.
- Not nephrotoxic.

Unfortunately, it is frequently not possible to find a suitable drug that fits these criteria, in which case dose adjustment is usually necessary. Two methods of dose reduction are used, either alone or in combination.
- Give a smaller dose at the same dose interval.
- Give the same dose at a longer dose interval.

It is possible to calculate a corrected dose/dose interval, but a more practical option is to use drug-dosing guidelines. The reader is referred to the sources on 🕮 p.205.

Renal impairment prolongs the half-life of any drug excreted by the kidney. The time to steady-state concentration is ~5 times the half-life.

Thus, just as in patients with normal renal function, a loading dose might be needed if an immediate effect is required. This is especially true if the dose interval has been ↑. The loading dose in patients with renal impairment is the same as in patients with normal renal function.

Certain drugs should always be checked if there is any suspicion of renal impairment (Table 10.7). In many instances, not only are these drugs primarily excreted by the kidneys, but some are also potentially nephrotoxic, such that accumulation could lead to further renal impairment. In addition, side effects caused by accumulation might be mistaken for disease deterioration, and the pharmacist should be alert to this and advise medical staff accordingly. Wherever possible, avoid using potentially nephrotoxic drugs in patients with renal impairment.

Remember that renal function might improve or further deteriorate according to the patient's condition and, consequently, doses may need to be readjusted accordingly.

Table 10.6 Normal creatinine clearances in infants and children

Age	Creatinine clearance (mL/min/1.73m^2)
<37wks gestation	<25
Neonate	15–35
1–2wks	35–60
2–4 months	60–80
6–12 months	80–110
12 months to adult	85–150

Table 10.7 Checklist of drugs requiring dose adjustment in renal impairment

Commonly used drugs for which dose reduction is always necessary in moderate or severe renal imirment[*]

- Aciclovir
- Aminoglycosides
- Capecitabine
- Cisplatin
- Imipenem
- Meropenem
- Methotrexate
- Penicillin
- Thiazide diuretics
- Vancomycin

Commonly used drugs for which dose reduction should be considered in moderate or severe renal impairment[*]

- Allopurinol
- Amoxicillin
- Cephalosporins
- Cyclophosphamide
- Flucloxacillin
- Digoxin
- Ethambutol
- Furosemide
- Lomustine
- Melphalan
- Opioids
- Quinolones
- Sulphonamides (including co-trimoxazole)

[*] These lists are not comprehensive—check specialist references (📖 p.205) for further information.

Drug dosing in renal replacement therapies

Renal replacement therapies are used in patients with chronic renal failure whose renal function is so poor that the kidneys are barely functioning. They can also be used temporarily in patients with acute renal failure. There are four types of renal replacement therapy in common use.
- Intermittent haemodialysis (HD).
- Continuous ambulatory peritoneal dialysis (CAPD).
- Continuous arteriovenous haemodialysis (CAVD).
- Continuous arteriovenous haemofiltration (CAVH).

Each method works on the principle of removing toxins from the blood by diffusion or osmosis across a semipermeable membrane into a dialysis solution. Therefore the factors that affect drug removal are much the same for HD, CAPD and CAVD. CAVH is a slightly different technique and is influenced by slightly different factors.

Dialysis-related factors

The following factors influence drug removal by dialysis or filtration:
- duration of dialysis
- blood flow rate in dialyser
- type of dialyser membrane
- flow rate and composition of dialysate.

However, these characteristics are difficult to quantify and therefore it is hard to predict exactly what effect they will have on drug removal. In CAPD, frequent exchanges (e.g. every 1–4h) ↑ drug clearance.

Drug-related factors

It is possible to judge whether or not a drug will be significantly cleared by dialysis according to the pharmacokinetic parameters. Factors that favour drug removal are as follows.
- Low molecular weight—removal ↑ as molecular weight falls below 500 Da.
- Low protein binding (<20%).
- Low volume of distribution (<1L/kg).
- High water solubility.
- High degree of renal clearance in normal renal function.

The exception is CAVH, where molecules with a higher molecular weight (up to that of insulin) are preferentially removed, but there is less removal of smaller molecules (e.g. K^+ and urea).

Drug dosing in renal replacement therapies

Accurately quantifying drug clearance during renal replacement therapies is of limited value. The equations tend to assume constant conditions, but in practice both patient and dialysis conditions can vary. For example, the patient's clinical status (e.g. BP or renal function) could change, which has an effect on drug clearance. In CAPD, peritonitis affects peritoneal permeability and thus clearance.

The most practical approach is to use empirical dosing according to theoretical GFR achieved by the dialysis technique used (Table 10.8). This should be backed up by close monitoring for drug response and toxicity, including TDM.

In patients receiving HD, drugs should be given after the dialysis session to avoid the possibility that the drug might be removed before it has time to act. Because CAVH and CAVD are continuous processes, doses do not need to be scheduled around dialysis sessions. The same is true for CAPD, but the dose might need to be titrated up or down if the frequency of exchanges is ↑ or ↓.

Table 10.8 Theoretical GFR in renal replacement therapy

Renal replacement therapy		Typical theoretical GFR achieved (mL/min)
HD	During dialysis	150–160
	Between dialysis periods	0–10
CAVD		15–20
CAVH		10
CAPD (4 exchanges daily)		5–10

Further reading

Ashley C, Currie A (eds) (2008). *The Renal Drug Handbook* (3rd edn). Abingdon: Radcliffe Medical Press.
Aronoff GR et al. (2007). *Drug Prescribing in Renal Failure* (5th edn). Philadelphia, PA: American College of Physicians.
Summaries of Product Characteristics.
South West Medicines Information Centre.

Drugs in pregnancy

A drug is defined as teratogenic if it crosses the placenta, causing congenital malformations. Teratogenic effects usually only occur when the fetus is exposed during a critical period of development. Even then, not all fetuses exposed will be affected—e.g. <50% of fetuses exposed to thalidomide developed congenital abnormalities.

Various textbooks and reference sources (see 🕮 p.193) give information on using drugs in pregnancy (Tables 10.9 and 10.10), but these sources do not always take into account all the relevant factors when assessing risk. To fully evaluate the risk/benefit of a drug in pregnancy, the following factors should be taken into account.

Other possible causes
- ≤10% of pregnancies result in an 'abnormal' outcome (including miscarriage and stillbirth), of which only 2–3% are caused by drugs or environmental factors.
- Maternal morbidity or an acute exacerbation/relapse of the disease could present a higher risk to the fetus than the drug.
- The underlying maternal disease might be associated with congenital abnormalities (e.g. epilepsy).
- Smoking and alcohol use during pregnancy can lead to congenital abnormalities, growth retardation, and spontaneous abortion.

Drug characteristics
- Most drugs cross the placenta.
- High molecular weight drugs do not cross the placenta—e.g. heparin and insulin.
- Non-ionized lipophilic drugs (e.g. labetalol) cross the placenta to a greater extent than ionized hydrophilic drugs (e.g. atenolol).
- A drug can cause fetal toxicity without crossing the placenta—e.g. any drug that causes vasoconstriction of the placental vasculature.

Timing
- If the drug is taken during the first 12 days (pre-embryonic phase), there is an 'all or nothing' effect—i.e. if most cells are affected, this leads to spontaneous miscarriage, and if a few cells are affected, this leads to cell repair/replacement and a normal fetus.
- Exposure during the first trimester (especially weeks 3–11) carries the greatest risk of congenital abnormalities.
- During the second or third trimester the main risks are growth defects or functional loss, rather than gross structural abnormalities. However, cerebral cortex and renal glomeruli continue to develop and are still susceptible to damage.
- Shortly before or during labour there is a risk of maternal complications (e.g. NSAIDs and maternal bleeding) or neonate complications (e.g. opioids and sedation).

Table 10.9 Some drugs that should be avoided* in pregnancy[1]

Drugs known to cause congenital malformations

- Anticonvulsants
- Cytotoxics
- Danazol
- Lithium
- Retinoids (systemic)
- Warfarin

Drugs that can affect fetal growth and development

- ACE inhibitors (after 12wks)—fetal or neonatal renal failure
- Barbiturates, benzodiazepines, and opioids (near term)—drug dependence in fetus
- NSAIDs (after 12wks)—premature closure of ductus arteriosus
- Tetracyclines (after 12wks)—abnormalities of teeth and bone
- Warfarin—fetal or neonatal haemorrhage

* Note that if the benefit clearly outweighs the risk (e.g. life-threatening or pregnancy-threatening disease), these drugs can be used in pregnancy.

[1] Welsh Medicines Resources Bulletin (2000) **7**: 1–5.

Table 10.10 Some drugs that have a good safety record in pregnancy

- Analgesics: codeine (caution near term) and paracetamol
- Antacids containing aluminium, calcium, or magnesium
- Antibacterials: penicillins, cephalosporins, erythromycin, clindamycin, and nitrofurantoin (avoid near term)
- Anti emetics: cyclizine and promethazine
- Antifungal agents (topical and vaginal): clotrimazole and nystatin
- Antihistamines: chlorphenamine and hydroxyzine
- Asthma: bronchodilator and steroid inhalers (avoid high doses in the long term), and short-course oral steroids
- Corticosteroids (topical, including nasal and eye drops)
- Insulin
- Laxatives: bulk-forming and lactulose
- Levothyroxine
- Methyldopa
- Ranitidine

Other considerations

- The presence or absence of teratogenic effects in animals does not necessarily translate to the same effects in humans. Think logically—if the agent causes tail shortening in rats, is this relevant in humans? Some studies use higher doses in animals than would be used in humans.
- Drugs associated with abnormalities at high doses/during the first trimester might be lower risk at low doses/during the second or third trimester (e.g. fluconazole).
- If treatment cannot be avoided during pregnancy, in preference use established drugs that have good evidence of safety. (NB: sometimes a lack of reports of teratogenicity for a well-established/frequently used drug may have to be taken as evidence of safety.)
- Some teratogenic effects are dose-related (e.g. neural tube defects with anticonvulsants). Higher doses or combining more than one drug with the same effect will ↑ the risk.
- Consider non-drug treatments (e.g. acupressure wrist bands for morning sickness) or whether treatment can be delayed until after pregnancy.

Maternal considerations

- Maternal drug-handling changes during pregnancy. Take special care with drugs that have a narrow therapeutic index.
- Remind the mother that some over-the-counter, herbal, and vitamin products should be avoided in pregnancy.
- Many women do not comply with drug treatment during pregnancy because of safety concerns, so discuss this with the mother and reassure her.

Handling potentially teratogenic drugs

There is little published evidence on whether occupational exposure to potentially teratogenic drugs can ↑ the risk of congenital abnormalities. In the absence of evidence or specific guidelines, sensible precautions should be taken to reduce the risk of exposure, especially by pregnant ♀ and ♀ planning a pregnancy. A risk assessment should be performed (using COSHH (Control of Substances Hazardous to Health) data as appropriate), and pregnant ♀ should be excluded from any task that poses even a low risk.

Handling blister-packed versions of a teratogenic tablet presents (virtually) no risk and film-coated or sugar-coated versions present a low risk. A high-risk procedure might involve preparation of cytotoxic infusions or handling crushed tablets of a known teratogenic drug. This type of procedure should not be carried out by pregnant ♀. ♀ (and ♂) of child-bearing potential (especially if planning a pregnancy) should take appropriate precautions (e.g. apron, mask, and gloves). Ideally, potentially teratogenic infusions should be prepared by centralized pharmacy reconstitution service, where the use of cytotoxic cabinets further ↓ the risk of exposure.

Further reading

Briggs GG, Freeman RK, Yaffe SJ (eds) (2008). *Drugs in Pregnancy and Lactation: A Reference Guide to Fetal and Neonatal Risk* (8th edn). Philadelphia, PA: Lippincott–Williams and Wilkins.

Folb PL, Dukes MNG (eds) (1990). *Drug Safety in Pregnancy*. Amsterdam: Elsevier.

Lee A, Inch S, Finnigen D (eds) (2000). *Therapeutics in Pregnancy and Lactation*. Abingdon: Radcliffe Medical Press.

Wolfson Unit Regional Drugs and Therapeutics Centre (Newcastle).

Toxbase drug monographs, including pregnancy risk (password required). www.toxbase.org. www.motherisk.org.

Drugs in breastfeeding

Breastfeeding has many advantages over bottle feeding. Even if the mother is taking a drug that is excreted in breast milk it can be preferable to continue breastfeeding. General principles to ↓ risk to babies are listed in Table 10.11.

The main questions to consider are as follows.

- Is the drug excreted into breast milk in quantities that are clinically significant?
- Do these drug levels pose any threat to the infant's health?

To answer these questions, the following factors must be considered.

Factors that affect drug transfer into breast milk

- **Maternal drug plasma level**—usually the most important determinant of breast milk drug levels. Drugs enter the breast milk primarily by diffusion. For most drugs, the level in the maternal drug compartment is directly proportional to the maternal plasma level. Thus, the higher the maternal dose, the higher is the drug level in the breast milk. Diffusion of drug between plasma and milk is a two-way process and is concentration dependent. At peak maternal plasma levels (T_{max}) drug levels in breast milk are also at their highest. As the level of the drug in the plasma falls, the level of the drug in breast milk also falls as drug diffuses from the milk back into the plasma. Thus drugs that only have a short half-life only appear in breast milk for a correspondingly short time.
  - During the first 4 days after delivery, drugs diffuse more readily into the breast milk because there are gaps between the alveolar cell walls in mammary capillaries. These gaps permit enhanced access for most drugs, in addition to immunoglobulins and maternal proteins. This results in ↑ drug levels in breast milk during the neonatal stage. After the first 4–7 days, these gaps close.
  - Some drugs pass into breast milk by an active process, such that the drug is concentrated in the milk. This occurs with iodides, especially radioactive iodides, making it necessary to interrupt breastfeeding.
- **Lipid solubility of the drug**—Fat-soluble drugs (e.g. benzodiazepines, chlorpromazine, and many other CNS-active drugs) preferentially dissolve in the lipid globules of breast milk. As a general rule, ↑ lipid solubility leads to ↑ penetration into milk. However, lipid solubility is not a good predictor of milk levels overall because fat represents a relatively small proportion of total milk volume.
- **Milk pH levels**—Breast milk has a lower pH than blood. Thus drugs that are weak bases (e.g. isoniazid and atropine-like drugs) are ionized in milk, which makes them more water-soluble and thus less likely to diffuse back into the plasma. This can lead to accumulation of these drugs in breast milk. Conversely, weakly acidic drugs (e.g. penicillins, aspirin, and diuretics) tend not to accumulate in breast milk.

Table 10.11 General principles to ↓ risk to breastfed babies

- Consider whether non-drug therapy is possible
- Can treatment be delayed until the mother is no longer breastfeeding or the infant is older and can tolerate the drug better?
- Use drugs where safety in breastfeeding has been established
- Keep the maternal dose as low as possible
- In preference, use drugs with a local effect (e.g. inhalers, creams, or drugs not absorbed orally, such as nystatin)
- Use drugs with a short half-life and avoid sustained-release preparations
- Avoid polypharmacy—additive side effects and drug interactions potentially ↑ the risk
- Advise the mother to breastfeed when the level of the drug in breast milk will be lowest. This is usually just before the next dose is due

- **Molecular size/molecular weight of the drug**—As a general rule, 'bulky' drugs do not diffuse across capillary walls because the molecules are simply too large to pass through the gaps.
- **Drug protein binding**—highly protein-bound drugs (e.g. phenytoin and warfarin) do not normally pass into breast milk in significant quantities because only free unbound drug diffuses across the capillary walls. Bear in mind that if a new drug is added that displaces the first drug from protein-binding sites, this could (at least temporarily) ↑ milk levels of the first drug.

Infant factors

- **Bioavailabilty**—drugs that are broken down in the gut or are not absorbed orally (e.g. insulin and aminoglycosides) should not cause any adverse effect because the infant's absorption of the drug is negligible, if any. Similarly, infant serum levels of any drug that has high first-pass metabolism are likely to be low. However, these drugs can sometimes have a local effect on the infant's gut, causing GI symptoms such as diarrhoea.
- **Infant status** must be taken into account. If the baby is premature or sick, they might be less able to tolerate even small quantities of the drug. Consider whether drug side effects could exacerbate the infant's underlying disease. For example, opioids in breast milk may be a higher risk for a baby with respiratory problems than for a healthy baby.
- **Metabolism and excretion** of some drugs is altered in infancy, especially in premature infants who might have impaired renal and hepatic function. Thus the drug effects can be greater than expected because the clearance of the drug is ↓. This can be especially marked for drugs with a long half-life.
- **Drugs that are often administered to infants** (e.g. paracetamol) are generally safe if absorbed in breast milk. As a general rule, <1% of the maternal dose reaches the infant. Thus, if the normal infant dose is >1% of the maternal dose, it is usually safe, but side effects can still occur (e.g. antibiotic-induced diarrhoea).

Other factors to consider

- Some mothers and healthcare workers assume that because the infant was exposed to the drug during pregnancy, it will be safe in breast-feeding. However, in pregnancy it is the maternal organs that clear the drug from the infant's circulation, but during breastfeeding the infant is clearing the drug. In addition, some adverse effects, such as respiratory depression, are not relevant during pregnancy but become relevant after delivery.
- Some mothers are resistant to using conventional medicines during breastfeeding because of perceived risks and decide to use alternative therapies. Mothers should be reminded that herbal or homeopathic medicines might be excreted in breast milk and cause adverse effects on the infant.
- Remember also to advise mothers that over-the-counter medicines, alcohol, and other recreational drugs may be excreted in breast milk.
- Some drugs can inhibit or even stop breast milk production. These includes bromocriptine and other dopamine agonists, diuretics, and moderate to heavy alcohol intake. Drugs that ↑ breast milk production (e.g. chlorpromazine, haloperidol, and other dopamine antagonists) may lead to concern from the mother that the baby is not taking the full amount.
- Sometimes breastfeeding might have to be interrupted or stopped completely if there is no alternative to administering a potentially risky drug. For short courses, it might be possible to stop breastfeeding temporarily. Using a breast pump and discarding the expressed milk until such time as it is safe to resume breastfeeding should encourage continued breast milk production. Some mothers might find bottle feeding difficult because of the more complex processes involved, cost, or cultural issues and might need extra support.

Further reading/information

Briggs GG, Freeman RK, Yaffe SJ (eds) (2005). *Drugs in Pregnancy and Lactation* (6th edn). Philadelphia, PA: Lippincott—Williams & Wilkins.
Hale TW (ed) (2004). *Medications and Mother's Milk*. Amarillo, TX: Pharmasoft Medical Publishing.
Lee A, Incha S, Finnigan D (eds) (2005). *Therapeutics in Pregnancy and Lactation*. Abingdon: Radcliffe Medical Press.
Trent and West Midlands Medicines Information Centre.

Drugs and dietary considerations

Dietary considerations may impact on drug therapy in various ways. In addition to drug–food interactions (see 📖 pp.20–1), food allergies or intolerances and cultural or religious dietary restrictions may have an impact on choice of drug therapy.

Food allergy or intolerance

Food and drink allergy is reported to affect 5% of children and 3–4% of adults in Westernized countries. It is important to distinguish between a true food allergy (i.e. symptoms of hypersensitivity occur after ingestion of the food) or intolerance (e.g. proven gluten intolerance) and a perceived food intolerance and consequent food exclusion on the part of the patient.

The most common food allergens in adults and children are:
- peanuts and other nuts
- wheat
- eggs
- milk
- soy
- fish and shellfish
- colouring agents.

In these instances a true hypersensitivity reaction, ranging from rash to anaphylaxis, could occur as a result of exposure to the allergen even in the extremely small quantities that might be present as excipients to the drug. Nut allergy is often potentially serious, with anaphylaxis being a risk. Some people will be so sensitive to nuts (especially peanuts) that topical exposure can lead to anaphylaxis. Pharmacists need to be aware that topical agents may contain nut oils, notably arachis (i.e. peanut) oil and sesame seed oil (to which there is often cross-sensitivity).

Food and drink intolerance can vary in severity, but exposure to the offending agent in a drug may lead to symptoms in some patients. Typical examples are:
- gluten (wheat, rye, barley, oats)
- lactose.

Pharmacists need to be aware of the possibility of food allergy or intolerance in their patients and should include questioning regarding this when taking a drug history. Listing drugs which may contain food allergens is beyond the scope of this section. If a patient reports significant symptoms as a result of exposure to a food or drink substance, pharmacists should check whether any new drugs contain the offending agent. This information can frequently be found in the summary of product characteristics (SPC), or contact the manufacturer for advice.

Egg allergy is often a cause for concern with vaccinations as some vaccines are derived from egg culture. The UK Department of Health advises that a history of hypersensitivity to eggs contraindicates influenza vaccine, and that a history of anaphylaxis to eggs contraindicates influenza and yellow fever vaccines. All other vaccines, including MMR (but check SPC as brand specific) are considered safe.

Cultural or religious considerations

Some drugs and formulation components (e.g. capsule shells) are derived from animal sources or may contain animal derivatives as excipients. This may affect drug choice for strict vegetarians or vegans and for those who avoid certain animal products for religious reasons. However, ingestion of the animal product may be permitted if it is for medical purposes or because it is not taken orally—e.g. Jewish law permits the use of heparins, even though they are of porcine origin, as they are not taken by mouth. It is important to remember that gelatin capsules are usually derived from animal sources. Lactose is a common excipient, but as it is milk derived it will be avoided by Jews who keep dietary laws strictly which prohibit consumption of milk and meat together.

Where alcohol is avoided for religious or cultural reasons, this may also affect the choice of drug or formulation as some liquid medicines and injections contain alcohol. Some individuals will also have concerns about the use of topical agents which contain alcohol as they could inadvertently ingest it by getting the alcohol-containing product on their hands.

Fasting for religious reasons (e.g. during Ramadan) may mean that patients miss both oral and parenteral medicines. Most religions exempt people who are sick from fasting, but patients who are well and on long-term therapy may wish to observe the fasts. Pharmacists can assist these patients by adjusting timings and frequency of medicines. Diabetics should be advised to be cautious about fasting, as it is difficult to maintain glycaemic control.

Further information

Drugs Derived from Pigs and their Clinical Alternatives: An Introductory Guide for Patients and Carers.
   www.mcb.org.uk/uploads/PBEnglish.pdf.

Glucose 6-phosphate dehydrogenase (G6PD) deficiency

G6PD is an enzyme that produces reduced glutathione, which protects red blood cells against oxidant stress. Exposure to an oxidant in G6PD-deficient individuals can lead to acute haemolysis of RBCs. G6PD deficiency is an X-linked genetic disorder. Thus ♂ are either normal or deficient, whereas ♀ are normal, deficient, or intermediate.

G6PD deficiency is distributed worldwide, with the highest prevalence in Africa, Southern Europe, the Middle East, Southeast Asia, and Oceania. Thus patients originating from any of these areas should be tested for G6PD deficiency before being administered an at-risk drug.

There are varying degrees of G6PD deficiency, with people of African origin generally having a lower level of deficiency (and therefore being more able to tolerate oxidizing drugs) and those of Oriental and Mediterranean origin generally having a high level of deficiency. Mild deficiency is defined as 10–15% of normal activity. Note that young red cells are not deficient in G6PD. Thus false-normal levels can occur during or immediately after an acute haemolytic attack, when new red cells are being produced.

Although many people remain clinically asymptomatic throughout their lives, they are all at risk of acute haemolytic anaemia in response to one of the following trigger events:
- infection
- acute illness
- fava (broad) beans
- oxidizing drugs.

A haemolytic attack usually starts with malaise, sometimes associated with weakness, lumbar pain, and abdominal pain. This is followed several hours or days later by jaundice and dark urine. In most cases, the attack is self-limiting, although adults (but rarely children) can develop renal failure.

Drug treatment in G6PD deficiency
- Patients in at-risk groups should be tested for G6PD deficiency. The normal range is 1.2–1.72 units/10^{10}RBC (3.2–6.4 units/gHb).
- Patients with severe deficiency should not be prescribed highly oxidizing drugs (Table 10.12), and drugs with a lower risk should be prescribed with caution.
- Patients with a lesser degree of deficiency may be able to tolerate even the drugs listed in the Table 10.12, but exercise caution.
- The risk and severity of haemolytic anaemia is almost always dose-related. Thus, even severely deficient patients can tolerate low doses of these drugs if there is no alternative. For example, for treatment of *Plasmodium vivax* or *plasmodium ovale*, a dose of primaquine 30mg once weekly for 8wks can be used instead of the usual dose of primaquine 15mg once daily for 14–21 days.

Table 10.12 Drugs to be used with caution in G6PD deficiency

Drugs with *definite* risk of haemolytic anaemia in most G6PD-deficient patients (avoid)
- Dapsone and other sulphones
- Methylthioninium chloride (methylene blue)
- Nalidixic acid
- Nitrofurantoin
- Primaquine
- Quinolones
- Sulphonamides

Drugs with *possible* risk of haemolytic anaemia in some G6PD-deficient patients (caution)*
- Aminosalicylic acid
- Amodiaquine
- Ascorbic acid
- Aspirin (doses >1g/day)
- Chloramphenicol
- Chloroquine[†]
- Dimercaprol
- Hydroxychloroquine
- Isoniazid
- Levodopa
- Menadione (water-soluble vitamin K derivatives)
- Penicillins
- Probenecid
- Pyrimethamine
- Quinidine
- Quinine[†]
- Streptomycin

*Use with caution; low doses probably safe.

[†]Acceptable to treat acute malaria at usual doses.

- Drug manufacturers do not routinely carry out testing to identify the potential risk of their drug to G6PD-deficient patients. Do not assume with new drugs that if there is no warning in the SPC, the drug is safe.

Treatment of a haemolytic attack
- Withdraw drug
- Maintain high urine output
- Blood transfusion, if indicated

Drugs in porphyria

The porphyrias are a group of rare hereditary metabolic disorders in which there are defects in the haem biosynthesis pathway. In the acute porphyrias (alanine (ALA) dehydratase deficiency, acute intermittent and variegate porphyrias, and hereditary coproporphyria) there is overpro-duction of porphyrin precursors as well as porphyrins which can lead to systemic symptoms including:

- acute (often severe) abdominal pain
- constipation
- nausea and vomiting
- hypertension
- tachycardia and cardiac arrhythmias
- muscle weakness and loss of sensation
- convulsions
- confusion, disorientation, hallucinations, paranoia
- hyponatraemia and hypokalaemia.

Numerous drugs have been linked to precipitating an acute porphyria attack, but these are mostly based on animal or *in vitro* studies. Pharmacists need to be aware of which drugs should be avoided and which are con-sidered safe in porphyria, as an acute attack is serious and potentially life-threatening. The Welsh Medicines Information Centre provides specialist advice on porphyria and publishes a list of drugs considered safe in acute porphyria.[1]

In serious or life-threatening conditions a drug should not be withheld just because it is not on the 'safe' list. If there is no alternative 'safe' drug, treatment should be commenced and urinary porphobilinogen measured regularly. If levels increase or symptoms of an acute attack occur the drugs should be stopped.

Patients with acute porphyrias need to be aware that drugs can precipitate an attack and to inform healthcare professionals that they have porphyria. The British Porphyria Association publishes a series of fact sheets for patients including advice on drugs.[2]

Treatment of an acute attack is symptomatic and supportive, ensuring that the drugs used are those considered safe in porphyria (Table 10.13). Specific treatment is with haem arginate, which replenishes the body's haem stores and so through negative feedback reduces the production of porphyrins and porphyrin precursors.

---

1 http://www.wmic.wales.nhs.uk/pdfs/porphyria/Porphyria_Safe_List_2010_with_letter_August%
202010.pdf.
2 www.porphyria.org.uk.

Table 10.13 Drug treatments in acute porphyria: symptomatic treatment

Condition	Drug category	Drug*
Abdominal pain	Analgesics	Aspirin
		Diamorphine
		Dihydrocodeine
		Ibuprofen
		Morphine
		Paracetamol
		Pethidine
Vomiting	Antiemetics	Chlorpromazine
		Ondansetron
		Prochlorperazine
		Promazine
Hypertension and tachycardia	Antihypertensives	β-blockers, e.g. atenolol, labetalol, propranolol
Neurosis, psychosis, and seizures	Sedatives, tranquillizers, and anticonvulsants	Chlorpromazine
		Clonazepam
		Lorazepam
		Promazine
Constipation	Laxatives	Bulk-forming (ispaghula)
		Lactulose
		Senna

* Drugs are listed alphabetically rather than preferred order of treatment. Management of symptoms should be individualized to meet the needs of the patient.

The non-acute or cutaneous porphyrias are associated with skin photosensitivity but do not show the serious systemic symptoms associated with the acute porphyrias. Thus it is not necessary to avoid exposure to 'unsafe' drugs in these conditions (with the exception of chloroquine and related drugs in antimalarial treatment and prophylaxis doses in patients with porphyria cutanea tarda). Patients should avoid exposure to the sun by sun avoidance and wearing appropriate clothing, as the majority of sun screens do not filter out the long UVA wavelengths and visible light which activate porphyrins.

Further reading

www.cardiff-porphyria.org—diagnostic and clinical advisory service.
www.wmic.wales.nhs.uk/porphyria_info.php.

Patient-specific issues

Medicines for children: introduction 206
Medicines for children: pharmacodynamics and
   pharmacokinetics 208
Medicines for children: licensing 210
Medicines for children: calculating children's doses 212
Medicines for children: adherence 214
'Pill school': teaching children how to take tablets and
   capsules 216
Medicines for elderly people: introduction 218
Medicines for elderly people: pharmacokinetics and
   pharmacodynamics 220
Medicines for elderly people: medication review 222
Dealing with injecting drug users in hospital 224
Discharge prescriptions for opioid-replacement therapy 229
Surgical patient and nil by mouth (NBM) issues 230

Medicines for children: introduction

Children represent a significant proportion of patients in both primary and secondary care. In the UK, the National Service Framework (NSF) for Children[1] lists a number of areas in which pharmacists can have an important role. These include the following areas.

- Developing and providing high-quality medicines information, especially with respect to unlicensed use or formulations.
- Promoting concordance.
- Ensuring good communication between primary and secondary care, especially with respect to unusual or unlicensed preparations.
- Advising on clinically appropriate, safe, and cost-effective use of medicines in children.

It is important to remember that children are not small adults, and neither are they a homogenous group. Drug handling in children can be quite different to that in adults and can also be different at different ages. For medical and pharmaceutical purposes, children are usually grouped according to the following ages:

- Premature—born before 40wks gestation.
- Neonate—≤4wks old (if premature, add the number of weeks premature, e.g. if born 2wks premature, the baby would be considered a neonate until it was 6wks old).
- Infant—4wks to 2 years.
- Child—2 years to (usually) 12 years.
- Adolescent—(usually) 12–18 years.

From 12 years old onwards, drug handling and dosing is usually the same as for adults, but adolescents require special consideration in terms of social and emotional needs.

1 http://www.dh.gov.uk/prod_consum_dh/groups/dh_digitalassets/@dh/@en/documents/digitalasset/dh_4090566.pdf.

Medicines for children: pharmaco-dynamics and pharmacokinetics

Virtually all pharmacokinetic parameters change with age. An understanding of how drug handling changes with age is essential to avoid toxicity or underdosing.

Tips on making medicine more palatable for children are given in Table 11.1

Absorption

GI absorption may be slower in newborns and infants than in adults. Newborns have a prolonged gastric emptying time. Lower levels of gastric acid in newborns might ↓ absorption of some drugs (e.g. itraconazole). Drugs that bind to calcium or magnesium should not be given at the same time as milk feeds.

Intramuscular absorption requires muscle movement to stimulate blood flow and so could be erratic in newborns who are relatively immobile. In addition, blood supply to the muscles is very variable.

Topical absorption of agents is enhanced in neonates and infants because the skin is thinner and better hydrated. This age group also has a proportionally larger body surface area for weight than older children. Thus, topical agents applied over a large area can provide a significant systemic dose.

Distribution

Total body water changes with age:
- premature—80% of body weight
- newborn—70% of body weight
- children—60–65% of body weight
- adults—60% of body weight.

This affects the volume of distribution of water-soluble drugs, and higher doses per kilogram might be required for premature or newborn infants.

Protein binding

In neonates, protein binding of drugs is less than in adults, but within a few months after birth it is similar to adult levels. ↓ protein binding might account for the ↑ sensitivity of neonates to some drugs (e.g. theophylline).

Metabolism

Premature and newborn infants metabolize drugs more slowly than adults. However, young children have a faster metabolic rate, which ↓ to adult levels with ↑ age. Thus doses of highly metabolized drugs are proportionally lower per kilogram for neonates and infants and higher for young children. As the child grows, doses should be frequently recalculated not only to allow for differing rates of drug metabolism, but also to allow for ↑ height and weight.

Premature infants and neonates have immature renal function, with the neonatal GFR usually ~30% of the adult rate. Thus doses should be ↓ accordingly. After infancy, plasma clearance of some drugs is significantly ↑ because of both ↑ hepatic elimination and ↑ renal excretion.

Table 11.1 Tips on making medicines more palatable

- Chill the medicine (but do not freeze it)[*]
- Take the medicine through a straw
- Use an oral syringe to direct the medicine towards the back of the mouth and away from the tongue (and therefore away from the highest concentration of taste buds)
- Chocolate disguises many flavours—try mixing the medicine with a small amount of chocolate milk, spread, or syrup[*]
- Coat the tongue and roof of the mouth with a spoonful of peanut butter or chocolate spread before taking the medicine.
- Suck an ice cube or ice lolly immediately before taking the medicine
- Brush teeth after taking the dose
- Eat strongly flavoured food after the dose—e.g. crisps, Marmite®, or citrus fruit (small amounts of these foods should not adversely affect drug absorption)

[*]Check drug compatibility and storage temperature requirements.

Medicines for children: licensing

Up to 40% of prescribing in children is unlicensed or 'off licence'—ie the drug is not licensed for use in that age range, route, dose or indication. Extemporaneous preparations and imported and specials products are effectively 'named patient' and thus unlicensed. Until such time as a wider range of formulations is available or drug manufacturers do the relevant trials to obtain licences for paediatric use or indications, this is an unavoidable practice. The Royal College of Paediatrics and Child Health and the Neonatal and Paediatric Pharmacists Group (NPPG) have issued a joint declaration stating the following:

> 'The informed use of unlicensed medicines, or of licensed medicines for unlicensed applications, is necessary in paediatric practice.'

Pharmacists should ensure that licensed preparations are used wherever possible. If there is no alternative, they should ensure that both prescribers and parents (and the child, as appropriate) are informed of unlicensed or off-label use. It is especially important to ensure that parents or carers do not feel that the medicine is 'sub-standard' or 'second best' because it is unlicensed. In general, it is not considered necessary to obtain formal consent for the use of unlicensed medicines in this context. The NPPG has produced leaflets suitable for parents and older children to explain the need to use unlicensed and off-label medicines. These are available on the NPPG website (see also 📖 p.214). Local guidelines on documentation and consent for use of unlicensed medicines should be complied with.

It is important that pharmacists ensure a continued supply of unlicensed, extemporaneous and special medicines by liaising with and providing product information to GPs and community pharmacists.

Medicines for children: calculating children's doses

A reputable reference source should be used for children's doses. Different sources quote doses in different ways and it is important to be clear how the dose is calculated to avoid the risk of overdose. Doses are usually quoted as follows:

- The total dose in mg/kg body weight per day, and the number of doses it should be divided into.
- The individual dose in mg/kg body weight per dose, and the number of doses that should be given each day.

Most doses are based on weight, although doses based on body surface area are more accurate because this takes into account the child's overall size (Table 11.2). Body surface area dosing is more frequent for drugs if accurate dosing is critical (e.g. cytotoxic drugs). Nomograms for calculating body surface area can be found in paediatric drugs handbooks, or the following equation can be used:

$$\text{body surface area (m}^2) = \sqrt{\frac{\text{body weight (kg)} \times \text{height (cm)}}{3600}}$$

Very rarely it is impossible to find a published and validated children's dose for a drug, in which case it can be estimated from the adult dose based on physiological or pharmacokinetic factors[1] or using approximate proportions (Table 11.3). This should only be used as a last resort. This method tends to give an underdose. Calculated doses should usually be rounded up, rather than down, and the dose titrated according to clinical response, as necessary.

1 Bartelink IH *et al.* (2006) Guidelines on paediatric dosing on the basis of development physiology and pharmacokinetic considerations. *Clinical Pharmacokinetics* **45**: 1077–97.

Table 11.2 Approximate surface area and weight[*]

	Weight (kg)	Surface area (m^2)
Newborn	3	0.2
1 year	10	0.5
3 years	15	0.6
5 years	20	0.7
9 years	30	1.0
14 years	50	1.5
Adult	70	1.7

[*]Note that many children in developing countries might only weigh 60–80% of the average weight.

Table 11.3 Estimating children's doses as a proportion of the adult doses[*]

Weight	Age	Proportion of adult dose
3–5kg	0–5 months	1/8
6–10kg	6 months–1 year	1/4
11–20kg	1–6 years	1/3
21–30kg	7–10 years	1/2
>30kg	11–15 years	3/4

[*]Note that this method tends to result in an underdose.

Medicines for children: adherence

Counselling on medicine use and adherence issues is important for children. Parents might be familiar with taking medicines themselves but this doesn't necessarily mean that they will cope with giving medicines to their child, especially if they are distressed by the child's diagnosis or the child is uncooperative. The toddler age group is often the most difficult because at this age they can be uncooperative but lack the language ability and insight needed for parents to reason with them.

- Wherever possible and within the child's level of understanding, pharmacists should aim to involve the child in discussions about their medicines.
- Ideally, counselling about medicine use and adherence should involve both parents (or two carers), especially if the therapy is complex and/or long term. As appropriate, also involve school nurses, for example, although it is best to avoid giving doses during school time if at all possible.
- The most appropriate delivery form should be selected. Most parents find an oral syringe easy to use but some children can object to this, and once measured the medicine might have to be transferred to a spoon.
- Parents and carers might find it easier to give the medicine mixed with a small amount of food or drink. They should be taught how to do this correctly so that the child takes the full dose. Medicines should not be added to baby's bottle feeds because the full quantity might not be taken.
- Be aware that some patient information leaflets might be for indications other than the one for which the medicine is being used.
- Explain to the child why they need to take their medicine in simple terms, allowing for any limitations on disclosure of the diagnosis—e.g. a child may not have been told that they have HIV but might have been told that they need medicine to help them fight infection.
- Encourage parents to involve the child in the administration process. From quite a young age (and with appropriate supervision and support), children can be taught to measure doses of liquid medicines, make up a dosette box, or even self-administer insulin.
- Help parents to think ahead to how medicines will be administered during the school day or on a school or youth organization residential event. Tailoring the regimen to once-daily or twice-daily dosing means that drug administration during school hours can usually be avoided.
- Adolescents might wish to discuss their medicines without their parents present. Non-adherence in adolescents is not uncommon as a way of expressing independence and requires sensitive handling.

Further reading

Paediatric Formulary Committee (2011). *British National Formulary for Children* London: Pharmaceutical Press. ℘ http://www.bnfc.org

Royal College of Paediatrics and Child Health and the Neonatal Paediatric Pharmacists Group (2003). *Medicines for Children*. London: RCPCH Publications Ltd.

Advice on administering medicines to children, formulae for extemporaneous preparation. ℘ http://www.pharminfotech.co.nz

Neonatal and Paediatric Pharmacists Group. ℘ http://www.nppg.scot.nhs.uk

National Paediatric Drug Information Advisory Line (DIAL). ℘ http://www.dial.org.uk

'Pill school': teaching children how to take tablets and capsules

Preparation

- Discuss the child's ability to swallow food, especially hard or chewy food, with the parents. Ask whether they think the child would be able to swallow tablets or capsules.
- Ask whether the child has had any previous experience of taking tablets and capsules and whether this was successful.
- Check any dietary issues with respect to the placebo capsules to be used, e.g. allergies to food colouring or consumption of gelatin products.
- Ask parents to ensure that the child has not eaten or drunk anything immediately before the session so that they are not too full to swallow the capsules or water.
- Arrange the appointment for a time when the child will be alert and cooperative—e.g. not straight after school or nursery when they may be tired.
- Advise parents and other healthcare workers not to tell the child in advance what the session is about because this might create anxiety and resistance.
- To avoid possible disruption, ensure that the child has been to the toilet before starting the session.

Equipment

- Prepare a series of capsule shells of different sizes containing sugar strands and place in bottles labelled with the sizes. Place some loose sugar strands in a bottle. Keep bottles and labels hidden from the child's view.
- Two cups (one for the child and one for you) and a bottle of water.
- Two small trays or containers (e.g. weighing boats), one on which to place capsules and one to use if the child spits out a capsule.
- Tissues for mopping-up purposes.

Environment

- The room should be quiet, without distractions such as books or toys.
- Have only one other person present (as a chaperone) and ask them to sit behind the child out of view. Advise them not to intervene at any stage. Ideally, this should not be a parent.
- Sit across the table from the child.

Process

- Explain the purpose of the session to the child in simple terms. Talk enthusiastically and mention good things about taking tablets or capsules—e.g. avoiding bad-tasting medicine.
- Show the bottle of sugar strands and place a few on the tray. Ask the child to show you that they can swallow these.
- Place two of the smallest capsules on the tray. Explain to the child that now you want them to try swallowing the sugar strands inside

a capsule. Explain how to swallow a capsule without chewing and demonstrate this.
  • Sit or stand upright.
  • Take a breath.
  • Put the pill in the middle of your tongue.
  • Take a mouthful of water and swallow.
  • Keep your head straight.
- Show the child that you have swallowed the capsule by opening your mouth and sticking out your tongue. Make the process fun, but be firm if necessary.
- Ask the child to show you that they can do the same with the other capsule.
- Get them to show you that their mouth is empty by opening their mouth and sticking out their tongue. Praise the child for their success.
- If the child has been successful, repeat the process with the next size of capsule, again demonstrating how to swallow it if necessary. State that it is the next capsule, not that it is larger. Give praise and encouragement at each stage.
- If the child has difficulties swallowing a capsule at any stage, get them to spit it out. Encourage them to try again with the same size of capsule.
- If the child is unsuccessful at the second attempt or if they refuse to try again, stop the session. Do not pressure the child because this could create an association between capsule taking and distress. Praise the child for trying hard.
- At the end of the session, if the parents have not been present, bring them into the room so that the child can demonstrate successful capsule swallowing.
- Give the parents a supply of the largest size swallowed and written instructions on how to take capsules for further practice at home.
- Explain to the child that the medicines they will take could look different to the sample capsules but they should be able to swallow them in the same way.

After the session
- Discuss the child's achievement with medical staff.
- Review current or planned medication to establish whether it can be dispensed as tablets or capsules of a suitable size and shape.
- Bear in mind that uncoated and/or round tablets are harder to swallow than capsules, coated tablets, or oval/capsule-shaped tablets.

Medicines for elderly people: introduction

Elderly people are high consumers of medicines, both prescribed and non-prescribed. In the UK, 50% of NHS drug expenditure is consumed by medicines for older people. Much prescribing for elderly people is done as 'repeats' and without regular review. This can frequently lead to inappropriate or unnecessary therapy, including prescribing for 'diseases' that are actually ADRs.

In the UK, the NSF for Older People[1] has a specific section on medicines management, with the following primary aims.

- Ensuring that older people gain maximum benefit from their medication to maintain or ↑ their quality and duration of life.
- Ensuring that older people do not suffer unnecessarily from illness caused by excessive, inappropriate, or inadequate consumption of medicines.

Elderly people are at ↑ risk of medication-related problems.

- ↑ risk of ADRs (many preventable) caused by polypharmacy, drug interactions, and changes in pharmacokinetics and pharmacodynamics.
- Underprescribing of some medicines—e.g. thrombolysis in MI.
- Non-adherence.
- Repeat medicines not being reviewed, leading to unnecessary long-term therapy and stockpiling.
- Difficulty in accessing the surgery and/or pharmacy.

1 http://www.dh.gov.uk/prod_consum_dh/groups/dh_digitalassets/@dh/@en/documents/digitalasset/dh_4071283.pdf.

Medicines for elderly people: pharmacokinetics and pharmacodynamics

Physiological changes that occur with age affect drug handling and sensitivity. Predicting at what age these changes become significant is almost impossible because people 'age' at different rates, depending on environmental, social, and other factors. However, the pharmacist should be alert to possible changes in drug handling and sensitivity in any patient >75 years of age.

Absorption

- Ageing rarely has a significant effect on absorption. Delayed gastric emptying ↑ time to peak concentrations (C_{max}) but is rarely clinically significant.
- ↓ production of gastric acid can lead to ↓ absorption of drugs that require an acid environment for absorption (e.g. itraconazole), but can slightly ↑ the amount absorbed of drugs that are broken down by gastric acid (e.g. penicillins).
- Bioavailability of levopdopa is ↑ in elderly people, possibly because of ↓ levels of dopa decarboxylase in the gastric mucosa.
- ↓ regional blood flow might ↓ the rate of absorption of drugs administered by the intramuscular or subcutaneous route, but the total amount absorbed is the same.

Distribution

- Lean body mass ↓ with age, leading to ↑ levels of drugs distributed in the muscle (e.g. digoxin).
- Adipose tissue ↑ up to the age of 85 years, leading to ↑ tissue levels and thus prolonged duration of effect of lipid-soluble drugs (e.g. diazepam). Patients >85 years tend to lose adipose tissue.
- ↓ in total body water leads to ↑ in the serum concentration of water-soluble drugs (e.g. gentamicin and digoxin).
- ↓ serum albumin leads to ↑ levels of free drug for highly protein-bound drugs (e.g. NSAIDs, sulphonylureas, and warfarin). In the acute phase, homeostatic mechanisms usually counteract the ↑ drug effects. ↑ level of free drug also means ↑ amounts for clearance, so the effect is rarely significant in the long term.

Metabolism

Elderly people can have up to a 40% ↓ in hepatic blood flow. Drugs with high first-pass metabolism can be significantly affected (see 📖 p.180). There might be up to 60% ↓ in metabolism of some drugs, such as NSAIDs and anticonvulsants, leading to ↑ concentration, duration of action, and possibly accumulation.

Excretion

The natural ageing process between the ages of 20 and 80 years leads to a 30–35% loss of functioning of glomeruli, with a consequent up to 50%

loss of normal renal function. Serum creatinine levels might be normal or near normal because of ↓ muscle mass, but creatinine clearance will be ↓. Acute illness and dehydration can cause a rapid decline in renal function, which can be exacerbated by the use of potentially nephrotoxic drugs, including high-dose antibacterials. Even a fairly well elderly patient may tolerate a combination of potentially nephrotoxic drugs (e.g. diuretic plus NSAID), but the addition of one more nephrotoxic drug (e.g. an antibacterial) can tip the balance towards renal impairment.

It is advisable to calculate the creatinine clearance (using the Cockroft and Gault equation (see Table 10.5)) for any patient >70 years who is prescribed renally cleared or potentially nephrotoxic drugs. Remember that drugs such as morphine have active metabolites that are renally cleared. Drugs that rely on excretion into the urine for their effect—notably nitrofurantoin—can be ineffective in elderly people.

Pharmacodynamic changes

As the body ages, there is a natural loss of function at a cellular level. This can lead to ↑ or ↓ drug sensitivity. Changes in receptor–drug interactions can occur—e.g. there is a ↓ response to both β-adrenoceptor agonists and β-adrenoceptor antagonists.

Homeostatic responses can be blunted in old age—e.g. postural hypotension is more likely to be caused by blunting of reflex tachycardia, and cardiac failure might result from fluid overload caused by over-enthusiastic rehydration or NSAIDs combined with ↓ cardiac output and renal function.

There is ↑ susceptibility to CNS effects of drugs. Even drugs that are not normally associated with CNS effects can cause such symptoms in the elderly, e.g. histamine H_2 receptor antagonists and diuretics. These effects can occur without changes in kinetics, probably because of ↑ CNS penetration or altered drug response. For example, confusion and dis-orientation are more common in elderly people receiving benzo-diazepines, antidepressants, and NSAIDs, even at standard doses. In addition, changes in kinetics can lead to CNS effects not usually seen in younger people—e.g. ↓ renal function can lead to confusion associated with ↑ levels of drugs such as ciprofloxacin and aciclovir.

Medicines for elderly people: medication review

See also 📖 *p.62.*

Regular medication review is an essential, but often overlooked, aspect of care of the elderly. Both hospital and community pharmacists are ideally placed to do this. Ideally, elderly patients should have their medication reviewed on admission to hospital, and in the community all patients >75 years should have their drugs reviewed at least annually. Prioritize those at highest risk of medication-related problems.

- Elderly patients taking four or more drugs.
- Elderly patients recently discharged from hospital.
- Elderly patients taking 'high-risk' medicines.
  - Hypnotics—drowsiness and falls.
  - Diuretics—dehydration, renal failure and confusion caused by hypokalaemia.
  - NSAIDs—fluid retention and GI bleeds.
  - Antihypertensives—falls resulting from postural hypotension.
  - Digoxin—nausea and vomiting. Confusion could be missed as signs of toxicity.
  - Warfarin—bruising and bleeding.

Other factors that can ↑ the risk of medication-related problems are as follows.

- Social—lack of home support.
- Physical—poor vision, hearing, and dexterity.
- Mental—confusion, depression, and difficulty in understanding instructions.

Elderly patients are often high users of over-the-counter medicines and the pharmacist should be alert to this. Many over-the-counter drugs can:

- be unnecessary
- ↑ the risk of drug interactions
- ↑ the risk of additive side effects
- be an indicator for ADRs to other medicines (e.g. high antacid consumption could point to NSAID-induced gastric irritation).

Medication reviews should include partners and carers (formal and informal) if possible, and the results should be fed back to the GP and other relevant healthcare workers. If patients are attending the clinic for a review, they should be asked to bring all medications with them ('brown-bag review'). This enables the pharmacist to check for the following.

- Stockpiling.
- Out-of-date medicines.
- Problems with reading or interpretation of medicine labels.
- Strategies for self-administration—e.g. marking containers or transferring medicines to other containers.
- Problems with manipulation—e.g. opening bottle caps or using technologically difficult products, such as inhalers or eye drops.
- Use of over-the-counter or herbal medicines.

The NO TEARS tool is useful model both for medication review and when considering initiating a new drug.[1]

- **N**eed and indication.
  - Is the drug really necessary?
  - Is it being used to treat an adverse effect?
  - Can it be stopped?
- **O**pen questions.
  - Ask non-directed questions about the medication.
    — Any problems?
    — Tell me how/when you take these medicines?
- **T**ests and monitoring.
  - Ensure that appropriate monitoring is being done for both desired effect and checking for ADRs.
    Where possible ensure that tests, such as TDM and INR, are done beforehand so that the results can be used to inform the review.
  - Check adherence.
- **E**vidence and guidelines.
  - Ensure that treatment is evidence-based and complies with up-to-date local and national guidelines.
- **A**DRs.
  - Ask about ADRs.
  - Check whether a medicine is being used to treat side effects and, if possible, stop or change the causative drug.
- **R**isk reduction and prevention.
  - Pay special attention to 'high-risk' drugs. Are they really necessary?
  - Could the dose be reduced?
  - If initiating a drug, start at the lowest dose and cautiously titrate according to the response.
- **S**implification and switches.
  - Could a change of drug or formulation simplify the regimen or make self-administration easier?

1 Lewis T (2004). Using the NO TEARS tool for medication review. *British Medical Journal*, **329**: 434.

Dealing with injecting drug users in hospital

Injecting drug users and people who misuse other drugs, including alcohol, can present behavioural, in addition to medical, challenges on admission to hospital. An awareness of the issues involved is important, but equally healthcare staff should not assume that all drug misusers are 'difficult' patients. Drugs of misuse include the following:

- opioids
- benzodiazepines
- other prescription or over-the-counter drugs (e.g. anticholinergics)
- cocaine
- cannabis
- alcohol.

Managing behaviour

- Don't assume that all drug misusers will misbehave. Treat the patient with respect, as you would any other patient. A suspicious or negative manner from the healthcare professional is more likely to generate negative behaviour from the patient.
- Remove temptation—ensure that all drug cupboards and trolleys are locked and drug deliveries are put away immediately.
- Use a firm no-nonsense approach. Guidelines or a contract for acceptable behaviour might be helpful (see 📖 p.75).
- Liaise with local addiction teams for advice and support.

Patients who misuse drugs on the ward

Healthcare professionals should be aware that patients (or their visitors) might misuse drugs on the ward. Indicators for this are as follows.

- Large numbers of visitors and/or visitors at odd times.
- Signs of intoxication or a behaviour change, often after receiving visitors or temporarily leaving the ward.
- Actual evidence (e.g. empty syringe).

Management depends on local policy, but this type of behaviour should not be tolerated. A senior doctor or nurse will normally be the member of staff who addresses this issue with the patient. Other healthcare staff should ensure that their dealings with the patient are consistent with agreed management policies. A suggested approach is as follows.

- Do not condone or tolerate the behaviour; make it clear that it is unacceptable.
- Give a warning that the behaviour will not be tolerated and the patient will be discharged if it is repeated.
- Consider limiting the number of visitors and the time during which they can visit.
- Involve hospital security or the police, especially if the safety of other patients or healthcare staff is compromised.
- Liaise with senior managers/hospital legal advisers to ensure that action taken is within the law.

Handling illegal drugs

Pharmacists could be asked to take possession of illegal drugs that ward staff have taken from a patient. This might include schedule 1 drugs, which normally require a license for possession. However, UK law allows pharmacists to take possession of illegal (including schedule 1) drugs for the following purposes:

• destruction of the drug.
• handing the drug over to the police.

In this situation, it can be difficult to maintain the patient's rights and confidentiality while remaining within the law.

If a sufficiently large quantity is involved, such that it is clear that the drug is not just for personal use, it might be deemed that the public interest outweighs patient confidentiality and the police should be called. The decision to involve the police should only be taken after consultation with senior management and legal advisers.

If the quantity involved is small and clearly for personal use, the drugs should be destroyed. The patient's authority is required to remove and destroy the drug, and if they refuse to hand it over, consideration should be given to discharging the patient or involving the police. Returning the drug to the patient is not an option, because this would make the pharmacist guilty of unlawful supply of a controlled drug.

Managing patients who are opioid dependent

Patients who are maintained on opioid-replacement therapy (e.g. methadone or buprenorphine) in the community should have this continued in hospital.

• Verify the dose independently—e.g. by contacting the GP, addictions service, or community pharmacist.
• Notify the community pharmacist of the patient's admission (to ensure the patient doesn't 'double up' by obtaining supplies from the community, in addition to the hospital supply) and discharge (to ensure that community supply is restarted).
• Liaise with the GP and addictions service to ensure a consistent approach.
• As a rule, it is best to avoid providing more than one or two doses of replacement therapy on discharge. Liaise with the GP/community pharmacist to ensure that valid prescription is available for therapy to be continued in the community after discharge.
• Avoid prescribing other opioids if at all possible, especially short-acting opioids (e.g. pethidine).
• Benzodiazepines should only be prescribed if medically indicated (e.g. for alcohol withdrawal). If night sedation is required, prescribe in accordance with local addictions service guidance.
• If a dose adjustment of the replacement therapy is required (e.g. because of drug interactions), liaise with the local addictions service.

Patients dependent on opioids who are not on replacement therapy require careful management.

• Methadone or buprenorphine should only be prescribed if there are objective signs of withdrawal (Table 11.4).

- The dose should be titrated according to objective withdrawal symptoms, not according to the patient's reported use of street opioids.
- A suggested regimen is as follows.

Day 1
- Objective signs of withdrawal—methadone 20mg single dose (stat).
- Further signs of withdrawal—methadone 10mg single dose can be repeated after 4h.
- Maximum dose of methadone in the first 24h is usually 40–50mg.

Day 2 onwards
- Total dose given in the first 24h should be prescribed as a single daily dose.
- Up to two additional doses of methadone (10mg) can be given every 24h if further objective signs of withdrawal occur. Rewrite the maintenance dose each day to include additional doses until dose titration is achieved.
- A dose of methadone 80mg daily is usually considered the maximum maintenance dose, but some centres use higher doses.
- At all times, doses should only be ↑ if there are objective signs of withdrawal. Bear in mind that methadone has a long half-life, and so it takes several days to reach steady-state concentrations.
- Additional doses should not be prescribed 'as required' (prn)—the patient should be assessed each time by a doctor and any extra doses (if needed) prescribed as a single dose.
- If the patient wishes to continue replacement therapy after discharge, they should be referred to the local addictions service as soon as possible.
- Patients who do not wish to continue replacement therapy might require a rapid reduction of the therapy before discharge. Note that these patients will usually return to using street opioids on discharge; thus the risk of withdrawal is minimal.

It is advisable for hospitals to produce written guidelines on opioid replacement therapy in consultation with the local addictions service. This ensures continuity of care and can also be a great help to junior doctors, who may be pressurized by patients to prescribe replacement therapy inappropriately.

Managing alcohol withdrawal
See 📖 p.610.

Management of concurrent illness
In general, concurrent illnesses in patients who misuse drugs should be managed in the same way as for any other patient. However, the following points should be considered.
- Avoid opioids, benzodiazepines, and other drugs that could be misused.
- Be aware that enzyme inducers and inhibitors can affect methadone levels.
- If the patient has a chaotic lifestyle, avoid drugs with a narrow therapeutic index—e.g. daily low molecular weight heparin is preferable to warfarin for deep vein thrombosis (DVT).

Table 11.4 Withdrawal scale from opiates

Methadone is indicated if score ≥7

Objective signs

Sweating		
	None	0 ☐
	Clammy	1 ☐
	Sweaty	2 ☐
	Running sweat	3 ☐
Retching		
	None	0 ☐
	Mild	1 ☐
	Moderate	2 ☐
	Vomiting and retching	3 ☐
Gooseflesh		
	None	0 ☐
	Some	1 ☐
	Moderate	2 ☐
	Severe, with piloerection and shivers	3 ☐
Lacrymation		
	None	0 ☐
	Watery eyes; no tears	1 ☐
	Some tears	2 ☐
	Crying	3 ☐
Score /12		
Record values of:		
Pulse (record value).	Below 80–0	☐
	Over 80	☐
BP (record value).		

Pain control

Pain should be managed in the same way as for any other patient. Many doctors assume that patients on opioid replacement therapy require less analgesia, and the patient might insist that they require extra analgesia because of tolerance. If the patient is experiencing pain, it is clear that the replacement therapy is not blocking all opioid receptors and analgesia is required. Ideally, opioids—both weak and strong—should be avoided. If an opioid is required, a long-acting opioid is preferred. Tramadol has no advantage over codeine in this setting.

Because buprenorphine is a partial antagonist, it can present a specific problem in patients who require opioid analgesia (e.g. postoperatively). It might be appropriate to convert the patient to an equivalent dose of morphine before surgery. The local addiction service should be contacted for advice.

Discharge prescriptions for opioid-replacement therapy

Injecting drug users who are stabilized with methadone (IV or oral) or buprenorphine (Subutex®) might require a supply on discharge from hospital. It is usually not advisable to give more than a 24–48h discharge supply, especially if the patient usually gets their supply on a daily basis from the community pharmacist. Sometimes there can be a delay before a prescription for a community pharmacy supply can be arranged (e.g. at weekends or on bank holidays). On these occasions, it might be appropriate to use a prescription issued by the hospital, which can be dispensed in the community (FP10(HP) in the UK).

Things to consider

- Could an alternative arrangement be made—e.g. could the patient attend the ward/out-patient clinic for a supply?
- In the UK, only Home Office registered doctors can prescribe diamorphine, cocaine, or dipipanone to injecting drug users, but any doctor can prescribe any other replacement therapy.
- Close liaison with the local addiction service/GP/community pharmacist is important to ensure continuity of care.

Writing the prescription (guidelines refer to UK law)

- Normal writing rules for controlled drug prescriptions apply.
- FP10(HP) prescriptions cannot be used for instalment prescribing. If a daily pick-up is required, a separate prescription must be written for each day.
- FP10(MDA)[1] prescriptions can be used by any doctor to write instalment prescriptions. The prescription must specify the total quantity required, the amount of the instalments to be dispensed, and the intervals to be observed between instalments.
- A maximum of 14 days' supply of schedule 2 controlled drugs can be prescribed by instalments for the treatment of substance misuse.
- FP10 prescriptions have a potential street value and may be sold to other injecting drug users. Consider posting or delivering the prescription to the community pharmacy, rather than handing it to the patient. Check normal practice with the local addiction service/GP.

---

1 HBP(A), HBP or GP10 in Scotland, WP10 (MDA) or WP10(HP)Ad in Wales.

Surgical patient and nil by mouth (NBM) issues

It is imperative that a comprehensive DHx is undertaken for all patients admitted to hospital for surgery. The DHx should include regular, if needed, and recently stopped or withheld medications. Over-the-counter and herbal products need to be documented.

- Medicines used to control life-threatening conditions should be continued.
- Optimize the treatment of chronic diseases before admission for surgery—e.g. for asthma and COPD.
- For surgical emergencies, e.g. abdominal aortic aneurysm (AAA), it might not be possible to optimize drug therapy preoperatively and the pharmacist needs to highlight any possible complications relating to a recently administered drug that otherwise should have been stopped or dose-modified.

In general, with the exception of those drugs noted in this section, few drugs need to be stopped before surgery.

NBM period

- Patients are at risk of aspirating their stomach contents during general anaesthesia. They are usually prevented from eating within 6h of surgery. However, clear fluids leave the stomach within 2h of ingestion, and thus free clear fluids that enable a patient to take routine medication are allowed up to 2h presurgery.
- After surgery, oral medicines can be restarted at their previous pre-operative dose as soon as the patient can swallow small amounts of fluid.
- If a patient is likely to be NBM for a long time (e.g. surgeon's plan and postoperative nausea and vomiting (PONV)), the drug can be given by an alternative route—e.g. rectal, transdermal, parenteral, or feeding tube delivery.
- Drugs with a long half-life (e.g. levothyroxine) or long duration of action (e.g. antidepressants) shouldn't cause a problem if they have to be omitted for several days.

Reviewing a patient's medication during the NBM period

The risks and benefits must be considered when deciding to continue or suspend medication. For example, the consequences of stopping long-term therapy for conditions such as osteoporosis or osteoarthritis in the NBM period might be considered non-problematic in the majority of patients.

To avoid interrupting appropriate long-term therapies, oral medicines can be administered with sips of clear oral fluid in the NBM period.

The anaesthetist should be contacted if there is any doubt about a patient's specific medication plan—e.g. if a drug is known to have potential interaction with anaesthetic agents.

There are a few significant interactions between drugs used during surgery and routine medications that require the drugs not to be administered concurrently. This is usually managed by the anaesthetist, by their choice of anaesthetic technique. Significant interactions are as follows.

- Enflurane can precipitate seizure activity in patients taking tricyclic antidepressants.
- Pethidine can precipitate fatal 'excitatory' reactions in patients taking monoamine oxidase inhibitors and can cause serotonin syndrome in patients taking SSRIs.
- The effects of suxamethonium can be prolonged by neostigmine.
- The metabolism of midazolam is significantly decreased by protease inhibitors and efavirenz.

Controversial therapy for surgical patients

Hormone-replacement therapy (HRT)

Women on HRT had an ↑ risk of developing venous thromboembolism (VTE) after major surgery compared with controls. The MHRA advise that there is no need to stop HRT unless patients have other predisposing risk factors for VTE; such patients require suitable thromboprophylaxis.

For patients with predisposing risk factors, HRT should be stopped 4wks before major surgery.

Combined oral contraceptives (see 📖 p.463)

Again, there is an ↑ risk of VTE in patients having therapy with COCs. Therapy should be discontinued 4wks before major elective surgery and all leg surgery. However, the risks and consequences of pregnancy versus VTE must be discussed with patients.

COCs should be restarted at the first menses that occurs at least 2wks after full mobilization.

Tamoxifen

Patients on tamoxifen therapy have a higher risk of VTE after surgery. However, tamoxifen treatment for breast cancer should be continued during surgery unless directed by the patient's oncologist, and close monitoring of VTE symptoms for 3 months post surgery should be planned.

Patients having tamoxifen treatment for fertility should have treatment suspended 6wks before major surgery.

Methotrexate

Fluid restriction, hypovolaemia, and renal hypoperfusion can result in ↓ clearance; it is advisable to suspend methotrexate for 2days before surgery and check renal function before recommencing therapy.

Monoamine oxidase inhibitors

MAOIs can result in hypertensive crisis if used concurrently with interacting drugs (e.g. pethidine, dextromethorphan, and pentazocine). They are usually withdrawn 2wks before surgery. However, the risk of psychiatric relapse must be considered. If necessary, MAOIs can be substituted with a short-acting form, such as moclobemide (which can be withheld on the morning of surgery). If withdrawal is not possible, avoid pethidine and indirectly acting sympathomimetics—use isoprenaline instead. Phentolamine can be used to ↓ BP in the event of a hypertensive crisis.

Corticosteroids

Stress caused by surgery is associated with ↑ cortisol production. Prolonged corticosteroid therapy, especially at high doses, can cause adrenal atrophy, an impaired stress response, and risk of hypoadrenal crisis, manifesting in circulatory collapse and shock.

The risk of HPA (hypothalmic–pituary–adrenal) axis suppression should be considered if patients have been on steroids for 1–2wks before surgery or within the last 6 months. The dose and duration of steroids determines the risk, in addition to the type of surgery. Therefore these patients will require IV hydrocortisone cover. The usual dose is 50–100mg of hydrocortisone given preoperatively, intraoperatively (if necessary), and every 6–8h for 2–3 days after surgery. Normal preoperative steroid doses should be restarted 2 days after surgery (no gradual dose reduction is needed from postoperative cover).

Lithium

Lithium prolongs the action of depolarizing and non-depolarizing muscle relaxants. Ideally, stop therapy 24–72h before major surgery, but therapy can continue during minor surgery. If it is not possible to stop therapy, ensure adequate fluid intake during and after surgery. Monitor U&E regularly; measure lithium blood levels if necessary.

Diuretics

Omit K$^+$-sparing diuretics on the morning of surgery because ↓ kidney perfusion in the immediate postoperative period can predispose to hyperkalaemia. Thiazide and loop diuretics need not be omitted. Any electrolyte imbalance should be corrected before surgery.

β-blockers

Anaesthesia and surgery can provoke tachycardia and ↑ BP in patients with hypertension. β-blockers can help to suppress these effects and therefore are usually continued perioperatively.

Antiplatelet drugs

Aspirin/clopidogrel should be stopped when the risks of postoperative bleeding are high or if the consequences of, even minor, bleeding are significant (e.g. retinal and intracranial bleeding). This must be balanced against the risk of precipitating thromboembolic complications if these drugs are stopped, particularly in patients with unstable angina. If low-dose aspirin or clopidogrel are stopped, this is generally 7–10 days before surgery to enable recovery of adequate platelet function. It is not usually necessary to stop dipyridamole before surgery, but if complete absence of antiplatelet effect is desired, it should be stopped 24h before surgery.

Anti-Parkinson's drugs

There is a small risk of arrhythmias or hypertension during anaesthesia in patients with Parkinson's disease. However, anaesthesia can worsen symptoms of Parkinson's disease after surgery and uncontrolled symptoms ↓ mobility and impede recovery. These drugs should be continued wherever possible. Procyclidine can be given by injection to relieve rigidity and tremor if the patient is unable to take oral medication after surgery.

Antipsychotics and anxiolytics

Generally these agents are continued to avoid relapse of the condition. Antipsychotics can ↓ anaesthetic requirements and potentiate arrhythmias. However, clozapine should be stopped 24h before surgery. Therefore if the patient is on the morning list, do not give medication on the day before surgery, in addition to the day of surgery itself. There are no withdrawal problems associated with doing this. If the patient is unable to take clozapine for >2 days because of being NBM, the drug must be gradually re-titrated up from the starting dose (12.5mg once or twice daily).

Oral hypoglycaemics

For major surgery, most patients with type 2 diabetes benefit from IV insulin therapy, especially if a prolonged NBM period is expected or if the stress from surgery has led to unacceptable hyperglycaemia.

However, the following guidance can aid your patient management.

- Glibenclamide—switch to a sulphonylurea with a shorter half-life 3 days before surgery or switch to soluble insulin.
- Gliclazide/glipizide/tolbutamide—omit therapy on the day of surgery.
- Metformin—to ↓ the risk of lactic acidosis, withdraw the drug 48–72h before surgery and restabilize 48h after surgery.

Pharmaceutical calculations

Concentrations 236
Moles and millimoles 238
Practical issues involving pharmaceutical calculations 240
Pharmaceutical calculations involving drug administration 242

Concentrations

Pharmaceutical preparations consist of a number of different ingredients in a vehicle. The ingredients can be solid, liquid, or gas.

'Concentration' is an expression of the ratio of the amount of an ingredient to the amount of product. Concentrations can be expressed in several ways.

- Solutions of solids in liquids, denoted by w/v.
- Solutions of liquids in liquids, denoted by v/v.
- Admixtures of liquids in solids (v/w) or solids combined with solids (w/w).

Concentrations are expressions of ratios and are written in different formats that can cause confusion. Formats traditionally used are as follows:

- amount strengths
- ratio strengths
- ppm (parts per million)
- percentage strength.

Amount strengths

A preparation contains 900mg of sodium chloride dissolved in water to make a final volume of 100mL. The concentration of this solution can be written as an amount strength in units of 900mg/100mL, 9mg/mL, 0.9g/100mL, or 9g/L.

Ratio strengths

Convention states that when ratio strength represents a solid in a liquid, involving units of weight and volume, the weight is expressed in grams and the volume in millilitres.

A 1 in 50 sodium chloride in water preparation is a solid in a liquid (w/v) ratio strength. This means that the solution contains 1g of sodium chloride made up to 50mL with water.

A 14 in 100 sulphuric acid in water preparation is a liquid in liquid (v/v) ratio strength, i.e. 14mL of sulphuric acid in 86mL of water.

Parts per million (ppm)

This expression is used when the ratio of ingredient to product is very small, by convention 1ppm weight in volume is 1g in 1000000mL. 1ppm weight in weight is 1mg per 1000000mg or 1g per 1000000g. In volume, it is 1mL in 1000000mL or 1L in 1000000L.

Percentage strength

'Percentage' in pharmaceutical calculations is quantified as the amount of ingredient in 100 parts of the product.

By convention, % w/v indicates the number of grams of ingredient in 100mL of product. Therefore 900mg of sodium chloride made up to 100mL with water can be expressed as 0.9g in 100mL and the percentage strength is 0.9% w/v.

A 1 in 1000 adrenaline injection is equivalent to 0.1% w/v or, by convention, 1g of adrenaline made up to 1000mL with water.

A 1 in 10000 adrenaline injection is equivalent to 0.01% w/v or, by convention, 1g of adrenaline made up to 10000mL with water.

Calculations

For example, how many millilitres of a 1 in 50 w/v solution are required to make 500mL of a 0.02% solution?

By convention, 1 in 50 means 1g in 50mL and 0.02% w/v means 0.02g in 100mL. Let the number of millilitres of the 1 in 50 solution be y and let the amount of ingredient in grams in 500mL of 0.02% solution be x. The amount of ingredient in grams in ymL of a 1 in 50 solution will also be x.

Setting up proportional sets

For 1 in 50:

Ingredient (g)	1	x	1g
Product (mL)	50	y	to 50mL

For 500mL of 0.02%:

Ingredient (g)	0.02	x	0.02g
Product (mL)	100	500	to 100mL

By 'spotting' $x = 0.1$; substitute into the first pair of proportional sets.
For 1 in 50

Ingredient (g)	1	0.1	1g
Product (mL)	50	y	to 50mL

By 'spotting' $y = 5$. Therefore 5mL of a 1 in 50 w/v solution is required to make 500mL of a 0.02% w/v solution.

Alternatively, how many grams in 500mL of 0.02% solution?

$$0.02\% = 0.02\text{g in }100\text{mL}$$
$$\text{in }500\text{mL} = 0.02 \times 5$$
$$= 0.1\text{g}$$

1 in 50 solution, by convention 1g in 50mL
Then, to calculate the volume containing 0.1g, 1/10 of 1g or 1/10 of 50mL = 5mL.

Moles and millimoles

The atomic and molecular weights of a drug can be used as methods of defining the amount of drug. The substance can be atoms, molecules, or ions; a mole is the weight expressed in grams. The mole is the SI base unit for the amount of a substance—e.g. the atomic weight of iron is 56 and 1 mole of iron weighs 56g.

The molecular weight of a drug (e.g. sodium chloride) is the sum of all the atomic weights of the individual atoms in the molecule. A molecule of sodium chloride consists of one sodium ion and one chloride ion :

- 1mole sodium ions weighs 23g
- 1mole chloride ions weighs 35.5g
- hence the molecular weight of sodium chloride is 58.5g

In the same way that the system of weights and volumes have multiples and subdivisions (e.g. milli, micro, and nano), so the mole has similar subdivisions and multiples:

- 1mole contains 1000 millimoles (mmol)
- 1mmol contains 1000 micromoles (mcmol)
- 1micromol contains 1000 nanomoles (nmol)
- 1nanomol contains 1000 picomoles (pmol)

Amount of substance concentration

In clinical chemistry, laboratory results are usually written in terms of mol/L (or mmol/L or micromol/L).

Example

How many millimoles of sodium chloride are there in a litre of sodium chloride 0.9% w/v?

First calculate the weight of sodium chloride in a litre:
0.9g in 100mL
=0.9g×10 in 1000mL
=9g in 1000mL.

For the molecule sodium chloride: 1mole = 58.5g
58.5g = 1000mmol
9/58.5 = x/1000
x = 9000/58.5
x = 153mmoL.

Alternatively, to calculate the number of millimoles contained in 1g of substance, use the following formula:

$$mmol = \frac{1000 \times number\ of\ specified\ units\ in\ one\ unit\ (atom,\ molecule\ or\ ion)}{atomic,\ molecular,\ or\ ionic\ weight}$$

Number of mmol of sodium in 1g of sodium chloride (molecular weight = 58.5):

$$mmol = \frac{1000 \times 1}{58.5}$$
$$= 17mmol\ in\ 1g\ or\ 153mmol\ in\ 9g$$

For $CaCl_2.2H_2o$ (molecular weight = 147)

$$\text{mmol of calcium in 1g } CaCl_2\,2H_2o = \frac{1000 \times 1}{147} = 6.8\text{mmol}$$

$$\text{mmol of chloride in 1g } CaCl_2\,2H_2o = \frac{1000 \times 2}{147} = 13.6\text{mmol}$$

$$\text{mmol of water in 1g } CaCl_2\,2H_2o = \frac{1000 \times 2}{147} = 13.6\text{mmol}$$

i.e. each gram of $CaCl_2.2H_2O$ represents 6.8mmol of calcium, 13.6mmol of chloride, and 13.6mmol of water of crystallization.

Practical issues involving pharmaceutical calculations

- Always work from a written master copy.
  - Calculate the amounts of ingredients for 200mL Chloral Mixture BP 1988:

Ingredients	Master formula	Scaled quantities
Chloral hydrate	1g	20g
Syrup	2mL	40mL
Water	To 10mL	To 200mL

- Use double checks: 1 is 1/10 of 10 and 20 is 1/10 of 200.
- Don't forget your units: 1g = 1000mg = 1 000 000micrograms.

Preparing dilutions

- Ensure correct choice of diluent.
- Calculate dilution factor.
- Correctly express the concentration of the diluted product on the label.

Example 1

Calculate the amount of benzalkonium chloride solution BP 2004 needed to prepare a 150mL of a solution of benzalkonium chloride 10% w/v. Benzalkonium chloride solution BP 2004 is a 50% w/v concentration.

Calculation of dilution factor
Method 1

$$\frac{\text{Strength of concentrate}}{\text{Strength of dilute solution}} = \text{dilution factor}$$

$$\frac{\text{Strength of concentrate}}{\text{Strength of dilute solution}} = \frac{50\% \text{ w/v}}{10\% \text{ w/V}} = 5 \text{ times}$$

$$\text{To prepare dilute solution} = \frac{\text{final volume}}{\text{dilution factor}}$$

$$150/5 = 30\text{mL of concentrate solution}$$

The diluted solution is obtained by using 30mL of BP solution and diluting with 120mL of water.

Method 2

Product of volume and concentration:
$V_c \times C_c = V_d \times C_d$ where
$V_c \times 50 = 150 \times 10$
$V_c = 150/5$
$V_c = 30$mL

V_c = volume of concentrated solution
C_c = concentration of concentrate
V_d = volume of diluted solution
C_d = concentration of diluted solution

Example 2

Calculate the quantity of potassium permanganate 0.25% w/v solution that is required to produce 100mL of a 0.0125% w/v solution of potassium permanganate.

Calculation of dilution factor

$V_c \times C_c = V_d \times C_d$

V_c = volume of concentrated solution	= unknown
C_c = concentration of concentrate	= 0.25%
V_d = volume of diluted solution	= 100mL
C_d = concentration of diluted solution	= 0.0125%

$V_c \times 0.25\% = 100\text{mL} \times 0.0125\%$
$V_c \qquad = 1.25/0.25$
$\qquad = 5\text{mL}$

Dilution instructions

5mL of potassium permanganate solution 0.25% w/v must be diluted to 100mL with water to produce a 0.0125% w/v solution.

Pharmaceutical calculations involving drug administration

Calculations

- Calculations usually involve fairly straightforward theory, but difficulties can arise as a result of interruptions, tiredness, or lack of experience.
- In preparing infusions, the mathematics normally involves translating units such as micrograms/kg body weight/min into a practical number of millilitres of diluted infusion solution per hour.

Examples

A patient requires a parenteral loading dose of 0.5mg of digoxin. Digoxin is available as an injection containing 250micrograms/mL. How many millilitres of injection will supply the required dose?

First convert mg to micrograms:

0.5mg = 500micrograms

Setting up a proportional set

| Weight of digoxin (mg) | 250 | 500 |
| Volume of injection (mL) | 1 | y |

250 multiplied by 2 gives 500, so 1 is multiplied by 2 to give y = 2.

Because the injection contains 250micrograms in 1mL, a 500micrograms dose will be provided in 2mL.

ITU prepare dobutamine as a standard concentration of 250mg in 50mL 5% dextrose solution. You need to confirm that the prescribed 5micrograms/kg/body weight/min dose for a 70kg patient is correctly delivered by the volumetric hourly rate set by the nurse.

Standard concentration = 250mg in 50mL (patient 70kg)

To calculate the hourly rate:	= 5micrograms × kg body weight × min
	= 5 × 70 × 60(min)
	= 21 000micrograms/h
Concentration of dobutamine (convert to micrograms)	= 250mg in 50mL
	= 250 × 1000 (micrograms) in 50mL
	= 250 000micrograms in 50mL
	= 5000micrograms in 1mL

Volume per hour requires 21 000micrograms to be administered
= (21 000micrograms/h)/(5000micrograms/mL)
= 4.2mL/h

Pharmaceutical care

The concept of pharmaceutical care 244
Core elements of pharmaceutical care 245
Medication problem checklist 246
Pharmaceutical care economics 248
Staffing 250
Standards for research 252

The concept of pharmaceutical care

Pharmaceutical care was probably first defined by Mikeal et al. in 1975 as 'the care that a given patient requires and receives, which assures safe and rational drug use'.[1] Hepler, in 1988, described pharmaceutical care as 'a covenantal relationship between a patient and a practitioner in which the pharmacist performs drug use control functions governed by the awareness of and commitment to the patients' interest'.[2] The term has caught the imagination of pharmacists and is frequently applied indiscriminately to describe pharmacy activities. The term 'patient-centred care' is gaining wider acceptance and is similar in principle.

Definition

The widely accepted definition by Hepler and Strand states 'Pharmaceutical care is the responsible provision of drug therapy for the purpose of achieving definite outcomes that improve a patient's quality of life'.[3] This definition built on earlier one describing pharmaceutical care as 'a practice in which the practitioner takes responsibility for a patients drug-related needs and is held accountable for this commitment'.[4] Early in these debates, the issue of drug-related morbidity was seen as a major problem and, in part, led to the final definitions outlined here.

Pharmaceutical care differs from traditional drug treatment because it is an explicitly outcome-orientated cooperative systematic approach to providing drug therapy directed not only at clinical outcomes, but also at activities of daily life and other dimensions of health-related quality of life. Historically, pharmacists have used a variety of methods to improve drug therapy, including formularies, drug-use reviews, prescriber education, and clinical pharmacy, but these have all been drug or prescription focused.

Pharmaceutical care involves the process through which a pharmacist cooperates with a patient and other professionals in designing, implementing, and maintaining a therapeutic plan that will produce specific outcomes for the patient. This, in turn, involves three major functions:
- identifying potential and actual drug-related problems
- resolving actual drug-related problems
- preventing drug-related problems.

1 Mikeal RL et al. (1975). Quality of pharmaceutical care in hospitals. American Journal of Hospital Pharmacy **32**: 567–74.
2 Hepler CD (1988). Unresolved issues in the future of pharmacy. American Journal of Hospital Pharmacy **45**: 1071–81.
3 Hepler CD, Strand LM (1990). Opportunities and responsibilities in pharmaceutical care. American Journal of Hospital Pharmacy **47**: 533–43.
4 Strand LM (1984). Re-visioning the professions. Journal of the American Pharmacy Association 100–258.

Core elements of pharmaceutical care

The pharmacist
- Collects and documents relevant information in a systematic, structured manner for the purpose of determining whether the patient is experiencing potential or actual drug-related problems.
- Identifies and lists the drug-related problems the patient is experiencing or is at risk of experiencing.
- Establishes and lists the desired therapeutic outcomes for each drug-related problem identified.
- Considers and ranks all the therapeutic interventions that might be expected to produce the desired therapeutic outcomes for each problem.
- Decides which therapeutic alternative to select and records the dosage regimen for each medication for each patient.
- Formulates and documents a pharmaco-therapeutic monitoring plan to verify that the drug-related decisions implemented have resulted in the outcomes desired and not in undesirable ADRs or toxicities.[1]

All must be in place for a comprehensive pharmaceutical care service. The only variable that affects the level of service is the patient's needs. This is assessed by determining the patient's risk factors. Patients who are considered at low risk might only require minimal intervention, whereas high-risk patients, by definition, require a higher level of pharmaceutical care.

Identifying risk in clinical practice
Risk factors fall into three distinct areas.
- Patients' clinical characteristics—these include physical and readily determined characteristics, such as age, gender, ethnicity, pregnancy status, immune status, kidney, liver and cardiac functions, nutritional status, and patient expectations.
- The patient's disease—some assessment of the rate and extent of harm caused by the disease and the patient's perception of these factors.
- The patient's pharmacotherapy—the risk is determined by an assessment of the toxicity of the drug therapy, the ADR profile, the route and techniques of administration, and the patient's perception of these three elements.

1 Strand LM (1991). Pharmaceutical care: challenge of implementation. *ASHP Annual Meeting* **48**: PI–28.

Medication problem checklist

The following list covers the range of potential medication problems that could be encountered by pharmacists seeking to deliver pharmaceutical care.

- Medications without medical indications.
- Medical conditions for which no medications are prescribed.
- Medications prescribed inappropriately for a particular medical condition.
- Inappropriate medication dose, dosage form, schedule, route of administration, or method of administration.
- Therapeutic duplication.
- Prescribing of medications to which the patient is allergic.
- Actual and potential ADRs.
- Actual and potential adverse clinically significant drug–drug, drug–disease, drug–nutrient, and drug–laboratory test interactions.
- Interference with medical therapy by social or recreational drug use.
- Failure to receive the full benefit of prescribed medication therapy.
- Problems arising from the financial impact of medication therapy on the patient.
- Lack of understanding of the medication therapy by the patient.
- Failure of the patient to adhere to the medication regimen.

There have been a number of attempts to formulate these problems into an easily remembered checklist. One of these is called PRIME, which is an acronym for Pharmaceutical Risks to patients, Interventions Mismatch between medications and indications, and Efficiency issues (Table 13.1). The key message behind these detailed checklists is that pharmacists must move from a prescription focus to a patient focus.

Table 13.1 PRIME pharmacotherapy problem types

Pharmaceutical—assess for incorrect factors, as follows

- Dosage
- Form
- Route
- Timing
- Duration
- Frequency.

Risks to patients—assess for risks, as follows

- Known contraindication
- Medication allergy
- Drug-induced problem
- Improper use (i.e. risk if misused)
- Common/serious ADRs
- Medication error considerations.

Interactions—assess for the following:

- Drug–drug
- Drug–disease/condition
- Drug–food
- Drug–laboratory test

Mismatch between medications and indications/conditions—assess for the following

- Medication used without indication
- Indications/condition untreated.

Efficacy issues—assess for the following

- Suboptimal selection of pharmacotherapy for indications
- Minimal or no evidence of therapeutic effectiveness
- Suboptimal pharmacotherapy (taking/receiving medications incorrectly)— e.g. patient preference considerations (undesirable prior experiences with medications or does not believe it works)
- Medications availability considerations (e.g. no access to medications)
- Compliance/administration considerations (e.g. inability to pay or unable to administer correctly or at all).

Pharmaceutical care economics

Clinical pharmacy services can be perceived as expensive by hospital managers. The reality is that clinical pharmacy can significantly improve patient outcomes and ↓ drug budgets. The following data are presented as a sample of what is available in the wider pharmacy literature and can be used to improve facilities and funding.

Clinical pharmacy interventions ↓ costs. In a large annual pharmacy staff survey, Bond[1] showed that each whole-time pharmacist ↓ the drug budget by approximately US $22 000 per hospital and that each US dollar spent on a pharmacist resulted in savings of just under US $50 in the drug budget. The same survey, in a different report,[2] also showed that although there was no association between number of medical staff and hospital mortality rates, pharmacists were one group demonstrating ↓ mortality rates as staffing levels ↑. The authors were unable to identify reasons for this finding but surmised that preventing adverse events could be significant. In yet another report on the same data the authors claim that hospitals that provide the services outlined in Table 13.2 within their pharmacy are associated with a reduction in deaths.

An Australian trial on fee for service[3] demonstrated savings in the intervention group. This was a randomized controlled trial of four parallel groups of community pharmacies conducted in 1996. The numbers in each group are small, but the authors claim that it was based on sufficient differences in intervention rates. The basic education covered drug information, attendance on hospital-ward rounds, basic therapeutics, and problem-solving. The advanced course included a weekend university-based course, covering complex medication reviews, attendance on ward rounds, advanced therapeutics, multiple coexisting disease states, and problem-solving. The cost was A$1500 per person.

Outcomes were based on cost savings or healthcare costs avoided based on healthcare costs, increased charges in medication costs, pharmacy times, and telephone calls. The savings were as follows (except in group D which showed an ↑ in costs).

- Group C   Professional fee + advanced education $85/1000 prescriptions
- Group B   Professional fee + basic education $26/1000 prescriptions
- Group A   No fee or education $14/1000 prescriptions
- Group D   Professional fee + no education $1/1000 prescriptions

The study is particularly interesting because a fee for services alone did not ↓ costs; the most effective contribution was a fee plus advanced education.

1 Bond CA *et al.* (1999). Clinical pharmacy services, pharmacist staffing, and drug costs in United States hospitals. *Pharmacotherapy* **19(12)**: 1354–62.

2 Bond CA *et al.* (1999). Health care professional staffing; hospital characteristics and hospital mortality rates. *Pharmacotherapy* **19**: 130–8.

3 Benrimoj SI *et al.* (2000). Economic impact of increased clinical intervention rated in community pharmacy. *Pharmacoeconomics* **18**: 459–68.

Table 13.2 Impact of pharamaceutical care on hospital deaths: reduction in mortality

Service	Reduction in mortality
Clinical research service	195 deaths/hospital/year
DI services	41 deaths/hospital/year
Drug-administration histories	128 deaths/hospital/year
Pharmacist on CPR team	18 deaths/hospital/year

Staffing

This information is provided to help clinical pharmacists make a case for establishing additional clinical services. There is good evidence that ↑ clinical pharmacy time has a major positive affect on budgets.

Work by Bond and Raehl[1,2] was referred to in the monograph on pharmaceutical care.[3] These authors have been responsible for regular useful publications in the USA. Bond and Raehl are based at the Texas Tech University Health Services Centre. Although the work is hospital-based, it does give an indication of the investment being made. The National Clinical Pharmacy Services study is seen as the largest hospital-based pharmacy database in the USA. The work involved a postal questionnaire to >3500 acute care hospitals with >50 beds. The percentages of patients receiving clinical pharmacy services was calculated for each hospital during a 10 year period from 1989 to 1998. Pharmacist numbers ↑ by 23%, pharmacy technician numbers ↑ by 43%, and pharmacy clerk numbers ↑ by 25%. This is in contrast with a rise in total hospital personnel of 55%. This represented an ↑ from 4.2(92.6) pharmacists per 100 occupied beds to 5.35(±2.7) pharmacists per 100 occupied beds in 1995—an ↑ of 5% per annum.[4]

Although 71% of hospitals surveyed stated that pharmacists had the authority to document pharmaceutical care in patient's notes, in practice this only happens in 31% of hospitals. When the levels of pharmaceutical care were analysed according to the training of the hospital, it was found that 64% of hospitals training PharmD students provided pharmaceutical care, which fell to 42% of hospitals who trained graduates and 33% of non-pharmacy-teaching hospitals.[5] By 1998, 52% of hospitals provided some level of pharmaceutical care and time spent had ↑ to a mean of 25min/patient/day.[3]

The authors analysed the total cost of care in relation to clinical pharmacy services for earlier (1992) data in a population of 1016 hospitals. Although the study was designed to show relationships rather than cause and effect, there is a strong hint that establishing additional clinical pharmacists is associated with ↓ total care cost; conversely, an ↑ in the number of dispensing pharmacists is associated with ↑ total cost of care.

1 Bond CA et al. (1999). Clinical pharmacy services, pharmacist staffing, and drug costs in United States Hospitals. *Pharmacotherapy* **19**: 1354–62.
2 Bond CA et al. (1999). Health care professional staffing, hospital characteristics and hospital mortality rates. *Pharmacotherapy* **19**: 130–8.
3 Raehl CL, Bond CA (2000). (1998). National Clinical Pharmacy Services Study. *Pharmacotherapy* **20**: 436–60.
4 Bond CA et al. (1999). Staffing and the cost of clinical and hospital pharmacy service in United States hospitals. *Pharmacotherapy* **19**: 767–81.
5 Raehl CL et al. (1998). Clinical pharmacy services in hospital educating pharmacy students. *Pharmacotherapy* **18**: 1093–102.

Standards for research

Pharmaceutical care is an obvious research area for pharmacists, but many of the publications in this area have been of poor quality. Two checklists are presented here in to aid those who read pharmaceutical care literature and those who undertake research into pharmaceutical care.

A review of pharmaceutical care by Kennie et al[1]. led to the authors to make 15 recommendations which are aimed at improving the quality of further research:

- Pharmacists must exercise discipline when using the term 'pharmaceutical care'.
- Database systems should take measures to ensure that pharmaceutical care research literature can be correctly and easily extracted.
- A standard reporting method should be adopted that clearly describes the pharmaceutical care process in the research methodology.
- Randomized controlled studies should be conducted to measure the affect of the provision of pharmaceutical care.
- Pharmaceutical care research should contain a clear description of the pharmacy practice setting and patient demographics.
- Consistent methods for data collection for different practice sites should be created and validated.
- Informed consent should be obtained for all patients involved in pharmaceutical research, and the procedure should be stated.
- A pharmacist's qualifications and/or certification in providing pharmaceutical care should be addressed and described.
- Pharmaceutical care research should not only emphasize the evaluation of patient outcomes, but must also first evaluate the structures that exist for the provision of pharmaceutical care.
- The three aspects of evaluation (i.e. structure, process, and outcome) should be linked when assessing the quality of pharmaceutical care.
- The economic impact of pharmaceutical care should be evaluated.
- Standards for pharmaceutical care research should be developed and accepted by the profession.
- Further pharmaceutical care research needs to be conducted, with an emphasis on community-based pharmacy.
- A pharmaceutical care research network should be developed to co-ordinate efforts and identify areas where research is required.
- Research should be conducted to determine the feasibility and extent of implementation of pharmaceutical care in various practice sites.

The authors concluded that few studies have evaluated the provision of pharmaceutical care in a defined population, and that the volume of research is painfully low.

1 Kennie NR et al. (1998). Critical analysis of the pharmaceutical care research literature. *Annals of Pharmacotherapy* **32**: 17–26.

Plumridge et al.[2] stated that research into patient perceptions and the patient–pharmacist relationship are needed, because these are critical success factors for pharmaceutical care. Patient understanding and involvement in the process are essential. Furthermore, reliable information is required about patients' willingness to pay for pharmaceutical care. Currently, a dilemma exists because pharmacists want to charge for services but cannot demonstrate improvements on clinical, economic, or quality-of-life outcomes.

When research is undertaken, the pharmaceutical care process used should be such that the study results can be critically analysed and the process replicated as necessary.

The authors made 13 recommendations for future research, which overlap with the previous list but are worth reproducing here.

- The paucity of published studies on the economic value of pharmaceutical care reinforces the requirement for additional well-conducted research in appropriate practice settings to address the high cost of drug-related morbidity and mortality. Descriptive reports, or inadequately conducted studies of the pharmaceutical care process do little to advance our present knowledge.
- Studies should use, and be refereed on, the correct definition of pharmaceutical care. If this is not done, the confusion that already exists with other pharmaceutical interventions will be exacerbated.
- The quality of pharmaceutical care requires the development of systems for documenting delivery processes and outcomes. Systems for documenting patient satisfaction are also required.
- Variable study design and lack of standardization in reporting causes difficulties in comparing study results. Uniformity is desirable for comparative purposes and to enable valid conclusions to be made.
- Comparative groups must be more fully described and consistent with intervention groups. Patients should be randomized.
- Evidence that external factors affecting outcomes have been controlled is desirable.
- Practice settings should be fully described to enable readers to understand the processes used, facilitate replication, and further develop future pharmaceutical care practice.
- All relevant direct and indirect costs should be considered. When this is achieved, attempts to use appropriate pharmacoeconomic methods (e.g. cost-effectiveness and cost–benefit analyses) can be considered. These will probably require specialist expertise.
- Structure and process should be described and appropriate outcome measures used. Process measures, intermediate outcomes indicators, and outcomes need to be correctly identified because these terms are often confused by researchers. If feasible, the link between structure, process, and outcomes should be evaluated.
- Outcomes must be identified in terms of the feasible effect of pharmaceutical care because certain outcomes can present difficulty in measurement (e.g. outcomes requiring years to observe, such as the treatment of osteoporosis).

2 Plumridge RJ, Wojnar Horton RE (1998). A review of the pharmacoeconomics of pharmaceutical care. *Pharmacoeconomics* **14**: 175–89.

- Research is needed to determine the value that specific interventions have on health outcomes so that effect is optimized. This includes identifying structures and processes that improve specific health outcomes and the types of outcomes that are most effected by pharmaceutical care programmes.
- Each study should attempt to address relevant pharmacoeconomic parameters, including clinical, economic, and quality of life.
- The potential for assessing opportunity costs, especially because healthcare resources are in cost-containment mode, should be considered. This is important in determining the best way of implementing pharmaceutical care as practice is evolving.

Medicines management

Medicines management 256
Evaluating new drugs 258
How to write a drug protocol 260
Unlicensed use of medicines 262
Drug and therapeutics committees 264
Patient group directions (PGDs) 266
Supplementary prescribing 268
Independent prescribing 272
Community (FP10) prescription use in hospitals 274
Electronic prescribing 276
Incident reporting 278
Medical representatives 279
Overseas visitors 280
Private patients 282
Professional supervision skills 283
National Service Frameworks (NSFs) 284
Appraisal 286
Confidentiality 288
Gene therapy 290
Pharmacogenetics 292
Standards of business conduct for clinical pharmacists 294
Waste management of medicines 296
Responsible pharmacist 300

Medicines management

Medicines management is made up of two components:
- clinical and cost-effective use of medicines
- safe and secure handling of medicines.

Each hospital should have a strategic plan for medicines management which reflects the following.
- The strategic direction for the local health economy.
- Priorities of the local population.
- Targets relating to NSFs and implementation of National Institute for Health and Clinical Excellence (NICE) guidance.
- Communication strategy for the dissemination of information.

Hospitals should ensure that the following systems are in place to ensure effective medicines management.
- Drug and therapeutics committee (or equivalent).
- Targeting clinical pharmacy activity to patients requiring early assessment following hospital admission.
- Patients should ideally have a complete DHx review within 24h of hospital admission.
- Acute medical admissions should be prioritized and, if possible, seen by a pharmacist.
- PODs should be used if they have been reviewed and considered suitable for continued use.
- As appropriate, all patients should be given the option of self-administering their own medicines while in hospital.
- Dispensing for discharge (or one-stop dispensing) systems should be in place to ensure that patients receive their discharge medication in sufficient quantity and in a timely manner, with the appropriate patient information leaflet.

The multidisciplinary team should be trained on medicines management.
- All doctors, nurses, pharmacists, and other relevant healthcare professionals should receive training on medicines management as part of their induction programme, including the legislative and GCP aspects of controls assurance (in particular, the safe and secure handling of medicines) and clinical and cost-effective use of medicines.
- Medicines management systems and policies should be incorporated into ongoing clinical training programmes.
- Information technology system support should be available to provide healthcare staff with accurate information on the use of medicines.
- The risk of medication errors occurring should be minimized.

Medicines management policies and procedures should be in place to minimize the risk of medication errors occurring during the medication process, i.e. for prescribing, dispensing, and administration.

Further reading

Department of Health (2003). *A Vision for Pharmacy in the New NHS*. London: Department of Health.

Audit Commission (2001). *A Spoonful of Sugar*. London: Audit Commission.

Smith J (2004). *Building a Safer NHS for Patients: Improving Medication Safety*. London: Department of Health.

Nursing & Midwifery Council (2010). *Standards for Medicines Management*. ℘ http://www.nmc-uk.org/Documents/Standards/nmcStandardsForMedicinesManagementBooklet.pdf

National Prescribing Centre. *Medicines Management*. ℘ http://www.npc.co.uk

National Prescribing Centre (2008). *Moving Towards Personalising Medicines Management: Improving Outcomes for People through the Safe and Effective use of medicines*. ℘ www.npc.nhs.uk/resources/personalising_medicines_management_web.pdf

Evaluating new drugs

New drugs appear on the market all the time and healthcare professionals are constantly bombarded with promotional material from the pharmaceutical industry. The pharmaceutical industry's business is to sell drugs—otherwise it would not survive—but promotional material should be reviewed with a critical eye.

Just because a drug has received regulatory approval, does not necessarily mean that it is a clinically significant advance, because regulatory authorities evaluate quality, safety, and efficacy, not therapeutic value. Assessments of the value of new drugs from Canada, France, and the USA have shown that, at best, only one-third offer some additional clinical benefit and as few as 3% are a major therapeutic advance.[1]

Premarketing trials are often placebo controlled, so they don't give comparative data. Ideally, the trial should compare the new drug with an established reference treatment. Even if the trial compares the new drug with a reference treatment, it might be too small or too short to provide meaningful data—in particular, rare ADRs or differences in response in subgroups of patients are unlikely to be identified.

Much of the data presented by the pharmaceutical industry is disease-orientated rather than patient-orientated, and this can make a difference to the patient outcome. For example, disease-orientated evidence (DOE) demonstrates that cyclo-oxygenase 2 NSAIDs cause fewer endoscopically detected ulcers than standard NSAIDs. However, many of these ulcers would not be clinically significant. A more relevant evaluation is to determine the difference between cyclo-oxygenase 2 NSAIDs and standard NSAIDs in causing symptomatic or bleeding ulcers. This latter approach is known as 'patient-orientated evidence that matters' (POEM) and is more relevant to clinical practice.

The STEPS acronym is a useful tool for evaluating new drugs.[2]

• **S**afety—evaluate the safety of the new drug versus a standard reference preparation, ideally using comparison studies that reflect the real-life situation. Pharmaceutical companies often highlight differences in ADRs that are relatively trivial or rare. Check especially for ADRs that would place the patient at particular risk, notably the following:
  • liver, kidney, or bone marrow toxicity
  • cardiovascular events
  • CNS events (e.g. fits)
  • significant skin or hypersensitivity reactions (e.g. Stevens–Johnson syndrome)
  • GI bleeding
  • congenital abnormalities.

1 Lexchin J (2004). Are new drugs as good as they claim to be? *Australian Prescriber* **27**: 2–3.
2 Preskorn SH (1994). Antidepressant drug selection: criteria and options. *Journal of Clinical Psychiatry* **55**(suppl A): 6–22, 23–4, 98–100.

Look at the frequency of these events versus the significance of the disease. A 5% risk of hepatotoxicity in a life-threatening disease is a more acceptable level of risk than if the disease is self-limiting.

- **T**olerability—are side effects likely to affect adherence? Look at drop-out rates in clinical trials. If there is a high drop-out rate because of ADRs versus the reference drug, this makes the new drug of less therapeutic value. If patients don't take the drug, it won't work!
- **E**ffectiveness—look at head-to-head trials of the new drug versus the reference drug, rather than comparing different trials. Ask 'Does this new drug work as well or better than the reference drug?'. The NNT is the best way of assessing therapeutic value. If the NNT of the new drug is the same or lower than the reference drug, it is worth considering.
- **P**rice—consider all the costs associated with the new drug versus the reference, not just the purchase price. This might include the following:
  - administration cost (e.g. IV giving sets)
  - monitoring costs
  - additional time/travel if patient has to attend more frequently at the start of therapy
- **S**implicity of use—is it relatively easy for the patient to use the drug? This includes considering the following:
  - dosage schedule
  - number of tablets
  - liquid versus tablets
  - parenteral versus enteral administration
  - special storage requirements (e.g. refrigeration).

WHO criteria for drug selection are listed in Table 14.1.

Table 14.1 WHO criteria for drug selection[1]

- On the WHO essential drug list
- Relevance to pattern of prevalent disease
- Proven efficacy and safety
- Evidence of performance in different settings
- Adequate quality, bioavailability, and safety.
- Favourable cost–benefit ratio, in terms of total treatment cost
- Preference for drugs that are well known or familiar to use and locally manufactured
- Single compounds

[1] World Health Organization (1988). *How to Develop and Implement a National Drug Policy.* (2nd edn). http://whqlibdoc.who.int/publications/924154547X.pdf.

How to write a drug protocol

Drug protocols are evidence-based documents that specify the indications for which a drug treatment can be prescribed within defined clinical settings. They help to ensure that drugs are used cost effectively and safely within the clinical setting.

The need for a drug protocol is usually highlighted for an area by the multidisciplinary team. Initially, the evidence base must be established. Literature searches, protocols from other hospitals or institutions, and information on local practice are used as the basis for the protocol.

Ensure that local practice is followed to implement new drug protocols. This might include approval by a hospital or primary care committee, such as a drugs and therapeutics or formulary committee.

A drug protocol should include the following.
- Drug name—international approved name and trade name.
- Formulation.
- Dose.
- Frequency of administration.
- Administration details.
- Side effects and their treatment.
- Dose reductions required for changes in organ function—e.g. impaired renal or liver function.
- Drug interactions.
- Indications for use.
- Place in therapy—e.g. if another option should be tried first (especially if use is restricted).
- Restrictions of use.
- Cost.
- References.

Stages of protocol development

Identification of need

A new or existing practice is recognized as being cumbersome, unsafe, or otherwise in need of revision. For example, a new use for a drug is developed that requires compounding in a specific way, additional monitoring, and adjunctive medication therapy. It has begun use with these orders written in longhand, but the inconsistency of this practice and increased likelihood of error make clear the need for a pre-written protocol.

Assignment of responsibility

A leader should be identified for the project. Although a group may be responsible for the final form, projects such as this typically require a leader who is responsible for moving the work along.

Gathering evidence and best practice

The leader and group obtain other similar protocols and enquire about their strengths and weaknesses. Other departments that will be affected by the protocol or whose work contributes to the project should be contacted with questions, although they may not need to sit on the committee. Literature searches are made to collect current evidence and best practices. These data should be reviewed and vetted, and the most useful results distributed to those working on the project, if applicable.

Draft compilation

After reviewing the available evidence, the leader or committee drafts a protocol. The protocol should be reviewed and revised by the committee or its writer until no major flaws remain. At times, substantive decisions must be delayed until the protocol can be reviewed by the next committee, or committee members from the next committee may be asked their opinion so that the protocol-drafting group can deliver a better result. After the draft has been rewritten and edited, the protocol is submitted to the appropriate hospital committee. After review by this committee, the protocol should assume a final or near-final form.

Education and roll-out

The completed protocol is often submitted to an education department to gain their expertise in training staff members. The date to begin using the protocol may also be set according to the time it will take for staff to be educated. It is important to remember that implementation of a protocol may need to be delayed after its approval if staff education is required. Staff members should be allowed to have the opportunity to familiarize themselves with a protocol before being expected to act on it.

It is imperative that pharmacists are able to review a protocol during its development. The protocol should be reviewed with great scrutiny because it will be used many times. A protocol containing drugs or focused on drug therapy should be reviewed for the following details.

- Generic and trade names for each drug, with emphasis on the generic name.
- Correct route, dose, and frequency for each medication.
- Frequency of administration.
- Dilution instructions for each drug present.
- All ambiguous statements clarified.
- Contraindications or reasons not to use drugs prominently placed.

Limitations

A protocol may not be made to deal with every eventuality. Rather, a well-designed protocol will succinctly provide a framework for dealing with a particular set of circumstances. Patients will inevitably fall outside these circumstances; thus a protocol should be developed with these limitations in mind so that it does not become inappropriately complex.[1]

1 American Society of Health-System Pharmacists (US). *Best Practices for Hospital and Health System Pharmacy 2011–2012.* ℘ http://store.ashp.org/Default.aspx?TabId=216&ProductId= 22953360

Unlicensed use of medicines

- The product licence of a medication defines the therapeutic purpose for which the product can be used.
- Unlicensed medicines have not been formally assessed through the licensing process for safety, quality, and efficacy. The risks associated with their use might not have been evaluated. Some unlicensed medicines may have been fully evaluated and licensed in another country, but not in the country of use.
- If a prescriber uses a licensed medicine for an unlicensed indication, this is outside its product licence and is sometimes referred to as 'off licence' or 'off label'.
- The same principles apply to unlicensed medicines as to licensed medicines used for unlicensed indications, e.g. in paediatrics (see 📖 'Medicines for children', p.210).
- Medicines that are not covered by a product license include the following.
  - Medicines prepared by a manufacturer but not on sale in this country. A specialist importer with the appropriate importing licenses can obtain these.
  - Medicines prepared for a specified patient in accordance with a prescriber's instructions. This includes any form of extemporaneous dispensing.
  - Unlicensed medicines obtained from a hospital or a commercial supplier with a special manufacturing license. These medicines are often known as 'specials'.
  - Repacked medicines—the product license regulates the container in which a medicine is sold. If a medicine is removed from its original container and repacked, it technically becomes an unlicensed product.
- Implications for the prescriber, pharmacist and nurses of prescribing, dispensing, and administering unlicensed medicines are as follows.
  - Prescribers need to be aware of the license status of medicines they prescribe. The responsibility of prescribing unlicensed medicines lies with the prescriber. The manufacturer takes no responsibility for any safety or efficacy of unlicensed medicines.
  - A pharmacist shares the responsibility with the prescriber, as the product purchaser, or if the pharmacist's actions or omissions have contributed to any harm.
  - Pharmacists should ensure that the prescriber is aware that they are prescribing an unlicensed drug, or a drug outside its license.
  - Nurses are responsible for administering medication that is administered outside of its license and must ensure that the relevant hospital or institution policies have been adhered to.
- A hospital or institution should have a clear written policy for the 'use of unlicensed medicines', outlining the responsibilities of all those involved in the prescribing, purchase, supply, and administration of this category of medicines. It should be a summary document, supported by standard operating procedures and making reference to existing

documents and sources of information. The drugs and therapeutics committee, or equivalent, should approve this.

The use of unlicensed medicines in a hospital or institution needs to be controlled and monitored. A risk assessment should be undertaken before an unlicensed medicine, or medicine outside its license, is prescribed. This is often done through the drugs and therapeutics committee, or equivalent.

- Written notification, signed by the prescriber and returned to the pharmacy department, is usually used. This usually includes the patient details, the name of the product and its specification, the reason for using an unlicensed medicine, and the prescriber's name and signature. The manufacturer, date ordered, quantity ordered, and batch number received are usually recorded in the pharmacy department. Check what documentation is used in your local hospital or institution.
- Some hospitals or institutions require that informed consent is obtained from patients for some unlicensed medicines to be supplied (e.g. thalidomide).
- Prescribing a medicine by a route for which it is not licensed is unlicensed but is often 'accepted practice' (e.g. subcutaneous cyclizine).

Further reading

Department of Health (2003). *A Vision for Pharmacy in the New NHS*. London: Department of Health.

Parkinson R et al. (2004). *Guidance for the Purchase and Supply of Unlicensed Medicinal Products: Notes for Prescribers and Pharmacists* (3rd edn). NHS Pharmaceutical Quality Assurance Committee.

Royal Pharmaceutical Society of Great Britain (2007). *Legal and Ethical Advisory Service Fact Sheet: Five. The Use of Unlicensed Medicines in Pharmacy*. http://www.rpharms.com/archive-documents/factsheet5.pdf

Medicines and Healthcare Products Regulatory Agency (MHRA). (2010) *Review of Unlicensed Medicines*. http://www.mhra.gov.uk/Howweregulate/Medicines/Reviewofunlicensedmedicines/index.htm

NHS Choices (2009). *Why are medicines licensed by the MHRA?* http://www.nhs.uk/chq/Pages/1004.aspx?CategoryID=73&SubCategoryID=101

Drug and therapeutics committees

Each hospital has a drug and therapeutics committee, or an equivalent committee. This committee is responsible for ensuring that the introduction of new drugs to the hospital formulary is cost-effective, safe, and has an acceptable evidence base. Before new drugs are bought by the pharmacy department and used in the hospital, they need to be approved by the drug and therapeutics committee using the principles of EBM. The ↑ cost of new drugs being licensed causes financial pressures on hospitals, which leads to some prioritization of drugs available for use.

Generally, the membership of a drug and therapeutics committee comprises representatives from the following disciplines.
- Medical staff—including medical director, surgeon, anaesthetist, clinical pharmacologist, and paediatrician.
- Nurse (chief nurse or nominee).
- Pharmacist—chief pharmacist and medicines management/formulary pharmacist.
- Finance (director or nominee).
- Commissioner.
- Primary care prescribing lead.
- Specialists—e.g. paediatrics, oncology, or clinical pharmacology.
- Public health.
- Medical microbiologist.
- Patient representative/lay member.
- Management.
- Administration.
- Executive board member (if not one of the disciplines already listed).
- Other members are co-opted, as needed.

The drug and therapeutics committee should have terms of reference and a membership list. There may be subcommittees, to whom decision-making may be devolved for some specialist areas (e.g. antimicrobials), which are responsible to the drug and therapeutics committee. In addition to making decisions on the introduction of new medicines into a hospital according to assessment of the clinical evidence, a drug and therapeutics committee can also have a role in the following areas.
- Maintenance and updating of a hospital formulary.
- Review of medicines expenditure.
- Horizon scanning of medicines to be licensed or those with national approval.
- Prioritization of new drugs.
- Overseeing safe medication practice systems, including maintaining policies and procedures for medicines, overseeing education and training for safe medication practice, and analysing medication error incident reports.

Evidence that is used by drug and therapeutics committees includes the following.
- Results of clinical trials.
- Scientific evidence.
- Cost-effectiveness.
- Safety.
- Effect of adopting a new drug.
- Pre-existing prescribing.
- Decisions of drug and therapeutics committees in other hospitals.
- Restrictions of use of a new drug.

Drug and therapeutics committees should meet regularly (monthly or bimonthly). Decisions made at the committee meetings are made available through minutes, newsletters, e-mail, or intranets.

Further reading

Fullerton DS, Atherly DS (2004). Formularies, therapeutics, and outcomes: new opportunities. *Medical Care* **42**(4 Suppl): III39–44.

Jenkings KN, Barber N (2004). What constitutes evidence in hospital new drug decision making? *Social Science Medicine* **58**:1757–66.

Martin DK *et al.* (2003). Priority setting in a hospital drug formulary: a qualitative case study and evaluation. *Health Policy* **66**: 295–303.

Schumock GT *et al.* (2004). Factors that influence prescribing decisions. *Annals of Pharmacotherapy* **38**: 557–62.

Department of Health. *A Vision for Pharmacy in the New NHS* (2003). London: Department of Health (℘ http://www.dh.gov.uk).

Patient group directions (PGDs)

Definition

- Written instruction for the sale, supply, and/or administration of a named medicine for a defined clinical condition.
- PGDs allow a range of specified healthcare professionals to supply and/or administer medicines, including PODs, directly to a patient with an identified clinical condition, without them necessarily seeing a prescriber. The healthcare professional working within the PGD is responsible for assessing that the patient fits the criteria set out in the PGD.
- Implementing PGDs might be appropriate both in circumstances where groups of patients might not have been previously identified (e.g. minor injuries and first-contact services) and in services where assessment and treatment follow a clearly predictable pattern (e.g. immunization and family planning).
- In general, a PGD is not meant to be a long-term means of managing a patient's clinical condition. This is best achieved by a healthcare professional prescribing for an individual patient on a one-to-one basis.
- Legal requirements and guidance on PGDs are set out in the circular HSC 2000/026.

Health professionals allowed to use PGDs

- Nurses
- Midwives
- Health visitors
- Optometrists
- Pharmacists
- Chiropodists
- Radiographers
- Orthoptists
- Physiotherapists
- Ambulance paramedics.

The pharmacist's role in PGDs

- Apart from developing practice using a PGD, pharmacists are expected to be involved in various aspects of PGDs.
- Development of a PGD for other healthcare professionals.
- Responsibility to ensure that only fully competent, qualified, and trained professionals operate within PGDs.
- Organization of arrangements for the security, storage, and labelling of PGD medicines. Such medicines would normally be expected to be supplied pre-packaged and robust reconciliation system for stock use is established.
- Checking that the use of the medicine outlined in a specific PGD is consistent with the summary of product characteristics, although off-licence use could be considered in exceptional circumstances, provided that it is justified by current best clinical practice.

Further reading

A Practical Guide and Framework of Competencies for All Professionals Using Patient Group Directions. ℘ http://www.npc.nhs.uk/non_medical/resources/patient_group_directions.pdf

National Electronic Library for Medicines. *Patient Group Directions (PGDs).* ℘ http://www.nelm. nhs.uk/en/Communities/NeLM/PGD

Department of Health website (UK) (℘ http://www.dh.gov.uk) has PGDs for drugs and chemical and biological counter-measures.

Supplementary prescribing

Pharmacists in the UK can train to become supplementary and/or independent prescribers. It is mandatory that specific supplementary and/or independent prescribing training is undertaken at a designated university, followed by a period of supervised practice. Supplementary prescribing is detailed here. For independent prescribing see 📖 p.272.

Definition

Supplementary prescribing is a '*voluntary partnership between an independent prescriber (doctor or dentist) and a supplementary prescriber to implement an agreed patient-specific clinical management plan with the patient's agreement*'.

There are some key principles that underpin supplementary prescribing. These principles emphasize the importance of the prescribing partners. The prescribing partners include the independent prescriber, the supplementary prescriber, and the patient.

- The independent prescriber is responsible for the assessment and diagnosis of patients, and deciding on the clinical management required, which includes prescribing.
- The supplementary prescriber is responsible for prescribing for patients who have been clinically assessed by the independent prescriber according to an agreed patient-specific clinical management plan.
- The patient must be treated as a partner in their care and be involved at all stages of decision-making, including the decision for part of their care to be delivered by supplementary prescribing.

The criteria that are set in regulations for lawful supplementary prescribing include the following.

- The independent prescriber must be a doctor (or dentist).
- The supplementary prescriber must be a registered nurse, midwife, pharmacist, or other healthcare professional (e.g. podiatrist, physiotherapist, optometrist).
- The patient must be involved in the decision for a supplementary prescriber to be involved in their care. The patient must be provided with written information, and informed consent must be obtained from the patient before supplementary prescribing starts.
- There must be a written clinical management plan relating to a named patient and to that patient's specific conditions. Both the independent and supplementary prescribers must record agreement to the plan before supplementary prescribing begins.
- The independent and supplementary prescribers must share access to, consult, and use the same common patient record.

There are no legal restrictions on the clinical conditions that supplementary prescribers can treat, and there is no specific formulary or list of medicines for supplementary prescribing. The independent and supplementary prescribers decide when supplementary prescribing is appropriate and when the clinical management plan is drawn up (Fig. 14.1). The medicines to be prescribed by the supplementary prescriber must be prescribed by an independent prescriber at NHS expense and referred to in the patient's clinical management plan. Some of the areas where supplementary prescribing might be of most benefit include the treatment of long-term medical conditions, such as asthma, coronary heart disease, or patients requiring anticoagulation.

Supplementary prescribers are able to prescribe the following
- All general sales list (GSL), pharmacy medicines, appliances and devices, foods, and other borderline substances approved by the advisory committee on borderline substances.
- All POMs.
- Controlled drugs.
- Medicines for use outside their licensed indications (i.e. 'off-label' prescribing), 'black-triangle' drugs, and drugs marked 'less suitable for prescribing' in the *BNF*.
- Unlicensed drugs that are part of a clinical trial which has a clinical trial authorization.

Benefits of supplementary prescribing include the following:
- Quicker access to medicines for patients.
- ↑ efficiency.
- ↓ in doctor's workload.
- Improved use of skill mix.

The supplementary prescriber should not be required to enter into a prescribing partnership that entails them prescribing any medicine that they do not feel competent to prescribe. It is recommended that supplementary prescribers prescribe generically if possible, except where this would not be clinically appropriate or if there is no approved generic name.

Further reading

Department of Health. *Supplementary Prescribing* ℜ http://www.dh.gov.uk/en/Healthcare/
   Medicinespharmacyandindustry/Prescriptions/TheNon-MedicalPrescribingProgramme/
   Supplementaryprescribing/index.htm

Hospital name and department
Clinical management plan

Name of patient:
Patient medication sensitivities/allergies:
Patient identification (e.g. ID number or, date of birth):
Independent prescriber(s): Name and profession
Supplementary prescriber(s): Name and profession

Condition(s) to be treated:

Might be specific indications or broader terms and might also include
treating side effects of specified drugs/classes of drug (e.g. treatment of
HIV and related opportunistic infections/complications or treatment of
side effects of antiretrovirals and other drugs used in treatment of HIV).

Aim of treatment:
Medicines that could be prescribed by supplementary prescriber:
 Preparation
 Drug names and preparations
 Can also be drug classes (e.g. antiretrovirals)
 Indication—does not have to be very specific
 Dose schedule—does not have to be very specific (e.g. could say 'as *BNF*')

Specific indications for referral back to the independent prescriber:

Guidelines or protocols supporting the clinical management plan:

Frequency of review and monitoring by:

 Supplementary prescriber

 Supplementary prescriber and independent prescriber

Process for reporting ADRs:

**Shared record to be used by independent prescriber and supplementary
prescriber:**

Agreed by independent prescriber(s): (signature and name)

Agreed by supplementary prescriber(s): (signature and name)

Date agreed with patient/carer:

Fig. 14.1 Example of a clinical management plan for supplementary prescribers.

Independent prescribing

Pharmacists in the UK can train to become independent prescribers when they are registered pharmacists, have at least 2 years experience practising as a clinical pharmacist, and have completed an independent prescribing education and training programme, which includes a period of supervised practice. Independent prescribing is detailed here. For supplementary prescribing see 📖 p.268.

The Department of Health defines independent prescribing as '*prescribing by a practitioner (e.g. doctor, dentist, nurse, pharmacist) responsible and accountable for the assessment of patients with undiagnosed or diagnosed conditions and for decisions about the clinical management required, including prescribing*'.[1]

The practitioner is required to assess the patient, interpret the assessment, and make a decision on the appropriate therapy including safety and a process for monitoring. Independent prescribing usually takes place as part of a multidisciplinary team using a single healthcare record, and the practitioner is accountable for their prescribing. Patients need to be informed that a non-medical practitioner is prescribing their medicine and give their consent. The pharmacist prescriber must ensure that their prescriptions are checked and dispensed by another pharmacist, in accordance with local clinical governance procedures that are in place for all prescribers.

Pharmacists are able to prescribe any licensed or unlicensed medicine for any medical condition for which they are competent and experienced to prescribe independently. At the time of publication the exceptions to this are that pharmacists are unable to prescribe controlled drugs independently. Pharmacists are able to prescribe licensed medicines for unlicensed indications, i.e. 'off label', independently if it is accepted clinical practice and supported by a local policy. Pharmacist prescribing must be in accordance with the RPSGB's *Medicines, Ethics and Practice—A Guide for Pharmacists*. Pharmacists are required to demonstrate Continuing Professional Development (CPD) in their area of prescribing practice. The RPSGB have published a clinical governance framework for pharmacist prescribers[2] and a Pharmacist Prescriber Pack.[3] Organizations should have a 'non-medical prescribing policy' in place to support pharmacist independent prescribing. Some specialist organizations also have guidance on pharmacist independent prescribing in a specialist area—e.g. the British Oncology Pharmacy Association (BOPA) *Guidance for the Development*

---

1 Department of Health (2006). *Improving Patients' Access to Medicines: A Guide to Implementing Nurse and Pharmacist Independent Prescribing within the NHS in England.* London: Department of Health.
2 Royal Pharmaceutical Society of Great Britain (2007). *Clinical Governance Framework for Pharmacist Precribers and Organisations Commissioning or Participating in Pharmacist Prescribing* (GB wide).
3 Royal Pharmaceutical Society of Great Britain. Pharmacist Prescriber Pack.

of Pharmacist Non-Medical Prescribing and Review of Patients Receiving Anticancer Medicines.[1.]

Benefits

The benefits of pharmacist independent prescribing are to improve patient care without compromising patient safety, make it easier for patients to get the medicines they require, increase patient choice, make better use of healthcare professional skills, and contribute to more flexible team-working in the NHS.

1 Faculty of Cancer Pharmacy and the British Oncology Pharmacy Association (2009). *Guidance for the Development of Pharmacist Non Medical Prescribing and Review of Patients Receiving Anti-cancer Medicines.* ℘ http://www.bopawebsite.org/contentimages/publications/Non_Medical_Prescribing_ Review_Best_Practice_Guidelines_FINAL.pdf

Community (FP10) prescription use in hospitals

Hospital out-patient departments can use community (FP10) prescriptions, according to local policy. In the UK, these are prescriptions that can be written by hospital doctors and dispensed by a community pharmacy, ↓ workload of busy pharmacy departments.

Who is it appropriate to use them for?
- Patients who are mobile and can easily get to a community pharmacy.
- Patients requiring an item that cannot be easily obtained by the hospital pharmacy.
- Patients who don't have time or would rather not wait in the hospital pharmacy.
- Patients on hospital transport who are unable to wait in the hospital pharmacy.

Who is it inappropriate to use them for?
- Patients requiring expensive items, unless they are part of a shared-care arrangement.
- Patients on clinical trials.
- Patients on drugs that are only available from hospitals.
- Patients requiring items that can be purchased without a prescription.
- Patients on complex therapy who may need counselling, but might miss out if they don't attend the hospital pharmacy.

Things to remember
- These prescriptions incur a dispensing fee for each item prescribed.
- Prescriptions are removed from the hospital and dispensed by community pharmacists and, as such, could be vulnerable to loss or tampering.
- The pharmacist who dispenses the prescription might not be familiar with prescribing habits or handwriting.
- It is very difficult for the dispensing pharmacist to contact the doctor in the event of error, omission, or illegible prescribing.
- The hospital is charged the commercial costs, in addition to the dispensing fees for the items prescribed. The resulting cost can be more expensive than if it were dispensed from the hospital pharmacy.
- The hospital is reimbursed for any prescription charge, so for cheaper items, they can be cheaper or issued without charge using an FP10 prescription.
- Drugs supplied are exempt from value added tax (VAT); hence it might be cost-effective to prescribe some drugs on FP10 prescriptions.

Electronic prescribing

Electronic prescribing systems are available commercially and are fully implemented by some hospitals and institutions, often linked to a patient management system. The NHS is aiming for all prescribing in secondary care within the UK to be undertaken electronically.

Some systems ensure a paper-free environment because an electronic prescription is used for patient care, electronic signatures are used for drug administration, and electronic transfer is used for ordering drugs from the pharmacy. Fully implemented electronic systems can mean that all patient records are electronic.

Electronic prescribing systems are often intelligent and flag areas of drug interaction, incorrect dosing, other prescribing errors, additional information required for safe drug administration, and formulary issues. These systems require input and maintenance by pharmacy and information technology teams.

High-risk areas, such as chemotherapy prescribing, should be implemented as a high priority. Most cancer hospitals and networks have implemented or are working towards implementing electronic prescribing systems for oral and injectable chemotherapy to minimize the risks associated with the prescribing and administration of these drugs for adult and paediatric patients.

Pharmacy staff using an electronic prescribing system require training in its use before working with the system. These systems have various levels of security, depending on the role of the professional in the use of the system. It is essential that there is good security for any electronic prescribing system, with frequent back-ups, and a system must be in place in case of system failure. Standard operating procedures should be in place for all aspects of the system.

Benefits

- Safer use of medicines.
- ↓ in medication errors.
- Improved quality and safety of prescribing.
- Improved safety of prescribing medication to patients with drug allergies.
- Prescriptions are legible.
- Accessibility of information between primary and secondary care.
- Improved patient compliance with protocols.
- Management of formulary compliance.
- Supports decision-making when prescribing.
- Implementation of policy decisions.
- Improved use of staff time.
- Pharmacy can make early identification of new scripts for screening and supply.
- Audit trail of transactions.
- Drug-usage reports for individual patients.
- Aids clinical audit.

Further reading

Smith J (2004). *Building a Safer NHS for Patients: Improving Medication Safety*. London: Department of Health.

Donyai P et al. (2008). The effects of electronic prescribing on the quality of prescribing. *British Journal of Clinical Pharmacology* **65**: 230–7.

Incident reporting

- Each hospital or institution should have a policy in place for reporting incidents. An incident reporting policy often covers all incidents, including adverse events, hazards, and near misses of an adverse event or hazard. Such a policy applies to all hospital staff. An induction programme to a hospital usually covers details of any local policy.
- An incident reporting program identifies, assesses, and manages risks that could compromise or threaten the quality of patient services or staff working in a safe environment, as part of the overall management of risk. It is a confidential process, and all staff should complete the appropriate documentation if they are involved in, or aware of, an incident.
- An 'incident' is usually defined as an event or circumstance that could have, or did, lead to unintended or unexpected harm, loss, or damage. Incidents might involve actual or potential injury, damage, loss, fire, theft, violence, abuse, accidents, ill health, and infection.
- It is necessary for incidents to be reported to ensure that the hospital can analyse the data for trends, causes, and costs. Action plans can then be developed to minimize future similar incidents. Reporting of incidents is also a mechanism for staff to have input into change of practice and procedures. Incident reporting follows a 'no-blame' culture.
- Medication incidents must be reported through this mechanism to ensure that there can be a review of trends, a root-cause analysis, arrangements for improvement, and a follow-up audit. This is a requirement of medicines management in hospitals.
- The types of incident that a pharmacist can report include medication errors and failure of systems or processes that affect patient care.
- In addition to reporting an incident, a pharmacist must also deal with an incident by communicating with the relevant members of staff involved (see 📖 p.72).

Further reading

Department of Health (2003). *A Vision for Pharmacy in the new NHS*. London: Department of Health.

National Patient Safety Agency. *National Reporting and Learning Service*. ℘ http://www.nrls.npsa.nhs.uk

Medical representatives

- Medical representatives provide information to healthcare practitioners, but their prime function is to promote and sell their products and services.
- Medical representatives should provide their services according to the Association of the British Pharmaceutical Industry (ABPI) code of practice (or similar). If the code of practice is breached, medical representatives can be reported to the director of the Prescription Medicines Code of Practice Authority (PMCPA).
- Most hospitals have a policy for dealing with medical representatives—check the local policy.
- Some hospitals do not allow medical representatives to leave samples. Check the policy for the local hospital before accepting trial samples from medical representatives.
- It is GCP for medical representatives to make an appointment before meeting with a member of staff. Some hospital policies restrict the grades of staff that are allowed to meet with medical representatives.
- Medical representatives are not allowed to promote unlicensed indications for their products or products that have not yet been licensed. However, they are allowed to answer specific questions on unlicensed use (see 📖 p.262).
- Hospital drug prices are confidential to the hospital and under no circumstance must they be revealed to a medical representative.
- Most hospitals limit the level of hospitality provided by representatives. For example, it is reasonable for representatives to provide food for a working lunch, but not expensive meals at a restaurant.

Further reading

Guidance Notes for Health Professionals, Understanding the ABPI Code of Practice for the Pharmaceutical Industry and Controls on the Promotion of Prescription Medicines in the UK.
🔗 http://www.abpi.org.uk

Overseas visitors

- The term 'overseas visitor' is used for patients who have fallen ill unexpectedly while visiting the UK and who, consequently, require standard NHS emergency care.
- People who do not normally live in the UK are not automatically entitled to use the NHS free of charge.
- Patients who are eligible for full NHS treatment include the following.
  - Anyone legally living in the UK for ≥12 months.
  - Permanent residents.
  - Students in the UK for >6 months.
  - Refugees or asylum seekers who have made an application to remain in the UK and are waiting for a decision on their immigration status.
  - People detained by the immigration authorities.
  - People from countries with a reciprocal agreement—e.g. European Union residents.
- Patients who are not eligible for full NHS treatment include the following.
  - Students on courses in the UK for <6 months.
  - Refugees or asylum seekers who have not yet submitted applications to the Home Office.
  - Those who have had an asylum application turned down and exhausted the appeals process.
  - Illegal immigrants.
- The NHS hospital is legally responsible for establishing whether patients are not normally resident in the UK.
- If patients are not eligible for free NHS care, the hospital must charge the patient for the costs of the NHS care.
- When the patient is charged depends on the urgency of the treatment needed.
  - For immediately necessary treatment, treatment must not be delayed or withheld while the patient's chargeable status is being established.
  - For urgent and non-urgent treatment, patients should pay a deposit equivalent to the estimated full cost of treatment in advance.
  - Any surplus can be returned to the patient on completion of the treatment.
- Treatment that is available to overseas patients free of charge is as follows.
  - A&E visits. However, treatment in other departments following an A&E visit (e.g. X-ray) is charged.
  - Emergency or immediately necessary treatment.
  - Treatment of sexually transmitted diseases (except HIV).
  - Treatment of diseases that are a threat to public health (e.g. tuberculosis (TB)) and acute treatment of all infectious diseases.
  - Family planning.
  - Compulsory psychiatric treatment.
- If an overseas visitor chooses to be treated privately, they are classed as an 'international private patient'. These patients are treated as private patients (see p.282).

Further reading

Department of Health (2007). *Implementing the Overseas Visitors Hospital Charging Regulations.* London: Department of Health.

Department of Health. *Overseas Visitors.* ℘ http://www.dh.gov.uk/en/Publicationsandstatistics/ Publications/PublicationsPolicyAndGuidance/DH_4080313

Department of Health (2010) *Overseas Visitors.* ℘ http://www.dh.gov.uk/en/Healthcare/ Entitlementsandcharges/OverseasVisitors/index.htm

Pollard AJ, Savulescu J (2004). Eligibility of overseas visitors and people of uncertain residential status for NHS treatment. *British Medical Journal* **329**: 346–9.

Private patients

In the UK, patients can choose to have treatment either from the NHS or privately. Private patients usually have private health insurance, which covers some, or all, of the costs of private treatment. Patients can be treated privately either in a private hospital or in NHS hospitals. Private patients treated in NHS hospitals are discussed in this section.

- NHS hospitals either have specific wards for private patients or private patients are treated on the same ward as NHS patients, often in a side room.
- Patients who are treated privately either have private health insurance or are paying themselves.
- Before the patient receives treatment, the private health insurance company must confirm what they will cover, according to the patient's insurance policy.
- Patients' drugs must be charged accurately to the private health insurance companies to ensure that the NHS generates income from using NHS facilities to treat these patients.
- If a patient is having private treatment, this should be annotated in some way on the patient notes or identification labels.
- Any prescription for a private patient must be annotated as 'private patient' to ensure that the pharmacy department can charge appropriately for the drugs.
- Private patients do not have to pay NHS prescriptions charges.
- Charging and systems can vary for in-patients and out-patients.
- An on-cost is usually added to the drug price when charging for private patients' drugs.
- Clinical pharmacists' input into patient care for drug review and counselling might be appropriate.
- Check what systems are in place for private patients' drugs in your hospital.
- Patients can choose to change from being a private patient to an NHS patient between consultations.

In 2009, the Department of Health issued guidance for patients to enable them to remain NHS patients, but to pay for additional private care, such as drugs, not available in or funded by the NHS.[1] The NHS continues to provide the care the patient is entitled to in the NHS, and the private care has to be delivered separately from the NHS care. Hospitals should have specific policies in place for patients requesting additional private care in accordance with this guidance.

---

1 Department of Health (2009) *Guidance on NHS patients who wish to pay for additional private care.* ॐ http://www.dh.gov.uk/en/Publicationsandstatistics/Publications/PublicationsPolicyAndGuidance/DH_096428

Professional supervision skills

- Start with goals or an action plan for the member of staff you are supervising.
  - These should be SMART—i.e. **S**pecific, **M**easurable, **A**chievable, **R**elevant,and **T**imescale.
  - Effective goals have five parts:
    — intentions
    — outcomes
    — methods and resources
    — midpoints and deadlines
    — action plans.
- Prioritize the workload with your staff.
- Set timelines.
- Time management—ensure that time is managed effectively.
- Listen effectively to your member of staff.
- Review and monitor action plans and progress at regular intervals.
- Support and coach, as necessary.
- Be available to discuss ways forward with the member of staff.
- Communicate the 'bigger picture', so that staff understand why tasks are being undertaken.
- Be honest.

Tips on day-to-day supervision

- Some of the professional supervision skills should be used on a daily basis to help with day-to-day supervision.
- Be aware of the workload to be covered that day and the staff available to undertake the work.
- If necessary, prioritize the day's work with the staff.
- Be available to trouble-shoot.
- Support the staff with the urgent and important work, if necessary.

National Service Frameworks (NSFs)

NSFs are national standards for specified clinical areas to ensure equality of NHS services throughout the UK. NSFs were developed by the Department of Health, with the help of external reference groups. These groups are made up of health professionals, service users and carers, health service managers, partner agencies, and other advocates. Usually, one new framework is developed each year.

National Service Frameworks:
• establish national standards and promote specific service models
• identify key interventions for a defined service or care group
• put in place strategies to support implementation
• establish ways to ensure progress within an agreed timescale
• are a measure to ↑ quality and ↓ variations in service within the NHS
• drive the delivery of the NHS modernization agenda.

Some examples of NSFs developed to date include the following:
• coronary heart disease
• cancer
• paediatric intensive care
• mental health
• older people
• diabetes
• long-term conditions (e.g. neurological)
• renal services
• children.

Opportunities for pharmacy

Some NSFs specifically mention pharmacy or medicine-related issues.
• Become familiar with the framework standards, and consider how to contribute to the achievement of the standards.
• A pharmacist should be involved with the local implementation team responsible for the development and delivery of a service plan and identifying what has to be done to implement the NSF.
• Decide on the services that can be initiated and the relevant links to the NSF standards.
• Identify links to the local delivery plan and other local priorities.
• Participate with an existing or developing service where possible.
• Identify the opportunities for pharmacy.
• Consult with other stakeholders who can influence the development of a proposed service.
• Identify training needs to provide a new service.
• Identify the outcomes proposed—are they realistic and measurable?
• Develop a business case which refers to the NSF, local priorities, and needs, and includes integration into local services.

Further reading

Stanley J (2004). Benchmarking the role of pharmacists in implementing NSFs. *Pharmacy Management* **20**: 2–5.

Appraisal

An appraisal meeting provides a formal opportunity for managers and staff to meet and discuss job performance, achievements against objectives previously set, future work objectives and priorities, career aspirations, and training and development needs. This process should ensure that staff are clear about what they are trying to achieve and why, and managers are clear on the progress being made by everyone in their department.

Definitions

- **Appraisal** is a dynamic ongoing process of performance management through objectives and staff development.
- **Performance management** is a system to align the work of individuals as closely as possible to the work of the organization.

The appraisal process

- Appraisal supports effective performance and personal development.
- Appraisals should take place annually, according to the local hospital policy.
- The line manager usually conducts the appraisal.
- Both the appraiser and the appraisee should prepare for the annual appraisal meeting. It is good practice to have at least 2wks notice to enable an individual to have time to prepare.
- In preparation for the annual appraisal, the appraisee should list their strengths and weaknesses, achievements, and performance highs and lows for the previous 12 months. There may be specific appraisal paperwork that needs completing by both the appraiser and the appraisee prior to the appraisal, according to local policy.
- The annual appraisal should be conducted to ensure an open two-way discussion, and usually lasts for ~2h.
- During the appraisal, the following areas are usually covered.
  - Introduction and purpose of an appraisal.
  - Review of the objectives set at the last appraisal, a discussion of which ones are met, and resolving difficulties with those that have not been met.
  - Review of an individual's work over the past year.
  - Outline and agree future objectives.
  - Review of individuals current knowledge and skills.
  - Prioritization of areas requiring development to improve effectiveness at work.
  - Agree a personal development plan for the next year.
  - Discussion of how an individual's objectives fit within the team and organization's objectives.
  - Discussion on how the organization/line manager can help the appraisee achieve their objectives.
  - Constructive feedback on performance.
  - Recognition of an individual's performance.
  - Discussion of any of the appraisee's concerns.
  - Review of job description and plans to update it accordingly.

- A paper record of the appraisal, which is signed by the appraisee and the appraiser, should be kept.

Review of performance should be continuous, and any concerns should be raised throughout the year and not left to the annual appraisal.

Further reading

Naisby A (ed) (2002). *Appraisal and Performance Management*. London: Spiro Press.
Chartered Institute of Personnel and Development (2010). *Performance Appraisal*. ℘ http://www.cipd.co.uk/subjects/perfmangmt/appfdbck/perfapp.htm

Confidentiality

Pharmacists and pharmacy staff are expected to maintain the confidentiality of any patient or customer they have contact with during the course of their professional duties. Information that should remain confidential includes the following:

- patient's identity and address
- diagnosis
- details of prescribed and non-prescribed medicines.

Pharmacists must also ensure that any written or electronic patient information is stored and disposed of securely and that electronic systems are password protected.

To avoid unintentional disclosure, it is important to develop good habits when dealing with patient information.

- Discussing a patient with colleagues is often necessary for patient care or training purposes, but be cautious about revealing names or other patient identifiers.
- Do not discuss patients in public areas—e.g. the lifts or the front of the shop.
- If talking about your work to family or friends, only talk about patients in very general terms.
- Ensure that written information (e.g. patient handover lists and prescriptions) is not left lying where other patients or the public can see it.
- If discussing medication with a patient, try to do this in a reasonably private area. If hospital in-patients have visitors, ask if the patient would like you to return when they have gone.
- Ensure that computers have passwords and always log off at the end of a session.

Disclosure of information

In certain situations, pharmacists might have to disclose confidential information. The UK pharmacy code of ethics allows this in the following circumstances.

- With patient consent or parent/guardian/carer consent for a child or adult not competent to give consent themselves. Information about adolescent patients should not normally be revealed without their consent.
- If required by law or statute.
- If necessary to prevent serious injury or damage to the health of the patient, a third party or the public health.

The RPSGB has published a fact sheet on confidentiality, which includes guidance on disclosure of information.[1] In addition, advice on disclosure of information if necessary to protect children and vulnerable adults can be found on the *Pharmaceutical Journal* website.[2]

Confidentiality when a friend, relative, or colleague is a patient

Pharmacists and pharmacy staff can be put in a difficult position in this situation, especially if others know that the patient is in their care. Well-meaning questions about the patient's welfare might be difficult to deal with without causing offence.

- Explain to the patient what level of involvement you have in their care and that you would have access to their medical notes. Ask whether they would prefer that another pharmacist deals with their care (although this might not always be feasible).
- If at all possible, discuss the situation with the patient and ask them what information they are willing for you to reveal to other friends, family, or colleagues.
- If the patient is unwilling for you to reveal any information, or if you are unable to discuss this with the patient, any enquiries should be dealt with by politely explaining that you cannot provide information about the patient. Bear in mind, however, that simply making this statement potentially discloses the fact that the individual is known to you as a patient.
- Try to avoid compromising your integrity by denying all knowledge of the patient, but in some situations this might be necessary.
- Inform the medical team that the patient is known to you socially.
- Personal information known to you because of your relationship to the patient should not be revealed to medical or nursing colleagues without the patient's consent.
- The patient might use your relationship to ask you to provide medical information that you would not normally reveal. Provide only the same information as you would to any other patient.
- If a colleague is a patient, be especially sensitive to any aspect of care that could breach confidentiality. As appropriate, you might need to consider the following.
  - Avoid writing your colleague's name on ward order sheets.
  - Use an agreed alias for labelling of medicines.
  - Label, dispense, and deliver medicines yourself.
  - Keep any written records separate from those to which other pharmacy staff have access.

1 RPSGB. http://www.rpsgb.org/pdfs/factsheet12.pdf
2 http://www.pjonline.com/libres/pdf/society/pj_20050806_childprotectionguidance.pdf

Gene therapy

The development of genetically modified viruses and advances in cloning and sequencing the human genome have offered the opportunity to treat a wide variety of diseases using 'gene therapy'. The term 'gene therapy' applies to any clinical therapeutic procedure in which genes are intentionally introduced into human cells. Gene therapy clinical trials have been undertaken in cystic fibrosis, cancer, cardiac disease, HIV, and inherited genetic disorders. Preparation of gene therapy products is a pharmaceutical preparation process that should be carried out under the control of a pharmacist in suitable facilities to minimize the risk of microbiological contamination and medication errors.

Gene therapy can be divided into two main categories: gene replacement and gene addition. Gene replacement tends to be used for monogenic diseases, in which a single 'faulty' gene can be replaced with a normal gene. For example, an abnormal cystic fibrosis transmembrane conductance regulator (CFTR) gene can be replaced in cystic fibrosis. Currently, the majority of gene therapy clinical trials use a gene- addition strategy for cancer, whereby a gene or genes can be 'added' to a cell to provide a new function, e.g. addition of tumour suppressor genes to cancer cells.

For gene therapy to be successful, a therapeutic gene must be delivered to the nucleus of a target cell, where it can be expressed as a therapeutic protein. Genes are delivered to target cells by vectors in a process called 'gene transfer'. The greatest challenge to gene therapy is finding a vector that can transfer therapeutic genes to target cells specifically and efficiently. Gene transfer vectors can be broadly divided into non-viral and viral systems. Non-viral vectors, such as liposomes, have limited efficiency. Genetically modified viruses have proved to be the most efficient way of delivering DNA. Viruses are merely genetic information protected by a protein coat. They have a unique ability to enter (infect) a cell, delivering viral genes to the nucleus using the host cell machinery to express those viral genes. A variety of viruses have been used as vectors, including retroviruses, herpes viruses, and adenoviruses. Many viral vectors have been genetically modified so that they cannot form new viral particles and so are termed 'replication-deficient' or 'replication-defective'. Replication-deficient viruses have had the viral genes required for replication and the pathogenic host response removed. This prevents the virus replicating and the potential for the therapeutic virus to reverse back to a pathogenic virus. The deleted genes are replaced by a therapeutic gene, thus allowing the delivery and expression of the therapeutic gene without subsequent spread of the virus to surrounding cells. Future gene therapy vectors will be able to replicate under genetically specified conditions.

There are potential infectious hazards with gene therapy, including possible transmission of the vector to hospital personnel. Therefore gene therapy products should be manipulated in pharmacy aseptic units, because of the uncertain effects of specific genes on normal human cells, potential for operator sensitization on repeated exposure, and the potentially infective nature of some products. Consideration has to be given to protecting both the product and the staff handling these agents. Some gene therapy agents might require handling in negative-pressure isolators in separate specific aseptic facilities.

A risk assessment should be made for each product, with input from the lead investigator or trust biological safety officer, because they should have a good understanding of molecular biology and virology.

Further reading

Stoner N (2009). Gene therapy applications. *Clinical Pharmacist* **1**: 270–4.

Watson M, Stoner N (2007). Safe handling of gene medicines. *European Journal of Hospital Pharmacy Practice* **13**: 24–6.

Vulto AG et al. (2007). European Association of Hospital Pharmacists (EAHP) guidance on the pharmacy handling of gene medicines. *European Journal of Hospital Pharmacy Practice* **13**: 29–39.

Stoner NS et al. (2006). Appendix 6—Gene therapy. In Beaney AM *Quality Assurance of Aseptic Preparation Services* (4th edn). London: Pharmaceutical Press.

Brooks G (ed) (2002). *Gene Therapy: The Use of DNA as a Drug*. London: Pharmaceutical Press.

Gene therapy advisory committee (GTAC). ℘ http://www.dh.gov.uk/ab/GTAC/index.htm?ssSourceSiteId=en

UK Health and Safety Executive (2000). *A Guide to the Genetically Modified Organisms (Contained Use) Regulations*. London: HSE Books.

Searle PF et al. (2002). Cancer gene therapy: from science to clinical trials. *Drug Delivery Systems and Sciences* **2**: 5–13.

Simpson J, Stoner NS (2003). Implications of gene therapy to pharmacists. *Pharmaceutical Journal* **271**: 127–30.

Stoner NS et al. (2003). Health and safety considerations for the administration of gene therapy within the clinical setting. *Journal of Oncology Pharmacy Practice* **9**: 29–35.

Pharmacogenetics

Pharmacogenetics is defined as the study of human genetic variation, which causes different responses to drugs. The differences in response can be both in the therapeutic effect and in ADRs.

For example, genetic make-up may determine variations in liver enzymes that are produced, which in turn affect drug metabolizm. One of the cytochrome P450 liver enzymes, CYP2D6, metabolizes drugs (e.g. β-blockers, antidepressants, and opioids) in the liver so that they can be eliminated. The level of this enzyme in the liver is genetically determined. Patients are classified as 'slow metabolizers' if they have low levels of CYP2D6 in the liver, which means that the drug is eliminated from the body more slowly, resulting in additional toxicity. 'Fast metabolizers' have a high level of CYP2D6 in the liver and therefore metabolize the drug more quickly, resulting in a possible reduced therapeutic effect. In practice, 'slow metabolizers' may require a lower dose of drug than 'fast metabolizers' for the same effect. An example of a drug metabolized through this mechanism is warfarin: 40% of the variability in warfarin levels is accounted for by the CYP2C9 enzyme.

Another example of genetic influence on drug response is via receptors. If drugs bind to specific receptors to generate a response and the number of receptors present is genetically determined, the response to the drug will vary according to the patient's genetics. This has enabled drug development to be much more targeted, so that only patients with specific characteristics receive the appropriate drugs. For example, breast cancer patients who have the HER2 receptor present on their breast cancer cells will be the only group of breast cancer patients who respond to trastuzumab. This highlights that in cancer patients, the presence or absence of some genes will determine the patient's response to some anti-cancer drugs.

Genetic testing of individuals is usually done from a saliva or blood sample. There will be issues regarding the quality of the tests, their initiation, communication to the patient, and the implication of the test to treatment. The general public would need to be more widely educated about pharmacogenetics and its implications. Tests would need to be rigorously evaluated. Currently there are some home test kits available, but the sale of these is not regulated. This means that some of the test kits available have no guarantee of being validated or of producing accurate results.

There are ethical issues that need to be considered in genotyping individuals. (The genotype is the genetic make-up of a cell or individual. Genotyping is the process of determining an individual's genotype using biological assays to find out the genetic make-up of an individual.) This could lead to discrimination of individuals who carry specific genes and affect the allocation of resources. For example, there is concern that some individuals may not be able to obtain insurance policies if their genetic test results are considered negatively. There is also concern about the privacy and confidentiality of genetic information, where it should be stored, and who would have access to it. Drug companies may only research drugs for diseases that are straightforward to treat, rather than those that could be used for rarer diseases. In addition, pharmacogenetic testing may predict for future risks of disease or raise implications for other family members, which adds to the ethical issues of informing patients and their families.

Pharmacogenetics will enable more cost-effective and targeted prescribing that will optimize the use of drugs, avoiding the prescribing of drugs that will be ineffective, and reduce the medical and financial impact of adverse drug reactions. This means that in the future patients will be prescribed drugs specific to their conditions, taking into account genetic factors when deciding on dosage regimens. However, targeted drugs may be more expensive. In addition, there may be a loss of any benefit of, for example, racemic mixtures.

Standards of business conduct for clinical pharmacists

Declaration of interests has become an integral part of professional life, and pharmacists are not exempt from showing that they are independent and unbiased. In addition, clinical pharmacists have access to valuable confidential data and can influence purchasing decisions that can have a major effect on a particular company's products. Therefore it is important that pharmacists are aware of relevant guidelines. In the UK, Department of Health guidelines have been produced on these issues and it is prudent to have a local policy designed using this or similar guidance.

The Department of Health guidelines cover the standards of conduct expected of all NHS staff, where their private interests could conflict with their public duties, and the steps that NHS employers should take to safeguard themselves and the NHS against conflict of interest.

Details can be found in the Code of Conduct for NHS Managers 2002; which is available on the Department of Health website.[1] Some key relevant issues are as follows.

- Avoid conflict of interest between private and NHS interests. It is a well-established principle that public sector bodies, which include the NHS, must be impartial and honest in the conduct of their business, and that their employees should remain above suspicion.
- NHS staff are expected to ensure that the interest of patients is paramount at all times, to be impartial and honest in the conduct of their official business, and to use the public funds entrusted to them to the best advantage of the service, always ensuring value for money.
- It is also the responsibility of staff to ensure that they do not abuse their official position for personal gain or to benefit their family or friends.
- Modest hospitality, provided that it is normal and reasonable in the circumstances (e.g. lunches in the course of working visits), are acceptable, although it should be similar to the scale of hospitality that the NHS, as an employer, would probably offer. Anything else should be declined.
- Casual gifts can be offered by contractors or others (e.g. at Christmas time). Such gifts should nevertheless be politely, but firmly, declined. Articles of low intrinsic value, such as diaries or calendars, or small tokens of gratitude from patients or their relatives, need not necessarily be refused.
- NHS employers need to be aware of all cases in which an employee or their close relative or associate has a significant financial interest in a business.

- Individual staff must not seek or accept preferential rates or benefits in kind for private transactions carried out with companies with which they have had, or might have had, official dealings on behalf of their NHS employer.
- All staff who are in contact with suppliers and contractors, in particular those who are authorized to sign purchase orders or place contracts for goods, are expected to adhere to professional standards of the kind set out in the ethical code of the Institute of Purchasing and Supply (IPS).[1]
- Fair and open competition between prospective contractors or suppliers for NHS contracts is a requirement of NHS standing orders and of EC directives on public purchasing for works and supplies.
- NHS employers should ensure that no special favour is shown to current or former employees in awarding contracts to private or other businesses run by them.
- NHS employees are advised not to engage in outside employment that could conflict with their NHS work or be detrimental to it.
- Acceptance by staff of commercial sponsorship for attendance at relevant conferences and courses is acceptable, but only if the employee seeks permission in advance and the employer is satisfied that acceptance will not compromise purchasing decisions in any way.
- Pharmaceutical companies, for example, might offer to sponsor, wholly or partially, a post for an employing authority. NHS employers should not enter into such arrangements, unless it has been made abundantly clear to the company concerned that the sponsorship will have no effect on purchasing decisions within the authority.
- Staff should be particularly careful of using, or making public, internal information of a 'commercial in confidence' nature, if its use would prejudice the principle of a purchasing system based on fair competition.
- Finally, many employers maintain a record of interests and pharmacists should cooperate with such practices.

---

1 Chartered Institute of Purchasing & Supply. ⅏ http://www.cips.org

Waste management of medicines

Pharmaceutical waste refers to the disposal of unwanted medicines, out-of-date or obsolete stock, sharps, and waste arising from diagnostic testing. The current regulations are detailed in the Hazardous Waste Regulations 2005, and further guidance specifically for community pharmacies are detailed in the Department of Health document *Environment and Sustainability Health Technical Memorandum 07-06: Disposal of Pharmaceutical Waste in Community Pharmacies*.

The legislation relevant to pharmaceutical waste derives mainly from European directives. The storage, carriage, processing, and supply of waste are all subject to stringent controls designed to minimize the negative effects of waste on the environment.

The Environment Agency or the relevant local authority is the enforcement authority for the legislation. Depending on the circumstances, and in cases of doubt, either can be contacted for advice. The Environment Agency helpline number is 08708-506-506.

Policies

Your hospital or community pharmacy must have a waste management policy that details general themes, including dealing with pharmaceutical waste such as cytotoxics. Key requirements that need specification in your policy are as follows.

- Detail how returned controlled drugs should be denatured and recorded—see Royal Pharmaceutical Society (RPS) on the denaturing of controlled drugs.
- Include a list of hazardous medicines that may be encountered in the pharmacy.
- Include instructions to staff on dealing with products other than medicines that are handed in to the pharmacy.
- Include instructions on identifying incompatible products such as flammable products and oxidizing agents.
- Include the protective measures to be adopted by staff when segregating controlled drugs and incompatible products.
- Include reference to monitored dosage system trays and the disposal of blister packs.
- Set out the retention and audit requirements for transfer notes, consignment notes, and quarterly returns.

The guidance also details the types of containers that need to be used for segregation and transportation of the different types of waste. For example:

- a purple-lidded sharps bin should be used for medicines or sharps contaminated with cytotoxic or cytostatic medicines
- a yellow-lidded sharps bin should be used for all other medicines or sharps contaminated with non-hazardous medicines
- other sharps (e.g. fully discharged syringes) may be disposed of in an orange-lidded sharps bin.

When completing any documentation needed for the transfer and transportation of waste from the pharmacy, pharmacies are advised to ensure that all waste coding and descriptions are robust and accurate, particularly with regard to the presence of medicinal waste and medicinally contaminated sharps.

Waste generated

The waste generated is likely to consist of the following.

Community pharmacy

- Pharmaceutical products returned from individuals and households as part of the essential services (i.e. the disposal of unwanted medicines—a service provided by all pharmacies).
- Out-of-date or obsolete stock.
- Needles and syringes.
- Waste arising from diagnostic testing such as blood glucose and cholesterol monitoring.

Hospital pharmacy

- Unwanted items from ward/department, including controlled drugs, PODs, fridge items, and hazardous, harmful, or toxic pharmaceuticals, require processing as many items can be recycled if storage conditions have been complied with.
- Otherwise waste will contain out-of-date dispensary stock, items that are not economically viable to recycle, and PODs that may have been returned to pharmacy for a variety of reasons.

Medicines brought into hospital by patients

Medicines brought into hospital by the patient are the property of the patient and should only be sent to pharmacy for destruction with the prior agreement from the patient or their agent. It is GCP to record the details of PODs sent to the pharmacy for destruction.

Carriage of waste and community pharmacy

Ensure that a carrier's licence is held if the pharmacy carries waste medicines from a patient's home or residential home to the pharmacy.

Handling waste within the pharmacy

The Hazardous Waste Regulations 2005 introduced significant changes for pharmacies. They required pharmacies to separate hazardous waste medicines from non-hazardous waste, if this is economically viable.

Staff safety is paramount. Handling of waste should be minimal and carried out with great care. Acceptance of waste other than medicines returned from households should not be undertaken.

It is not absolutely necessary for pharmacies to separate hazardous waste medicines from non-hazardous waste medicines before they are sent to a suitably authorized waste contractor for incineration. However, whenever waste that may contain some hazardous waste medicine is sent for incineration, it is required to be consigned as though it were hazardous and needs to be accompanied by a hazardous waste consignment note.
▶ Under the Hazardous Waste Directives, only cytotoxic or cytostatic medicines are classified as hazardous waste.

As an aid to pharmacists, a suitable starting point for identifying hazardous medicines is to adopt the list of hazardous drugs provide by the National Institute for Occupational Safety and Health (NIOSH).

Liquid medicines

Liquids should generally not be decanted and mixed. Where liquid medicines are being discarded, they should be retained within their individual containers and placed in the waste bins provided for the purpose.

If the waste contractor has provided a waste bin specially designed for liquids and suggests that the liquid medicines can be emptied from containers and mixed in the waste bin, the pharmacist has a duty of care to ensure that only compatible products are mixed

Empty medicine containers that have held liquids must be disposed of as waste medicines for incineration as it is not possible to ensure that the contents have been completely removed (containers cannot be rinsed into the sewerage system). If residues of liquid controlled drugs are present, these should be emptied, as far as possible, and denatured before the container is placed in the waste container.

If segregation is not being undertaken, purple-lidded burn bins should be used for all pharmaceutical waste, including cytotoxic agents and antibiotic products.

Transfer of waste to a waste carrier

A consignment note is required to list the hazardous medicines that are being consigned so that they can be handled safely and disposed of appropriately (no list of individual non-hazardous medicines is required). Refer to *Health Technical Memorandum 07-06* for details of completing required documentation.

Radioactive waste

Radioactive waste is governed by the Environmental Agency, which issues organizations with certificates of authorization that regulate the routes of disposal, limits of disposal, and type of radioactive material disposed of.

Disposal and destruction of controlled drugs

A controlled drug ceases to be classified as a controlled drug after it has been rendered irretrievable, i.e. all controlled drugs that are disposed of should be unrecognizable as controlled drugs (Misuse of Drugs Act 1971).

Hospital only—controlled drugs must be returned to pharmacy

All controlled drugs (e.g. expired stocks, PODs, and excess stock) must be notified to the pharmacist responsible for the ward/unit/ department. These controlled drugs must not be destroyed on the ward.[1]

The pharmacist must return the controlled drugs to the pharmacy to either the pharmacy controlled drug record book for destruction (in the case of expired stock or PODs) or the pharmacy controlled drug record book (in the case of excess stock of controlled drugs, which can be entered back into pharmacy stock).

---

1 Royal Pharmaceutical Society of Great Britain (2005). *The Safe and Secure Handling of Medicines: A Team Approach.* ⅗ http://www.rpharms.com/support-pdfs/safsechandmeds.pdf

Departments who do not receive a pharmacy visiting service must either arrange for a pharmacist to come to the ward or agree a mutually convenient time for the nurse to take their controlled drugs and the controlled drug record book to the pharmacy, where a pharmacist will sign for their return.

Records of CD destruction

In both cases outlined, an entry must be made in the ward controlled drug record book or the patient's own controlled drugs record book on the appropriate page for the drug in question, specifying 'destruction' or 'return to pharmacy', the quantity involved, the new stock balance and the signatures of the two persons involved.

Prefilled PCA/PCEA/epidural syringes and opiate infusions

Part contents of opiate infusions/PCA/PCEA/epidural syringes that were initially set up and issued in theatres but are no longer needed must be destroyed on the ward where the patient resides.

Opiate infusions/PCA/PCEA/epidural syringes containing residual unused injections must be emptied into an in-use sharps bin, in addition to the empty syringe. Empty bags can be disposed of in a clinical waste bag according to procedure for disposing of empty infusion bags. This must be witnessed by a second person. One of the two witnesses should be the nurse looking after the patient.

Responsible pharmacist

The responsible pharmacist

The responsible pharmacist regulations came into effect on 1 October 2009. Prior to this date, in order to conduct a retail pharmacy business lawfully the Medicines Act 1968 specified that there had to be a pharmacist in 'personal control'. 'Personal control' meant that the pharmacist needed to be physically present in the pharmacy. Furthermore, sales of prescription and prescription-only medicines had to be under the supervision of a pharmacist. However, the Medicines Act did not define 'supervision', although it was interpreted as needing a pharmacist to be able to 'intervene and advise'.

It was recognized that, to improve the range of services available in pharmacies, pharmacists must be able to work more flexibly and be allowed to undertake their role out of the pharmacy for a limited period to make better use of their clinical training and the skills of pharmacy staff, and hence the concept of the responsible pharmacist was developed.

The Health Act 2006 amends relevant sections of the Medicines Act 1968. Instead of requiring a pharmacist in 'personal control', there must be a 'responsible pharmacist' in charge of each registered pharmacy.

Responsible pharmacists—community pharmacists

The responsible pharmacist has to:
• secure the safe and effective running of the pharmacy, including during periods of absence;
• display a notice with their name, registration number, and the fact that they are in charge of the pharmacy at that time;
• complete the pharmacy record to identify who the responsible pharmacist was for a pharmacy at any one time;
• establish (if not already established), maintain, and keep under review procedures for safe working.

Responsible pharmacists—hospital pharmacists

The responsible pharmacist changes to the Medicines Act only affect those hospitals that have registered all or part of their pharmacy premises with the General Pharmaceutical Council.

Hospitals may choose to have registered pharmacy premises for a number of reasons including the following.
• Operation of a retail pharmacy, which allows dispensing of prescriptions that have not originated within their hospital and selling prescription medicines to visitors and staff.
• To allow the dispensing of private prescriptions when consultation is not covered as part of the business of the hospital.
• To allow for self-prescribing by medical staff.

If you have a registered pharmacy within the hospital, the law and standards for responsible pharmacists will apply. This means that the registered pharmacy is required to have a responsible pharmacist when it is operating as a pharmacy business. As a hospital pharmacist you are advised to check with your chief pharmacist for clarity concerning responsible pharmacist requirements within your pharmacy.

Requirements of responsible pharmacist legislation

The law covers four key areas.

- Have a responsible pharmacist to secure the *safe and effective* running of the pharmacy.
- Conspicuously display to the public the name and registration number of the current responsible pharmacist.
- Maintain a pharmacy record detailing who has been the responsible pharmacist at any particular time.
- Maintain and operate pharmacy procedures on a range of specified matters.

The responsible pharmacist is the pharmacist appointed by the employer, who is responsible for securing the safe and effective running of the pharmacy at that time. The responsible pharmacist continues to be responsible for securing the safe and effective running of the pharmacy during any periods of absence.

If there is more than one pharmacist working in the pharmacy at any one time, only one can be the responsible pharmacist. A pharmacist cannot be the responsible pharmacist for more than one pharmacy at any one time.

A hospital department has to be registered with the Council for 3 years before EU-trained pharmacists can assume responsible pharmacist responsibility.

Absence of the responsible pharmacist

A responsible pharmacist can be absent from the pharmacy for a maximum of 2 hours during the business hours of the pharmacy when the pharmacy is operational. The responsible pharmacist continues to be responsible for the safe and effective running of the pharmacy throughout this absence. A responsible pharmacist must comply with the conditions for absence, which are as follows.

- They remain contactable throughout their absence.
- They return with reasonable promptness.
- In the event that they cannot remain contactable, they must arrange for another pharmacist to provide advice during their absence.

Examples of standard operating procedures that need to be established

- Medicine management that describes procedures for ordering, storage, preparation, sale and supply, delivery, and disposal.
- Advice about medicinal products that includes:
  - staff training to be undertaken to provide advice.
  - those products for which staff may/may not provide advice.
  - when staff should refer to a pharmacist and what to do if a pharmacist is not physically present.
- Pharmacy staff listing based on competency.
- Management of records including controlled drugs, invoices, training details.
- Arrangements during absence.
- Change of responsible pharmacist.
- Complaints and incidents procedures.
- Changes to the pharmacy procedures and how staff are notified.

Research

Audit and research *304*
Writing a research proposal *306*
Citations in documents and articles for publication *309*
Personal bibliographic databases *310*

Audit and research

Research on humans should be subject to ethical committee review. Sometimes there is a blurred distinction between audit or quality assurance activities and research. Pharmacists need to consider projects carefully and ensure that they comply with local requirements. The following may help to distinguish research from audit and quality assurance.

Audit (which might not need to go to ethics committee review)
- Measures the process and outcome of care.
- Is not randomized.
- Is usually initiated and conducted by those providing the clinical service.
- Involves review of recorded data by those entitled to have access to such data.
- May include patient questionnaires.

Research (which should go to ethics committee review if it involves patients or volunteers)
- Randomized studies.
- Data collection if outside personnel can access sensitive information about patients.
- Interventions involving contact with patients by a health professional previously unknown to them.
- Questionnaires asking for personal data or sensitive sociodemographic details.
- If there is an intention to publish data as research.
- If pharmaceutical data are collected (other than post-marketing surveillance).
- If patients or volunteers have any procedure or treatment additional to normal medical care.
- If patient samples of any sort are taken additional to normal medical care.

Writing a research proposal

Structure of a research proposal

- Title of project
- Purpose of project
- Background of project
- Central research question(s)
- Research design
- Data analysis
- Timetable
- Research staff required
- Resources required
- Proposed budget
- References

Title of project

- Descriptive
- Clear
- Succinct
- Use recognizable keywords
- Comprehensible (to non-specialists)
- Should not imply an expected outcome

Examples

- 'A randomized controlled trial of amitriptyline in chronic pain'
- 'A controlled evaluation of advice giving for low back pain'
- 'A descriptive study of the needs of patients on an orthopaedic surgery ward'

Purpose of the project

- Why undertake the project?
- Who will benefit?
- Academic potential/contribution?
- Clinical potential/contribution?
- Patient potential/contribution?
- What gaps are likely to be filled?

Background of project

- Literature review
- Critical appraisal of literature/evidence
- Establish scientific adequacy of evidence
- Establish clinical and social adequacy of evidence
- Identify positive evidence and the potential to support, replicate, or challenge it
- Identify negative evidence and the potential to support, replicate, or challenge it
- Identify uncertain evidence and the potential to clarify, support, or reject it
- Identify lack of evidence and potential to remedy this
- Justify research questions

Research questions
- Clear
- Specific
- Distinctive
- Comprehensible (to self and others)
- Answerable
- Feasible (scientifically and financially)

Research design
- Type of design:
  - randomized controlled trial
  - matched comparison
  - cohort study
  - single case study
  - descriptive/ethnographic
- Sampling frame
- Sample selection criteria
- Baseline and follow-up strategy
- Measures/data to be collected (methods/outcome/satisfaction/costs)
- Access to data arrangements (Data Protection Act might apply)
- Ethical considerations—research often requires approval from an ethics committee or equivalent body (see 📖 p.304)

Data analysis
- How data will be stored:
  - manually and computerized
  - coded
  - entered
  - confidentiality and anonymity
- How data will be retrieved from computer?
- How data will be manipulated:
  - descriptive versus inductive
  - univariate/bivariate/multivariate analysis
  - tests of significance
  - qualitative data handling
- Which statistical/epidemiological package (e.g. SPSS/EpiInfo/NUDIST)?
- Data presentation strategy
  - report writing strategy (eg report/journal publications/book/meeting presentation/poster)

Timetable
- Preparation time
- Start/baseline data collection
- Follow-up data collection
- End of data collection
- Data retrieval time
- Data manipulation and analysis
- Report preparation, writing, and dissemination
- Do not underestimate the time involved—be realistic and keep to the schedule

Research staff required
- Self
- Research assistants
- Interviewers
- Secretarial/administrative support
- Data entry, retrieval, and handling staff
- Consultancies (statistician/specialist advice/support)

Resources required
- Staff
- Accommodation (office space and storage space)
- Equipment:
  - computer hardware/software
  - telephones/fax/email
  - furniture/filing cabinets/storage
  - audio/video recording machinery
  - specialist/technical equipment
- Laboratory time/access
- Books, journals, and library services
- Printing and stationery
- Postage
- Travel—both staff and reimbursement for participants in the study
- Overheads (staff and agency)

References
Provide supporting references in a standard format, such as Vancouver (see 📖 p.309).

Citations in documents and articles for publication

A variety of styles are used to cite publications in the medical literature. Editors of several medical journals have established guidelines for the format of manuscripts submitted to their journals. This group, known as the International Committee of Medical Journal Editors (ICMJE), has broadened its focus beyond manuscript and reference formatting to include ethical principles related to publication in biomedical journals. Many journals now follow ICMJE's *Uniform Requirements for Manuscripts Submitted to Biomedical Journals: Writing and Editing for Biomedical Publication* (www. icmje.org/). Review of the *Uniform Requirements* is beyond the scope of this book but it should be consulted by those preparing materials for publication.

The commonly used methods of citation are listed here with examples. For further details see the BMA website.[1]

Harvard style

In the Harvard style references are cited using the author–date system. For example:
- Journal/book articles—in the text:
  - Davies and Mehan (1988) have argued …
- Journal/book articles—in the reference list:
  - Davies, P.T. and Mehan, H. (1988). Professional and family understanding of impaired communication. *British Journal of Disorders of Communication* **23**, 141–51.
- Books—in the text:
  - Davies (1983) has argued that …
- Books—in the reference list:
  - Davies, PT (1983). *Alcohol Problems and Alcohol Control in Europe.* London: Croom Helm.

List all authors (up to a maximum of six) in the reference list.

Vancouver style

In the Vancouver style references are cited using the author–number system:
- Journal/book articles—in the text:
  - Onghena and Van Houdenhove[4] have argued …
- Journal/book articles—in the reference list:
  - 4. Onghena P, Van Houdenhove B. Antidepressant induced analgesia in chronic pain: a meta-analysis of 39 placebo controlled studies. *Pain* 1992 May; **49**(2): 205–19.
- Books—in the text:
  - Colson and Armour[5] have argued …
- Books—in reference list:
  - 5. Colson JH, Armour WJ. *Sports Injuries and their Treatment* (2nd rev. edn). London: S Paul; 1986.
  - List all authors (up to a maximum of six) in the reference list.

1 ᪣ http://www.bma.org.uk/library_services/ask_for_help/libraryreferencestyles.jsp

Personal bibliographic databases

Personal bibliographic databases are simply structured database files with some useful features that enable references to be quickly stored, retrieved, or inserted into word-processed documents. The basic layout of the database is designed to handle information published in various formats (e.g. journal articles or books) and the fields are set up to hold that information. There are additional fields that include sections for keywords and reference numbers. The simplest use of the database is to manually add information into the fields in a logical sequence. The data are held as records that can then be searched using a variety of options, such as author, date of publication, or keywords. It is then a simple task to assign a number to the record that matches a number added to a stored original article (e.g. in numerical order of the collection) and subsequently to retrieve the hard copy of a reference by searching for keywords, for example. Databases of many thousands of papers can be built up in this way and single articles identified in seconds. For example, a single reference in a ProCite® database of 20 000 records can be found in <5 seconds.

There are some useful additions that make this type of software particularly valuable. First, searches that have been carried out electronically using a database, such as MEDLINE, can be downloaded directly into the personal bibliographic database using a linking software package, such as Bibliolinks. Translators are available for most of the commonly used databases, and this facility enables a database of useful information to be created quickly without re-keying the information. The full record is usually imported, including the abstract, thus extending the search possibilities within the personal database.

Secondly, all the software packages have the means for either simple or complex searches. In ProCite® the following options are available.

To search a database, it is possible to build a 'search expression' in the text box. You can type the text or use the 'Fields', 'Operators', and 'Terms' buttons to help build your search expression. For example, you could enter: AUTHOR = Smith and KEYWORDS = Asthma.

It is possible to search by date, or a range of dates. You can save your search expression with the 'Expressions' button, so you can perform the same search again after more records are entered, or you can save the list of records that results from your current search by highlighting them and using the 'Group' menu to save them to a 'Group'.

The third key feature is the ability to link a manuscript to the database to generate a reference list. This task, which is usually time-consuming and tedious, is quickly performed because the word-processing package interacts to find the references mentioned, marks the text in the appropriate way (e.g. superscript number), and produces the reference list. Various styles of reference are available, so if your manuscript in Vancouver style, for example, is rejected by your favourite journal, it can be submitted to another journal that might require Harvard formatting with ease.

Author Analytic (01): Carroll, D.// Jadad, A.// King, V.// Wiffen, P.// Glynn, C.// McQuay, H.

Article Title (04): Single-dose, randomized, double-blind, double-dummy cross-over comparison of extradural and i.v. clonidine in chronic pain

Journal Title (03): Br J Anaesth
Date of Publication (20): 1993
Volume Identification (22): 71
Issue Identification (24): 5
Page(s): 665–9
ISSN (40): 0007–0912
Notes (42): HC

Abstract (43): We studied 10 patients with chronic back pain who had claimed benefit with a previous extradural dose of clonidine 150 micrograms combined with local anaesthetic. We compared a single dose of clonidine 150 micrograms given by either the extradural or i.v. route in a double-blind, randomized, double-dummy and cross-over fashion, with 80% power to detect a difference in the analgesic effect of the two routes. Pain intensity, pain relief, adverse effects, mood, sedation and vital signs were assessed by a nurse observer. I.v. clonidine produced significantly ($P < 0.04$) greater analgesia than extradural clonidine in one of the five analgesic outcome measures. Clonidine given by either route produced statistically significant sedation and significant decreases in arterial pressure and heart rate. In this study, extradural clonidine had no significant clinical advantages compared with i.v. clonidine; clonidine 150 micrograms by either route produced a high incidence of adverse effects.

Keywords (45): Yes/Chronic non-malignant pain/Pharmacolgical intervention/Adult/Aged/Analgesia, Epidural/Clonidine administration and dosage/Clonidine adverse effects/Double Blind Method/Injections, Intravenous/Middle Age/Pain Measurement/Back Pain drug therapy/Clonidine therapeutic use/Comparative Study/Female/Human/Male/Support, Non U.S. Gov't

Fig. 15.1 Example from ProCite®.

The reference shown in Fig. 15.1 appears as follows when presented in Vancouver format:

Carroll D, Jadad A, King V, Wiffen P, Glynn C, McQuay H (1993). Single-dose, randomized, double-blind, double-dummy cross-over comparison of extradural and i.v. clonidine in chronic pain. *Br J Anaesth* **71**(5): 665–9.

It is beyond the scope of this book to recommend a particular package, but a number of are available, including Reference Manager®, ProCite®,

Idealist®, and EndNote®. Other less well-known packages include Papyrus®, Citation 8®, and RefWorks®. Some are web-based applications, i.e. the reference database is accessible from any computer that has access to the internet. Other programs store the reference databases on the user's computer or a portable storage device and are accessible whether internet access is available or not.

Most reference manager software products offer a trial period. It is recommended that prospective buyers define their own needs and find the product that is best suited for them.

Therapy-related issues: gastrointestinal system

Diarrhoea 314
Constipation in adults 318
Management of nausea and vomiting 322
Dyspepsia, peptic ulcer disease, and gastro-oesophageal
   reflux disease 326
Pharmaceutical care in gastrointestinal stoma patients 334

Diarrhoea

Description and causes

- 'Diarrhoea' is a term generally understood to mean an ↑ frequency of bowel movement relative to normal for an individual patient.
- The normal bowel habit in Western society lies somewhere in the range between two bowel actions/week and three bowel actions/day.
- The mechanisms that result in diarrhoea are varied and include ↑ secretion or ↓ absorption of fluid and electrolytes by cells of the intestinal mucosa and exudation resulting from inflammation of the intestinal mucosa.
- Diarrhoea is a non-specific symptom that is a manifestation of a wide range of GI disorders, including inflammatory bowel disease, irritable bowel syndrome, GI malignancy, a variety of malabsorption syndromes, and acute or subacute intestinal infections and infestations.
- Diarrhoea can be an unwanted effect of almost any drug, particularly those listed in the next section.

Medications commonly causing diarrhoea

Osmotic (drugs that create a hypertonic state in the intestine)
- Acarbose, magnesium salts, and antibiotics.

Secretory (↑ intestinal ion secretion or inhibit normal active ion absorption)
- Antineoplastics, digoxin, metformin, NSAIDs, misoprostol, and olsalazine.

Disturbed motility (leading to shortened transit time)
- Erythromycin, levothyroxine

Exudative (drugs that cause inflammation and ulceration)
- Antineoplastics, NSAIDs, and simvastatin

Malabsorption or impaired digestion of fat or carbohydrates
- Aminoglycosides, colestyramine, metformin, orlistat, and tetracyclines

Microscopic colitis (drugs causing a submucosal band of collagen in the intestine, resulting in a watery diarrhoea)
- Cytotoxic agents, budesonide, carbamazepine, ciclosporin, co-beneldopa, ranitidine, and simvastatin.

All patients presenting with diarrhoea should be questioned about the relationship between symptoms and changes in medications.

If an underlying cause of diarrhoea can be identified, management is directed at the cause rather than the symptom of diarrhoea.

Treatment

Chronic diarrhoea

The treatment of chronic diarrhoea depends on controlling the underlying disease.

Acute diarrhoea

Fluid and electrolyte therapy

Even in the presence of severe diarrhoea, water and salt continue to be absorbed by active glucose-enhanced sodium absorption in the small intestine. Oral replacement solutions are effective if they contain balanced quantities of sodium, potassium, glucose, and water. Glucose is necessary to promote electrolyte absorption.

Proprietary soft drinks and fruit juices may be inadequate treatment for individuals in whom dehydration poses a significant risk—e.g. the elderly and patients with renal disease.

In adults, an oral rehydration solution should be considered for patients with mild to moderate dehydration (loss of <6% of body weight). Solutions should be made up freshly according to manufacturers' recommendations, refrigerated, and replaced every 24h.

Several proprietary rehydration products are available and are made up according to brand recommendations. The recommended range of concentrations for rehydration solutions for use are as follows:

- sodium 50–60mmol/L
- potassium 20–35mmol/L
- glucose 80–120mmol/L.

For adults, encourage 2–3L of rehydration solution orally to be taken over 24h. This will provide 100–180mmol of sodium and 40–105mmol of potassium. Once rehydration is complete, further dehydration is prevented by encouraging the patient to drink normal volumes of an appropriate fluid and by replacing continuing losses with an oral rehydration product.

Drug therapy

Antimotility drugs may be of symptomatic benefit in adults with mild or moderate acute diarrhoea. Their most valuable role is in short-term control of symptoms during periods of maximum social inconvenience (e.g. travel and work). They are contraindicated in patients with severe diarrhoea, and in patients with severe inflammatory bowel disease or dilated or obstructed bowel. However, antimotility drugs are also sometimes useful for control of symptoms if treatment of the underlying cause is ineffective or the cause is unknown. Antimotility drugs are never indicated for management of acute diarrhoea in infants and children <12.

If an antimotility drug is considered appropriate, it is reasonable to use one of the following regimens.

- Loperamide 4mg orally initially, followed by 2mg orally after each unformed stool (maximum of 16mg/daily).
- Diphenoxylate 5mg + atropine 0.05mg orally three to four times daily initially (↓ dose as soon as symptoms improve).
- Codeine phosphate 30–60mg orally up to four times daily.

Adsorbents, such as kaolin and activated charcoal have not been shown to be of value in the treatment of acute diarrhoea. They could interfere with absorption of other drugs and should not be used.

Antibacterials are rarely indicated in uncomplicated infective diarrhoea, except to treat properly diagnosed enteric infections such as dysentery and antibacterial-associated colitis.

Diarrhoea can reduce the absorption of medicines. Drugs that may be affected clinically significantly include antiepileptics, modified release formulations, antidiabetic agents, anticoagulants, antimalarials, anti-retrovirals, and oral contraceptives.

Constipation in adults

Description and causes of constipation in adults

- Defined as a ↓ frequency of defecation.
- The normal frequency of bowel motions in western countries varies from three times/day to twice/wk.
- A person might complain of constipation for the following reasons.
  - Defecation occurs less frequently than usual.
  - Stools are harder than usual.
  - Defecation causes straining.
  - Sense of incomplete evacuation.

There are a large number of causes of constipation, ranging from common dietary problems to mechanical obstruction, including the adverse effects of many commonly used drugs. One of the most common causes is a low-residue diet.

Some medications commonly causing constipation

- Aluminium- and calcium-containing antacids
- Amiodarone
- Anticholinergic agents (e.g. tricyclic antidepressants, antipsychotics and antispasmodics, antiparkinsonian agents)
- Clozapine, olanzapine, risperidone and quetiapine
- Iron preparations
- Diuretics
- Lithium
- NSAIDs
- Opioids
- Calcium-channel blockers

Changing or stopping these drugs might be all that is required to restore normal bowel function.

Most of the factors predisposing to constipation are potentially magnified or compounded in the older patient. In this group, particularly, prolonged constipation can lead to faecal impaction, causing urinary and faecal overflow incontinence. The latter is sometimes misdiagnosed and treated as diarrhoea. It is an avoidable cause of hospital admission.

Treatment of constipation in adults

Patients, especially if ambulant and otherwise healthy, should be encouraged to control their bowel activity by attention to diet and exercise. The diet should contain adequate amounts of fibre and fluid. Physical exercise has been shown to ↓ intestinal transit time and is believed to stimulate regular bowel movements.

If these measures are ineffective, intermittent or regular use of a laxative might be necessary (Table 16.1). The duration of treatment with laxatives should be limited to the shortest time possible. The undesirability of long-term laxative use should be explained to the patient.

Diet

The major lifestyle factor leading to constipation is inadequate dietary fibre intake. Dietary fibre consists of plant complex carbohydrates that escape digestion in the small intestine and are only partly broken down by bacterial enzymes in the large intestine. The ingestion of dietary fibre ↑ stool bulk by ↑ both solid residue and stool water content. This results in ↓ intestinal transit time and ↓ water absorption in the large bowel, resulting in stools that are softer, wetter, and easier to pass.

The recommended amount of dietary fibre is 30g/day. The fibre content of the diet should be built up gradually to avoid adverse effects, such as bloating or flatulence. Patients should be encouraged to choose a wide variety of fibre sources (e.g. wholegrain or wholemeal products such as breads, cereals, pastas and rice, fruits and vegetables, legumes, seeds and nuts) rather than adding a few very high fibre foods (e.g. unprocessed bran) to the diet. Ensure that adequate fluid intake is encouraged.

Drug therapy

There is little clinical evidence on which to judge the relative effectiveness and tolerability of individual laxatives. Therefore choice should be based on symptoms, patient preferences, side effects, and cost of medicines.

First-line therapy

If dietary management is not sufficient, bulk-forming agents are the laxatives of choice for mildly constipated individuals. Provided that good fluid intake is maintained, use the following agents:

- oral bulk-forming agents

The effect of bulk-forming laxatives is usually apparent within 24h, but 2–3 days of medication might be required to achieve the full effect.

Second-line therapy

- Osmotic laxative—lactulose syrup 10–30mL orally twice or three times daily. Lactulose syrup contains free lactose and galactose and therefore it should be used with caution in patients with diabetes mellitus and is contraindicated in galactosaemia. The laxative can take 48h to work, so it must be taken regularly.
- Stimulant laxative—senna 7.5mg or bisacodyl 5mg, one or two tablets daily (interchangebly). The agents used for second-line therapy can also be used as first-line therapy in acute illness or for hospitalized patients.
- Although stool-softening agents, such as docusate salts, are often used in the treatment of constipation, they have limited effectiveness as monotherapy.

Third-line therapy

If constipation is resistant to the first- and second-line therapies, there should be a re-evaluation of the underlying cause(s), including impaction. For further therapy, use one of the following regimens:

- Magnesium sulphate 5–15g (5–15mL) orally in water daily.
- A stimulant agent (e.g. senna 30mg or bisacodyl 20mg) orally daily at night.

If required, consider the following regimens.

- Glycerin suppository rectally (allow to remain for 15–30min).
- Phosphate enema rectally.

Magnesium salts should not be used in pregnant women or patients with impaired renal function.

Fourth-line therapy

In a minority of patients all three therapies are unsuccessful and repeated enemas, macrogols (polyethylene glycol, e.g. Laxido® or Movicol®, sodium phosphate or sodium picosulphate bowel preparations) and/ or manual evacuation might be required, sometimes after admission to hospital. Laxido®/Movicol®, 1–3 sachets daily in divided doses usually for ≤2wks; each sachet should be dissolved in 125mL of water.

Opioid-induced constipation

When an opioid is first prescribed, either lactulose and senna or co-danthrusate (one or two capsules) at night should be added as a prophy-lactic measure. (Sometimes the dosage must be ↑ to two capsules twice daily acutely, and then reduced to one or two at night).

If the patient is already constipated, ↑ the dosage to co-danthrusate two capsules at night; adjust the dose according to response, up to a maximum of three capsules three times daily.

If the maximum dose is ineffective, ↓ the dose by 50% and add an osmotic laxative—e.g. lactulose 20–30mL twice daily or Movicol® one sachet twice daily.

Table 16.1 Laxative choice

Constituent(s), form, and preparation	Dose (adult dose, unless otherwise specified)	Time to onset
Bulk-forming laxatives		
Note: it is recommended that bulk-forming agents be taken with adequate fluid		
Ispaghula granules	1 sachet or 5mL spoonful, twice daily	Usually 24h, 2–3 days for full effect
	Child 6–12yrs: 50% adult dose	
Sterculia	1–2 heaped 5mL spoonfuls twice daily	Usually 24h, 2–3 days for full effect
	Child 6–12yrs: 50% adult dose	
Osmotic laxatives		
Lactulose syrup	15–30mL daily, in one or two doses initially	1–2 days
	Child, <1yr: 5mL	
	Child, 1–6yrs: 10mL	
	Child, 7–14yrs: 15mL daily initially	
Magnesium sulphate mixture	5–15mL in 250mL water	1h

Table 16.1 (*Contd.*)

Constituent(s), form, and preparation	Dose (adult dose, unless otherwise specified)	Time to onset
Macrogols	1–3 sachets in 125mL water daily	1h
Phosphate enemas	See product information	2–5min
Stool-softening laxatives		
Docusate tablets	200mg twice daily	1–3 days
Arachis oil (rectal) (contraindicated in peanut allergy)	See product information	1 day
Stimulant laxatives		
Bisacodyl 5mg tablets	1–2 tablets daily	6–12h
Bisacodyl 10mg suppositories	1 suppository daily	15–60min
Senna 7.5mg tablets	2–4 tablets daily Child >6 years: 50% adult dose	6–12h
Co-danthrusate (opioid-induced constipation)	1–3 capsules at night	6–12h
Lubricant laxatives		
Glycerol/glycerin suppositories	1 suppository, as required	15–30min
Liquid paraffin oral emulsion	10–30mL at night	8–12h

Note: prolonged use of liquid paraffin oral emulsion can cause deficiency of fat-soluble vitamins and is associated with lipoid pneumonia

Bulk-forming combined with stimulant laxatives

Note: it is recommended that bulk-forming agents be taken with adequate fluid

| Frangula+sterculia granules | 1–2 heaped teaspoonsful once or twice daily | 6–12h |

Management of nausea and vomiting

Nausea and vomiting are common and distressing symptoms, which can lead to the following clinical conditions:
- poor hydration and nutrition
- weight loss
- depression
- ↑ length of stay
- poor adherence to oral medicines.

Causes of nausea and vomiting
- Chemical:
  - exogenous—e.g. microbial toxins and drugs
  - endogenous—e.g. uraemia and hypercalcaemia.
- CNS:
  - emotional and anxiety
  - CNS lesions
  - vestibular
  - ↑ intracranial pressure.
- Obstructive:
  - constipation
  - GI tumours

Factors that can ↑ the risk or severity of nausea and vomiting include the following:
- ♀
- tendency to nausea and vomiting (e.g. motion sickness and drug intolerance)
- non-smoker
- history of migraine
- pain
- anxiety.

Management of nausea and vomiting requires accurate diagnosis of the cause and knowledge of control pathways and the ways in which anti-emetics work.

Four steps to managing nausea and vomiting
- Identify the cause—this is not always easy because nausea and vomiting are often multifactorial, but it is important because antiemetics are not equally effective against all types of nausea and vomiting. Take an accurate and detailed history, including prescribed and over-the-counter drugs.
- Remove or correct cause if possible—e.g. stop NSAIDs or prescribe laxatives if constipated.
- Treat according to cause—start an appropriate treatment according to the diagnosis (Table 16.2). About 10% of cases require more than one drug. These should preferably be from different groups (but anti-cholinergics antagonize the prokinetic effect of metoclopramide and domperidone). Parenteral administration is frequently more appropriate than oral. See Table 16.2 for recommended drugs.

Table 16.2 Treatment of nausea and vomiting

Cause	First-line drug group	First-line treatment	Second-line treatment	Other treatment
Obstruction	Anticholinergic*/antihistamine	Cyclizine	Hyoscine	Dexamethasone Antihistamine Laxatives
Gastric stasis	Prokinetic	Metoclopramide[†]	Domperidone	Antacid Dexamethasone
Gastritis	Prokinetic	Metoclopramide[†]	Cyclizine Domperidone	Antacid Ranitidine Proton-pump inhibitor
Chemical	Dopamine antagonists	Prochlorperazine Haloperidol	Levomepromazine Granisetron/ondansetron/tropisetron Nabilone	Dexamethasone Acupressure (e.g. Sea Band®)
CNS	Antihistamine/anticholinergic	Cyclizine	Hyoscine	Dexamethasone
Psycho-logical Emotional	Anxiolytic	Diazepam	Midazolam Levomepromazine Lorazepam	Reassurance

*Note that anticholinergic side effects can ↑ obstruction.

[†]At high doses, metoclopramide acts as a 5-HT$_3$ antagonist.

- Specialist advice should be sought for patients with chemotherapy-induced nausea (see 📖 p.478) or radiotherapy-induced nausea and vomiting or bowel obstruction.
- Review frequently and regularly—if nausea and vomiting persist, change from oral to parenteral administration, ↑ dose, or try drugs from a different therapeutic class. Allow a 24h trial of each intervention before trying another option.

Postoperative nausea and vomiting (PONV)

PONV is a highly undesirable complication of surgery, which can occur in up to 50% of cases. In addition to the consequences already described, severe retching and vomiting postoperatively can put tension on suture lines, cause haematomas below surgical flaps, and ↑ postoperative pain.

Additional risk factors for PONV are as follows.

- Use of inhalation anaesthetics.
- Duration of anaesthesia.
- Use of opioids.
- Use of nitrous oxide.
- Abdominal surgery, notably laparoscopic procedures.
- Perioperative dehydration.

For non-emergency surgery, good preoperative care can ↓ the risk of PONV.

- Identify risk factors and correct or minimize wherever possible.
- Assess unavoidable risk factors:
  - if one risk factor or less, no prophylaxis is required;
  - if two or more, risk factors are present give prophylactic anti-emetics preoperatively;
  - for patients at high risk of PONV, give two antiemetics from different classes preoperatively.

If the patient experiences PONV despite prophylaxis, give an additional antiemetic from a different class.

Drug points

- Avoid metoclopramide in younger patients (≤20 years), because of ↑ risk of dystonic reactions.
- Domperidone does not cross the blood brain–barrier and so is a suitable alternative to metoclopramide in young (♀) patients.
- Long-term metoclopramide, prochlorperazine, and haloperidol can cause extrapyramidal side effects in older patients.
- Levomepromazine should be administered in low doses and titrated cautiously because it is sedative and hypotensive at higher doses.
- Anticholinergics antagonize the prokinetic effect of metoclopramide and domperidone.
- Anticholinergics can cause a 'high' in some patients; avoid in patients with a current or past history of drug misuse.
- Tolerance to opioid-induced nausea and vomiting usually develops after 7–10 days. A prophylactic antiemetic should be used initially and the continued need reviewed after 7–10 days.

Dyspepsia, peptic ulcer disease, and gastro-oesophageal reflux disease

Dypspesia

- Broad range of symptoms related to dysfunction of the upper GI tract from oesophagus to duodenum. Also described as bad indigestion or heartburn.
- Symptoms include upper abdominal pain or discomfort, acid reflux, fullness, bloating, wind, nausea/vomiting, early satiety, flatulence. It affects 40% of the UK population a year.
- Conditions associated with dyspeptic symptoms include gastro-oesophageal reflux disease (GORD), which accounts for 25–50% of cases, peptic ulcer disease (PUD), gastritis, oesophagitis, gastric, pancreatic, or oesophageal cancer, biliary disease, liver cirrhosis, CRF, Crohn's disease.

GORD

- Acid pepsin or bile reflux into oesophagus from the stomach due to reduced sphincter tone, hiatus hernia, or abnormal oesophageal clearance.
- Symptoms include heartburn, acid regurgitation, and sometimes dysphagia.
- GORD can be complicated by strictures, ulceration, aspiration, Barrett's oesophagus, and adenocarcinoma.

PUD

- Discontinuity/breach in the entire thickness of the gastric or duodenal mucosa of >5mm in diameter with associated inflammation. Commonly involves the stomach (gastric ulcer (GU)), duodenum (duodenal ulcer (DU)), and oesophagus.
- In GU, symptoms of upper abdominal pain are precipitated by eating and weight loss is common. 5% of GU are malignant.
- In DU, symptoms of pain are usually nocturnal, before meals, and are relieved by food or antacids. Weight gain is common.

Pathology of ulcer formation

- Due to imbalance of injurious and protective factors
  - **Injurious factors:** pepsin, bile reflux, gastric acid, *Helicobacter pylori*, rapid gastric emptying, lifestyle (e.g. stress, alcohol, smoking,
  - obesity, fatty diet, chocolate, caffeine,) comorbidities, drugs (e.g. NSAIDs, aspirin, clopidogrel, corticosteroids, SSRIs, calcium-channel antagonists, nitrates, bisphosphonates, theophylline, potassium chloride SR).
  - **Protective factors:** mucus, bicarbonate, prostaglandins, mucosal renewal, mucosal blood flow.
- Acid secretion is under nervous and hormonal control.
- The most common factors contributing to ulcer formation are *H.pylori* and NSAIDs. They are independent risk factors for bleeding and ulceration.

Helicobacter pylori

- *H.pylori* found in gastric antrum predisposes to duodenal ulceration (majority of cases). Infection of proximal stomach predisposes to gastric ulceration.
- Eradication reduces recurrence of gastric and DUs and risk of re-bleeding
- Urea breath test—used to confirm presence of *H.pylori* prior to pre-eradication treatment or post-eradication if symptoms persist or there are complications (e.g. haemorrhage). Proton pump inhibitors (PPIs) should be stopped 2wks prior to test (false positives) and antibacterials 4wks prior to test. Biopsy and stool antigen tests are alternative methods for detecting *H.pylori*.

NSAIDs

- Increased risk during first month of use, elderly, female, high dose/potency, PUD history, smoking, other antiplatelets or anti-coagulants, comorbidities (e.g. rheumatoid arthritis (RA) (5-fold increase), cardiac (2–5-fold increase).
- Corticosteroids alone are insignificant ulcer risk but potentiate NSAIDs.
- SSRIs potentiate NSAIDs and increase risk of bleed 6-fold.
- Topical and E/C NSAIDs can also cause ulceration.
- COX-2 inhibitors have equal efficacy to non-selective NSAIDs but are not without ulcer risk. PPI cover is still recommended in high-risk patients. They are also associated with increased risk of thrombotic events (e.g. MI, stroke).

Referral for endoscopy

- Endoscopy is indicated in patients with the following.
  - Significant upper GI bleed.
  - Dyspepsia associated with alarm symptoms (urgent) defined as any age with any of the following: chronic GI bleeding, weight loss, progressive dysphagia, persistent vomiting, iron-deficiency anaemia (if not on NSAIDs and no menorrrhagia), epigastric mass.
- Consider if >55 years old *and* persistent symptoms despite *H.pylori* testing and acid suppression plus one or more of the following: continuing need for NSAIDs, previous GU or surgery, raised risk of anxiety of gastric cancer.

Treatment options

- Lifestyle—e.g reduce alcohol, stop smoking, stress relief, weight loss.
- Drugs.

Antacids/alginates

- Symptomatic relief of PUD especially ulcer dyspepsia and gastro-oesophageal reflux. Not effective in severe disease—do not affect acid secretion.
- Cheap and simple; available OTC. Take when symptoms occur or are expected.

- Some have high sodium content (caution liver disease, hypertension, pregnancy). Aluminum-based—constipating; magnesium-based—diarrhoea. Liquids better than tablets.
- Added ingredients include alginates (Gaviscon®, Rennie®), which form a raft over stomach contents and may help in reflux oesophagitis, or simethicone (Infacol®, Asilone®) which is an antifoaming agent to relieve flatulence.

Proton pump inhibitors (PPIs)

These include lansoprazole, omeprazole, pantoprazole, rabeprazole, esomeprazole. Most effective drugs for PUD/GORD—faster healing rates than H_2 antagonists.

Act by blocking acid pump (H^+/K^+-ATPase) of gastric parietal cell and cause almost total acid suppression for >24h. Inactive pro-drugs with high affinity for acidic environments. Different PPIs bind different sites on the proton pump which may account for variation in potency.

- Indications for oral PPIs.
  - *Short-term treatment*—reflux oesophagitis, benign gastric and duodenal ulcer, *H.pylori* eradication, NSAID-associated ulceration, high-output stomas (e.g. ileostomy). Therapeutic trial in cardiac patients (recommend 2wks and review).
  - *Long-term treatment/prophylaxis*—maintenance therapy with PPIs is usually limited to patients with Barrett's oesophagus, hyper-secretory conditions (e.g. Zollinger-Ellison syndrome), complicated oesophagitis (strictures, ulceration, haemorrhage), oesophageal reflux that relapses on stopping therapy. *For these indications, full treatment doses may be needed long term.*
  - High risk factors for GI bleeding that require long-term NSAID use (e.g. the elderly).
  - There is no indication for PPI cover in patients prescribed cortico-steroids alone.
- PPIs are generally well tolerated. Haematological effects are rare. There is a reported association with increased risk of hip fracture rates and long-term PPI use. Caution should be taken in severe liver disease, pregnancy, and breastfeeding.
- PPIs may mask the symptoms of gastric cancer and particular care is required in those presenting with 'alarm features'. In such cases gastric malignancy should be excluded before treatment is commenced.
- Co-administration of PPIs and antibacterials increases risk of *Clostridium difficile* 2–3-fold. Review all PPIs on admission, especially if high risk of *C.difficile*-associated diarrhoea (CDAD).
- Drug interactions—PPIs reduce conversion of clopidogrel, a pro-drug, to its active form by competively inhibiting CYP450 2C19. This leads to reduced effectiveness of clopidogrel and increases risk of MI, stroke, etc. The interaction is not seen with H_2 antagonists or pantoprazole which are not metabolized by this enzyme.
- PPIs should be reviewed regularly to ensure that patients are not continued unnecessarily.
- NICE recommends that the least expensive appropriate PPI (within its licensed indications) should be used.

H_2 antagonists

These include ranitidine, cimetidine, nizatidine, famotidine
- Act by blocking histamine receptors on gastric parietal cell, preventing acid secretion into stomach.
- Indications are broadly similar to PPIs, but as PPIs have generally superseded H_2 antagonists the latter are usually only used if PPIs are not tolerated or where drug interactions are an issue.
  - Melaena.
  - Prophylaxis in ITU/hepatic coma/obstetrics.
- More effective than antacids. If once-daily dosing give at night. Side effects rare (<3%). Cimetidine can cause impotence, confusion, and gynaecomastia
- Interactions: CYP450—cimetidine (e.g.warfarin, theophylline, phenytoin); ranitidine (theophylline).
- Dose reduction in renal failure, pregnancy.

Motility enhancers

These include metoclopramide and domperidone. Dopamine receptor antagonists that stimulate gastric emptying and small bowel transit, improve gastro-oesophageal sphincter control, increase oesophageal clearance of refluxed acid. May be of benefit in GORD and in functional dyspepsia unresponsive to PPI/H_2A.

Sucralfate

Complex of aluminium hydroxide and sulphated sucrose which has mucosal protective properties but minimal antacid properties. Used as stress ulcer prophylaxis, GU < DU, chronic gastritis. Side effects are constipation, aluminium toxicity, bezoar formation—care in ITU patients.

Bismuth chelate (tripotassium dicitratobismuthate, Denoltab®)

- Ulcer healing properties comparable to H_2 antagonists, but not in maintaining remission. Used in H.pylori regimens—toxic to H.pylori.
- Blackens stools and tongue and may accumulate in impaired renal function.
- Counselling required with respect to timing with milk and antacids.

Misoprostol

Synthetic prostaglandin E_1 analogue with antisecretory and protective properties (stimulates mucus and bicarbonate secretion). Promotes GU and DU healing and prophylactic option for NSAID-associated ulcers (when NSAIDs cannot be withdrawn). Side effects—diarrhoea (at dose required), uterine contractions, colic. Take with/after food.

Treatment

H.pylori eradication therapy

- Long-term healing of GU and DU can be achieved by eradicating H.pylori. H.pylori should be confirmed first.
- Several equally effective regimens available—no large randomized comparable trials; 85% eradication with published regimens.
- 5–20% of patients will not respond because of poor compliance and/or bacterial resistance.

- PPI should usually only be continued if there has been a gastric bleed or perforation.
- 7-day triple-therapy regimes commonly used consisting of a PPI and antibacterials.
- 14-day triple regimes offer higher eradication rate but are offset by more ADRs and poor compliance. 2-week dual regimens are licensed but have poor efficacy and are not recommended.
- Antibacterial-associated CDAD is an uncommon risk.
- Typical regimen—7 days of:
  - omeprazole 20mg bd (any PPI)
  - clarithromycin 500mg bd
  - amoxicillin 1g bd or metronidazole 400mg bd (if penicillin allergic).
- If any of the antibacterials have been used for other infections use the others in combination.
- Resistance to amoxicillin is rare, unlike clarithromycin and metronidazole.
- Tinidazole is an alternative to metronidazole.
- PPI should be continued for a further 3wks if ulcer is large or complicated by haemorrhage or perforation.
- Always give these regimes orally or via a nasogastric tube. Do not start the eradication therapy until the patient can take the full 7-day course by these routes. There is no place in therapy for intravenous *H.pylori* eradication regimens.
- Patient counselling on *H.pylori* eradication should include purpose, dose and frequency, duration (complete the course), avoidance of alcohol with metronidazole (sickness and headache), common side effects. Also advise on general lifestyle changes.

NSAID-induced ulceration
- Withdraw NSAID/COX-2 if possible and substitute with simple analgesia or use lowest dose possible.
- Full-dose PPI or H_2 antagonist for 2 months.
- Eradicate *H.pylori* if present
- Long-term prophylaxis with PPI, misoprostol, or ranitidine 300mg bd if NSAID cannot be withdrawn.
  - Prophylaxis indicated in patients at risk of ulceration on NSAIDs (e.g. elderly, history of PUD) or on other medications with GI risk (e.g. anticoagulants, antiplatelets, etc.)

Complications of PUD
- GI haemorrhage 10% (5–10% morbidity and mortality)
- Perforation—peritonitis 7%
- Pyloric stenosis/obstruction
- Chronic iron-deficiency anaemia
- Penetration—damage to other organs
- Gastric cancer—MALT lymphoma
- Oesophageal—strictures, cancer

Upper GI bleed

- **Haematemesis**—bleed proximal to duodenal–jejunal junction.
  - Large volume, bright red—*rapid, large bleed*
  - Small amount, dark red, 'coffee grounds'—*small bleed altered by gastric acid.*
- **Melaena**—proximal to and including caecum. Black tarry appearance, >60mL blood.
- PUD is most common cause of upper GI bleed—up to 50% due to chronic PUD
- Risk ratio: 3-fold increase if taking NSAIDs.
- Risk of mortality from upper GI bleed assessed via the Rockall score.[1]
- If large bleed or clinical signs of shock, restore blood volume and blood pressure.
- Stop NSAIDs/aspirin, review anticoagulants, SSRIs, aspirin, cortico-steroids.
- **Endoscopy** will define cause of bleeding in most patients and therefore is the best treatment. Perform within 24h. Emergency scope and/or surgery candidate if continued bleeding, re-bleed. Consider antibacterial prophylaxis if heart valves etc. Test for *H.pylori.*

Endoscopic therapy

The most effective intervention for those at highest risk of re-bleed and death from PUD.

- Actively bleeding lesion, non-bleeding visible vessels/adherent clot to ulcer:
  - injection sclerotherapy: adrenaline 1:10 000—*vasoconstriction*
  - heater probes/argon plasma gas—*thermal coagulation*
  - endoclips—*ligation.*
- Uncontrolled bleeding/perforation:
  - arterial embolization
  - surgery—under-running (DU), excision/partial gastrectomy (GU).
- Varices—banding, sclerotherapy, trans-intrahepatic portal systemic shunt, balloon tamponade, cyanoacrylate.

Drug therapy

Aims to stabilize clots, and reduce the risk of further bleeding in high-risk patients and the need for surgery. Most deaths from upper GI bleeding are due to respiratory, cardiac, or renal decompensation. Mortality 10–14%.

- PPIs
  - Several reviews have found PPI treatment significantly reduced re-bleeding, surgical interventions and requirement for further endoscopic treatment but it is unclear what effect it has on mortality.

1 Rockall TA *et al.* (1995). Incidence of and mortality from acute upper gastrointestinal haemorrhage in the United Kingdom. *British Medical Journal* **311**; 222–6.

- No conclusive data on optimum dose of PPI for effectively reducing re-bleeding although national published guidance (SIGN, BNF, and British Society of Gastroenterology recommend high-dose continuous infusion of PPI *post-endoscopic intervention* for major bleeding peptic ulcers (active bleed or non-bleeding visible vessel)—e.g. omeprazole 80mg stat followed by 8mg/h for 72h then po ± *H.pylori* eradication
- Pantoprazole/omeprazole is currently unlicensed for this indication but used in practice. Esomeprazole is licensed.
- There is evidence to show that IV PPI prior to endoscopy has no effect on re-bleeding, need for surgery, or risk of death.
- Ranitidine IV no longer has a place in management.
- Somatostatin and octreotide—poor trial data.
- Tranexamic acid (antifibrinolytic) may be of value in patients with risk of high mortality (Rockall score >3) and confirmed peptic ulcer.
- Can improve clot stability and ↓ risk of re-bleed.
- Terlipressin—variceal bleed (see 📖 p.183).

Further reading

NICE (2004). *Clinical Guideline 17. Dyspepsia: Management of Dyspepsia in Adults in Primary Care.* 🖰 http://www.nice.org.uk/nicemedia/pdf/CG017NICEguideline.pdf
NICE *Gastrointestinal Bleeding: The Management of Acute Upper Gastrointestinal Bleeding* (in progress). 🖰 http://guidance.nice.org.uk/CG/Wave21/1
SIGN (2008). *Guideline 105 Management of Acute Upper and Lower Gastrointestinal Bleeding.* 🖰 http://www.sign.ac.uk/guidelines/fulltext/105/index.html
British Society of Gastroenterology: 🖰 http://www.bsg.org.uk

Pharmaceutical care in gastrointestinal stoma patients

A GI stoma is a surgically created permanent opening between the GI tract and the skin. These stomas can be temporary or permanent. A stoma may be formed during surgery for cancer, inflammatory bowel disease, or trauma. Patients with GI stomas are susceptible to certain conditions such as ↑ output and dehydration or ↓ output and obstruction, but the presence of a stoma can also influence the choice of drug therapy as it may affect the pharmacokinetics of the chosen formulation.

Dietary advice for stoma patients is provided by specialist dieticians and stoma therapists. Long-term vitamin B_{12} supplementation will be required in patients with an ileostomy because of loss of the terminal ileum.

Management of constipation

Constipation in colostomy patients is usually managed by manipulation of the diet and fluid intake. If drug therapy is considered necessary, its effect should be monitored closely to avoid high output and dehydration. Sodium docusate or balanced osmotic laxatives such as Movicol®/Laxido® are suitable. Lactulose should be avoided as flatulence makes management of the stoma bag difficult.

Laxative enemas and suppositories can be administered via the colostomy but should only be carried out by experienced practitioners. After insertion of the suppository a dressing has to be placed over the stoma to allow the suppository to dissolve; this takes ~20min. The stoma appliance can then be applied. This is a time-consuming method of medication administration.

Constipation is highly unlikely in ileostomy patients, and a lack of output from an ileostomy is usually an indication of obstruction and should be referred for expert management. Laxatives should never be used in ileostomy patients.

Management of a high-output stoma

A normal stoma output will depend on the position of the stoma along the GI tract and the clinical condition of the patient. Colostomy output is usually formed stools. Ileostomy output is more liquid and usually ~1L/day. When output is ↑ the patient will lose different electrolytes depending on the site. Colostomy patients will lose K^+ and fluid; ileostomy patients will lose fluid, Na^+, Mg^{2+}, and possibly Ca^{2+}.

Primary therapy is aimed at removing the cause of the ↑ output such as infection or bacterial overgrowth, but drug therapy should also be reviewed as a possible cause of rapid gut transit. Once any causative factors have been removed or treated, the ongoing output is controlled using loperamide and/or codeine. The dose used depends on the site of the stoma and the output. For colostomy patients a regular dose of loperamide 2mg 1–3 times daily can be effective. For patients with high-output ileostomies or those with a shortened length of gut, loperamide doses of up to 24mg four times daily have been used. This should be under expert supervision. For very-high-output patients a PPI may also be added to reduce the fluid and acid production of the stomach. Not only does this reduce the volume, but it also reduces the acidity and increases the transit time. Occasionally a high-strength salt solution such as 'St Mark's rehydration solution'[1] or oral rehydration sachets (e.g. Dioralyte®) made to double strength can be used to encourage salt and water reabsorption in the small bowel. The sodium concentration should be >90mmol/L.

Octreotide is not considered effective in management of high-output stomas and is usually considered as a last resort. This should be used in specialist centres only.

High-output ileostomy management
- Expert dietetic advice.
- High-dose loperamide—e.g. 6–24mg four times daily 30min before meals.
- High-dose PPI—e.g. omeprazole 40mg twice daily.
- Codeine phosphate 30–60mg four times daily 30min before meals.
- High-strength salt solution.

Bowel preparation in stoma patients
Bowel preparation is rarely used prior to surgery or procedures now. However, if necessary standard therapies can be used in colostomy patients. Bowel preparation should never be used in ileostomy patients; a clear liquid diet in the 24 hours prior to the procedure is sufficient in these patients.

Medication choice in patients with GI stomas
Where possible modified and slow-release preparations should be avoided as these patients tend to have a reduced GI transit time and the formulation may not have time to release the dose. For ileostomy patients the transit time can vary on a daily basis and variability of absorption can be a problem. Conventional release preparations should be first choice. There is no advantage in using liquid preparations, and occasionally the high sugar or sorbitol content can ↑ the output.

Medication that affects gut transit time should be used with caution and output monitored closely—e.g. metoclopramide, domperidone, or erythromycin in patients with an ileostomy; opiates and ondansetron in patients with a colostomy.

Patients should be counselled on any medication that may colour stool output (e.g. iron preparations) as this can be distressing.

---

1 ℘ http://www.nelm.nhs.uk/en/NeLM-Area/Evidence/Medicines-Q--A/What-is-St-Marks-Electrolyte-Mix-solution/?query=%22St+Mark's%22&rank=100

Therapy-related issues: cardiovascular system

Angina *338*
Tolerance to nitrate therapy *341*
Heart failure *342*
Drug interventions for severe heart failure *348*
Acute cardiogenic pulmonary oedema *350*
Treatment of hypertension *352*
Understanding anticoagulation *356*
Clinical use of anticoagulants *358*
Warfarin dosing *362*
Counselling patients treated with warfarin *364*
Reversing the effects of warfarin (or other vitamin K
    antagonists) *366*
Out-patient anticoagulation clinics *368*
Acute coronary syndrome *370*
ST-segment elevation myocardial infarction (STEMI) *372*
Drug treatment in acute coronary syndromes *378*
Cardiopulmonary resuscitation *382*

Angina

Definition

Angina is defined and diagnosed by clinical criteria. Cardiac pain is retro-sternal, intense and gripping, constricting or suffocating, and diffuse rather than sharp.

Pain can radiate to one or both arms, neck, jaw, or teeth. However, it can be difficult to distinguish angina from severe dyspepsia, so other signs need to be considered to help differential diagnosis, such as whether pain comes on acutely following exertion and is relieved within a few minutes by resting or sublingual nitrates.

The underlying pathology is usually, but not always, coronary athero-sclerosis. Smoking, hyperlipidaemia, hypertension, obesity, and diabetes mellitus are risk factors that accelerate coronary atherosclerosis.

Types of angina

- Stable angina is induced by effort and relieved by rest.
- Unstable angina (crescendo) is angina of ↑ frequency or severity, which occurs at minimal exertion and ↑ with ↑ risk of MI.
- Decubitus angina is precipitated by lying flat.
- Variant (Prinzmetal) angina is caused by coronary artery spasm.

In stable angina, the problem is chronic atherosclerotic obstruction which is slowly progressive, although the onset of symptoms is often sudden. Severe obstructive coronary atherosclerosis restricts myocardial blood flow, whereas exercise or emotional stress creates a demand for more blood flow, which cannot be achieved because of the obstruction.

Anginal pain signals temporary myocardial ischaemia, which subsides promptly with rest because the ↑ demand subsides.

Not all patients experience typical chest pain. Some experience atypical pain, shortness of breath, or light-headedness.

Aims of treatment

- To relieve or prevent pain.
- To slow progression of atherosclerosis.
- To improve prognosis.

Assess the occurrence of pain in relation to the patient's lifestyle. Drug therapy should be initiated immediately, and risk factors should be assessed.

Attention to good drug adherence/concordance is important, and potential obstacles to this should be considered.

Advice should be given regarding regular moderate exercise and avoidance of heavy, sudden, and unaccustomed exertion and acute emotional stress, if practicable.

Acute attack

The patient should stop activities as soon as pain is felt. To shorten the attack, use one of the following regimens.

- Glyceryl trinitrate (GTN) spray 400micrograms metered-dose sublingually—repeat the dose once after 5min if pain persists (maximum of two metered doses).
- GTN tablet 500micrograms sublingually—repeat every 3–5min up to a maximum of 1500micrograms. (It is important that patients are made aware of the limited 8wk shelf-life of opened containers.)

Note: avoid nitrates if the patient has used sildenafil (Viagra®) in the previous 24h, or tadalafil (Cialis®) or vardenafil (Levitra®) in the previous 5 days.

The patient should sit or lie down, particularly when first using GTN, because of the possibility of hypotension.

If pain persists after three tablets taken over 15min or two sprays at 5min intervals, the patient should be advised to call an ambulance for transfer to the nearest hospital.

Continuing therapy

The aims of continuing therapy are to ↓ myocardial ischaemia, hence ↑ effort tolerance, and to prevent the development of acute coronary syndrome, arrhythmia, and death. Antiplatelet therapy ↓ the incidence of ischaemia at rest and the risk of MI or death. β-blockers enhance effort tolerance by ↓ the onset of myocardial ischaemia. Either of the following regimens can be used for continuing therapy:

- aspirin 75–300mg oral daily
- clopidogrel 75mg daily (if intolerant of aspirin).

The therapies described are given in addition to one of the following regimens:

- Atenolol 25–100mg oral daily.
- Metoprolol 25–100mg oral twice daily.

Nitrates can be used prophylactically before exertion that is likely to provoke angina.

For patients in whom a β-blocker alone does not prevent angina, add a dihydropyridine calcium-channel blocker and/or a nitrate and/or nicorandil, as follows

- Amlodipine 2.5–10mg oral daily or nifedipine controlled-release 30–60mg oral daily.
- Isosorbide mononitrate 30–120mg oral daily in divided doses or GTN 5–15mg transdermally (apply for a maximum of 16h in a 24h period).
- Nicorandil 5mg oral twice daily, ↑ after a week to 10–20mg twice daily.

For patients in whom there is a contraindication to a β-blocker, substitute a calcium-channel blocker, preferably a long-acting non-dihydropyridine and/or a nitrate and/or nicorandil, as follows.

- Diltiazem 30–120mg oral three times daily; diltiazem controlled-release 180–360mg oral daily; verapamil 40–120mg oral twice or three times daily; verapamil sustained-release 160–480mg oral daily; or amlodipine 5–10mg oral daily.
- Isosorbide mononitrate 30–120mg oral daily in divided doses or GTN 5–15 mg transdermally (apply for a maximum of 16h in a 24h period).
- Nicorandil 5mg oral twice daily, ↑ after a week to 10–20mg twice daily.

Choice of calcium-channel blockers

When calcium-channel blockers are used without a β-blocker, the agents of choice are verapamil or diltiazem which slow the heart rate. In general, verapamil should not be administered in combination with β-blockers because of the risk of severe bradycardia, and diltiazem should be administered with caution in combination with a β-blocker for the same reason. Dihydropyridine calcium-channel blockers can be administered in combination with β-blockers.

Amlodipine, which has a very long half-life, and the once-daily form of nifedipine can be used alone for angina, but caution should be exercised because of the possibility of ↑ sympathetic tone and heart rate secondary to arteriolar dilatation.

Tolerance to nitrate therapy

Tolerance to all forms of nitrate therapy develops rapidly. Sustained-release isosorbide mononitrate administered once daily and a GTN patch worn for <16h/day avoid this complication by allowing a nitrate-free period. The commonly used regimen of isosorbide dinitrate three or four times daily results in rapid development of tolerance.

In patients who have a low ischaemic threshold, rebound ischaemia can develop during the drug-free interval when the GTN patch is not worn. This problem might be less common during the low-drug-concentration period with sustained-release isosorbide mononitrate. Therefore this might be useful for patients with a very low ischaemic threshold.

It should be noted that a combination of long-acting nitrate regimens (e.g. sustained-release isosorbide mononitrate plus transdermal GTN) results in the rapid development of tolerance and should be avoided.

Heart failure

Heart failure is mainly a disease of the elderly. It can be predominantly left ventricular, with pulmonary congestion and dyspnoea, or predominantly right ventricular, with ↑ venous pressure, peripheral oedema, and hepatic congestion. Usually both forms coexist in the classical syndrome of congestive or biventricular heart failure.

Heart failure is generally a consequence of myocardial damage, leading to ↓ systolic function. Underlying causes and/or precipitating factors include the following.

- Hypertension.
- Coronary artery disease.
- Valvular heart disease.
- Hypertrophic cardiomyopathy.
- Hyperthyroidism can cause heart failure, particularly in association with rapid atrial fibrillation (AF).
- Alcohol abuse.
- Pericardial effusion.
- Obstructive sleep apnoea.

Non-drug interventions

Physical activity
Patients should be encouraged to be active if symptoms are absent or mild. However, bed rest might have a marked diuretic effect and, in general, patients should be rested if symptoms are severe. When confined to bed, they should receive heparin prophylaxis.

Weight reduction
Obesity is a risk factor for heart failure and left ventricular hypertrophy. Weight reduction should be advised for obese patients.

Sodium restriction
The use of diuretics avoids the need for strict sodium restriction in many patients with heart failure. However, excessive salt ingestion can precipitate or exacerbate heart failure and a no-added-salt diet (60–100mmol/day) should be recommended. More severe salt restriction might be necessary in patients with severe heart failure.

Water restriction
In patients with severe heart failure the ability to excrete a free water load is diminished. The combination of ↓ sodium intake, potent diuretics, and continued water intake often leads to dilutional hyponatraemia. Liberalizing salt intake or ↓ diuretic dosage is usually inappropriate, because these patients are often still oedematous. Water intake should be limited to ≤1.5L/day in patients with hyponatraemia, particularly those in whom serum sodium concentration falls below 130mmol/L.

Oxygen
Patients with acute pulmonary oedema are hypoxaemic and require O_2. Carbon dioxide (CO_2) retention is not usually a problem, except in patients with cor pulmonale or very severe pulmonary oedema.

Pleurocentesis and pericardiocentesis

Occasionally, patients with heart failure have significant pleural effusions which might require pleural aspiration. Pericardial aspiration should be performed in patients who have compromised circulatory function resulting from pericardial effusion and cardiac tamponade.

Drug interventions for mild to moderate heart failure

Optimization of therapy can take several months and requires close monitoring of symptoms, fluid status, renal function, and electrolyte levels.

ACE inhibitors improve prognosis in all grades of heart failure and should be used as initial therapy in all patients.

Angiotensin II receptor antagonists offer a potential alternative therapy in patients who are intolerant of ACE inhibitors, except if there are contraindications to either class of drug.

ACE inhibitor therapy

Virtually all patients with clinical heart failure should receive an ACE inhibitor as initial therapy (Table 17.1). Asymptomatic patients should also receive an ACE inhibitor if there is significant left ventricular dysfunction (i.e. left ventricular ejection fraction is <40%).

Most symptoms and signs of heart failure are caused by retention of salt and water and the consequent ↑ in cardiac filling pressures. Diuretics should be added to ACE inhibitor therapy to help control congestive symptoms and signs. If the patient's response to ACE inhibitor monotherapy is inadequate, add a diuretic and/or ↑ the dose of ACE inhibitors. Virtually all patients with clinical heart failure require combination therapy with an ACE inhibitor and a diuretic.

Table 17.1 Dosing regimens for ACE inhibitors in heart failure

Drug	Initial dose	Maintenance range
Captopril	6.25mg twice daily	50mg 3 times daily
Enalapril	2.5mg daily	20mg daily in 1–2 doses, maximum 40mg
Lisinopril	2.5mg daily	20–40mg daily
Perindopril	2mg daily	4–8mg daily
Ramipril	1.25mg daily	5–10mg daily

Angiotensin II receptor antagonists

Some patients are unable to tolerate ACE inhibitors because of adverse effects, such as cough or skin rashes. In these patients, angiotensin II receptor antagonists should be used to provide an alternative mechanism of inhibiting the renin–angiotensin system. However, if a patient has experienced angioedema with an ACE inhibitors, angiotensin II receptor antagonists are also contraindicated. They probably provide the same benefits as ACE inhibitors with regard to control of heart failure and improvement in prognosis.

If progressive worsening of renal function is the principal reason for stopping an ACE inhibitor, angiotensin II receptor inhibitors are likely to produce the same effect on renal function.

Diuretic therapy

- Diuretics should be added to ACE inhibitor therapy to control congestive symptoms and signs. Close monitoring of weight, renal function, and electrolytes is required.
- Loop diuretics are commonly used, particularly for heart failure of moderate severity; thiazides produce a gradual diuresis and are effective for mild heart failure. Caution: if thiazide and loop diuretics are combined, there is a considerable synergistic effect and the combination should be reserved for severe heart failure.
- In patients with normal renal function, the combination of ACE inhibitor, diuretic, and a K^+-sparing diuretic or K^+ supplement is occasionally needed.
- In patients with renal impairment, if diuretics are used with an ACE inhibitor, K^+-sparing diuretic or K^+-supplementation is usually not necessary and could cause life-threatening hyperkalaemia.
- If hypokalaemia proves difficult to correct, hypomagnesaemia may be present.

Spironolactone

Has been shown to decrease mortality in patients with NYHA III–IV at doses of 25mg daily who are already receiving standard therapy. As spironolactone is an aldosterone antagonist, it prevents this hormone's mechanism which causes sodium and water retention.

β-blocker therapy

Recent clinical trials have demonstrated beneficial effects of β-blockers in patients with systolic heart failure and low ejection fraction, with improvement of heart failure, left ventricular ejection fraction, and prognosis. The benefits of β-blockade, proven in clinical trials, included ↓ in all-cause mortality, sudden death, and hospitalization rates for heart failure and reversal of some degree of heart damage. Carvedilol and bisoprolol are currently licensed in the UK for chronic heart failure.[1,2,3]

There are two clinical situations in which β-blockers have been used for some time.

- After stabilization of acute heart failure in patients with AF, to control rapid ventricular rate.
- In patients with primarily diastolic heart failure, to improve diastolic filling.

1 CIBIS-II Investigators (1999). The Cardiac Insufficiency Bisoprolol Study II (CIBIS-II): a randomized trial. *Lancet* **353**: 9–13.
2 MERIT-HF Study Group (1999). Effect of metoprolol CR/XL in chronic heart failure: Metoprolol CR/XL Randomized Intervention Trial in Congestive Heart Failure (MERIT-HF). *Lancet* **353**: 2001–7.
3 Krum H *et al.* (2003). Carvedilol Prospective Randomized Cumulative Survival (COPERNICUS) Study Group. Effects of initiating carvedilol in patients with severe chronic heart failure: Results from the COPERNICUS Study. *JAMA* **289**: 712–18.

β-blocker therapy in patients with heart failure can be extremely difficult to manage. Initiation and up-titration should be undertaken in consultation with a specialist.

Patients with systolic heart failure are often very sensitive to β-blockers. Major complications include worsening of heart failure, severe hypotension, and bradyarrhythmias. These complications are caused by β-blockade, leading to withdrawal of sympathetic nervous system support for the failing heart. These complications may be minimized by the following strategies.

- Starting therapy with extremely low doses.
- ↑ the dose very gradually.
- Monitoring the patient frequently, by weighing daily.
- Adjusting the dose of other medications, such as diuretics and ACE inhibitors, to compensate for any tendency to ↑ heart failure.
- Avoiding simultaneous addition of vasodilator drugs.
- Excluding patients with extremely severe heart failure and those whose heart failure is not well controlled on other therapy.

The best advice is 'start low and go slow'. Use one of the following regimens.

- Bisoprolol 1.25mg once daily (the dose can be doubled every 2–4 weeks, provided that the patient is stable, with the aim of ↑ the dose to 10mg once daily).
- Carvedilol 3.125mg twice daily (the dose can be doubled every 2–4wks, provided that the patient is stable, with the aim of ↑ the dose to 25mg oral twice daily).
- Metoprolol 12.5mg twice daily (the dose can be doubled every 2–4wks, provided that the patient is stable, with the aim of ↑ the dose to 100mg oral twice daily).

It seems probable that standard β_1-blockers, such as metoprolol, provide similar benefits to the newer β-blockers, such as bisoprolol and carvedilol, and therefore might be much more cost-effective. However, both bisoprolol and carvedilol offer the advantage of lower-strength tablets for initiation of therapy. Moreover, they are the only β-blockers explicitly approved for use in heart failure.

Digoxin therapy

There are two indications for the use of digoxin in patients with heart failure:

- in patients with AF, to control rapid ventricular rate.
- in patients with sinus rhythm (SR), if heart failure is not adequately controlled by optimal doses of ACE inhibitors and loop diuretics.

If the patient has not been taking digoxin, give the following dose regimen.

- Digoxin 62.5–500micrograms oral daily, according to age, plasma creatinine, and plasma digoxin level.

In patients with normal renal function, the half-life of digoxin is ≥24h. Following initiation of therapy or change in the digoxin dose, the patient will require ≥5 days (five half-lives) to achieve a steady state. In patients with impaired renal function, the half-life of digoxin might be greatly prolonged.

Patients take much longer to reach steady state, and require ↓ in the maintenance dose. Monitoring of digoxin plasma level is recommended.

If the patient requires more rapid digitalization (e.g. AF with rapid ventricular rate), give the following dose regimen.

- Digoxin 500micrograms–1mg oral immediately, followed by 250–500micrograms oral every 4–6h (up to 1.5–2mg in the first 24h) followed by digoxin 62.5–500micrograms oral daily, according to age, plasma creatinine level, and plasma digoxin level.

Caution: elderly patients are susceptible to digoxin toxicity, partly because of ↓ renal clearance and partly because their cardiac tissue is more sensitive to the drug's action. Therefore loading and maintenance doses generally need to be lower.

Drug interventions for severe heart failure

Patients with severe symptomatic heart failure should be hospitalized, and require bed rest. Therapy will include all of the following drug regimens:

- maximum tolerated dose of an ACE inhibitor orally
- ↑ dose of furosemide, up to a maximum of 500mg/daily
- low-dose spironolactone, 25mg/daily (range 12.5–50mg/daily).

Low-dose spironolactone (25mg/daily) when added to therapy with a loop diuretic and an ACE inhibitor, improves prognosis in patients with severe heart failure, without a major risk of hyperkalaemia or dehydration.

In patients with severe refractory oedema due to severe heart failure, K^+-sparing diuretics, such as amiloride and spironolactone (which are weak diuretics), can facilitate diuresis when used in combination with loop diuretics. They are also much more effective than K^+ supplements in maintaining the serum K^+ level.

All K^+-sparing diuretics can cause severe life-threatening hyperkalaemia, particularly in patients with renal impairment or those taking K^+ supplements or an ACE inhibitor.

The combination of an ACE inhibitor, loop diuretics, and spironolactone can cause severe dehydration and/or hyperkalaemia.

If heart failure is poorly controlled, consider adding one of the following regimens.

- Bendroflumethiazide 2.5mg oral (use a single dose initially and repeat in 2–7 days, depending on diuretic effect).
- Spironolactone—↑ doses to 100–200mg daily.
- One of the following three (only when the patient is stable on optimal doses of ACE inhibitor and combination diuretic therapy).
  - Bisoprolol 1.25mg oral once daily (the dose can be doubled every 2–4 weeks, provided that the patient is stable, with the aim of ↑ the dose to 10mg oral once daily).
  - Carvedilol 3.125mg oral once daily (the dose can be doubled every 2–4wks, provided that the patient is stable, with the aim of ↑ the dose to 25mg oral twice daily).
  - Metoprolol 12.5mg oral once daily (the dose can be doubled every 2–4 weeks, provided that the patient is stable, with the aim of ↑ the dose to 100mg oral twice daily).
- If the patient has not been taking digoxin, add digoxin.
- If the patient has been taking digoxin, check the trough plasma digoxin level not less than 6h after the latest dose and consider ↑ the maintenance dose to achieve a plasma level in the high therapeutic range, provided that there are no symptoms or signs of toxicity.)
- If the patient is confined to bed, give prophylactic heparin as well.

Useful additional therapies in severe heart failure

Nitrates/GTN

Nitrates cause prompt, but temporary, lowering of pulmonary venous pressure. Patients with heart failure associated with hypertension or ischaemia are particularly likely to benefit.

GTN is the preferred IV vasodilator therapy, usually in the setting of an intensive care or coronary care unit. Normally, IV therapy is required for only a short period; prolonged infusion rapidly induces tolerance. Use GTN 10micrograms/min IV and ↑ the dose according to the clinical response, but maintain the systolic BP (SBP) >90mmHg.

Warfarin

Warfarin is recommended for patients who have heart failure with AF and in those with previous systemic embolism and severe left ventricular systolic dysfunction. The INR should be maintained between 2 and 3. It might be less stable in the presence of heart failure, making warfarin therapy more difficult to control.

Patients who have underlying ischaemic or hypertensive heart disease and who are not on warfarin should take low-dose aspirin.

Patients with very severe heart failure might benefit temporarily from further intensive measures. These should only be employed if there is some transient exacerbating factor (e.g. myocardial ischaemia, infection, or surgery) or if some remedial measure (e.g. cardiac transplantation) is planned.

Sodium nitroprusside

Sodium nitroprusside can also be used. It is generally administered with BP monitoring using an arterial line. It is particularly effective for patients with heart failure associated with severe hypertension. If treatment is continued for >24h, monitor thiocyanate and cyanide levels to avoid toxicity. Use sodium nitroprusside 0.3micrograms/kg body weight/min IV initially and ↑ by 0.3micrograms/kg body weight/min every 5–10min to maintain SBP at <90mmHg. Do not use for >3 days.

Other therapies

Short-term catecholamine inotrope administration can cause temporary improvement. However, therapy with positive inotropic drugs has been associated with ↑ mortality. Use dobutamine 2.5–10micrograms/kg body weight/min IV.

Increasingly, patients presenting with severe heart failure are taking a β-blocker. In these patients, the dose of β-blocker should be ↓ or the drug should be completely withdrawn. If temporary IV inotropic support is required, the phosphodiesterase inhibitor milrinone can be used and is effective in ↑ contractility even in the presence of β-receptor blockade.

Finally, an intra-aortic balloon pump might occasionally be required, and cardiac transplantation should be considered in younger patients with severe refractory heart failure. Ventricular-assist devices can provide a bridge to transplantation and, perhaps, even a long-term alternative.

Acute cardiogenic pulmonary oedema

- A medical emergency requiring urgent treatment in hospital. Initially, the patient should receive O_2 4–6L/min through a mask and furosemide 20–80mg IV (repeated 20min later, if necessary).
- Larger doses might be required, particularly in patients on pre-existing diuretic therapy or with impaired renal function. If the response to IV furosemide is inadequate, consider morphine with or without nitrates.
- Morphine 2.5–10mg IV (use the lower end of the range in the elderly).
- If pulmonary oedema is severe, not responding, or associated with ischaemia or significant hypertension, add GTN 10micrograms/min IV and ↑ according to clinical response, but maintain SBP >100mmHg.
- If the patient is in AF with a rapid ventricular rate and has not been taking digoxin, add digoxin 500micrograms oral or IV and repeat at 4h and 8h, if necessary. Administer digoxin 500micrograms oral the following day, followed by digoxin 62.5–500micrograms oral daily, according to age, plasma creatinine level, and plasma digoxin level.
- If the patient is not in AF, withhold digoxin until acute pulmonary oedema is controlled, when a maintenance dose of digoxin can be commenced or restarted.
- If pulmonary oedema remains severe and does not respond to treatment, add continuous positive airway pressure ventilation (CPAP) to improve oxygenation.
- If pulmonary oedema is severe and not responding to diuretics and vasodilator therapy, consider adding either of the following regimens.
  - Dobutamine 2.5–10micrograms/kg body weight/min IV.
  - Milrinone 50micrograms/kg body weight IV slowly over 10min, followed by 0.375–0.75micrograms/kg body weight/min IV, adjusting the dose according to clinical and haemodynamic responses up to a maximum of 1.13mg/kg body weight daily.
- See Table 17.2.

Treatment of hypertension

High BP is characterized by elevated arterial BP and ↑ risk of stroke, MI, renal failure, heart failure, or other vascular complications.

High BP is one of many risk factors for cardiovascular disease. Currently, there is a shift from consideration of individual risk factors, such as BP, to overall cardiovascular risk. Normal BP is defined as <130/85mmHg. BP is ↑ by drugs such as the following:

- NSAIDs (including cyclo-oxygenase-2 (COX-2) inhibitors)
- corticosteroids
- oral contraceptives
- topical or oral decongestants
- excessive liquorice or salt intake.

Assessment and management of other cardiovascular risk factors, particularly smoking and diabetes mellitus, is an important part of management. These factors can modify the overall cardiovascular risk substantially. Lipids and blood glucose might need checking after changes of therapy (e.g. initiation of diuretics).

Non-pharmacological measures to reduce both BP and cardiovascular risk should be introduced in all patients with hypertension. These might be the only interventions necessary in some patients. Effective measures include the following.

- Weight reduction in overweight patients.
- ↓ of heavy chronic or intermittent alcohol intake (defined as >3units/day in ♀ or >5 units/day in ♂).
- Regular physical activity.
- Moderate sodium restriction (e.g. no-added-salt diet).
- Management of sleep apnoea.
- Stress reduction.

Obstructive sleep apnoea is a strong independent risk factor for stroke and cardiovascular events. Effective management ↓ BP and can reverse these risks, but this has not been formally demonstrated.

Patients should be vigorously encouraged to stop smoking, and hyperlipidaemia should be managed. Management of cardiovascular risk factors, in addition to good glycaemic control, is particularly important in hypertensive patients with diabetes mellitus.

Drug treatment

If the non-pharmacological measures described do not achieve risk factor and BP goals, drug treatment should be commenced (Table 17.2).

In patients with no other risk factors, treatment should be commenced at systolic BP levels >160mmHg and at diastolic BP levels ≥100mmHg. Patients at raised CVD risk (10-year risk of CVD ≥20%, or existing CVD or target organ damage) with persistent BP >140/90 mmHg.

See NICE Clinical Guideline 127[1] and refer to British Hypertension Society guidelines[2] for when to initiate antihypertensives when risk factors (e.g. risk of coronary events, diabetes or end-organ damage) are present.

The six major drug groups used at present are diuretics, β-blockers, ACE inhibitors, angiotensin II receptor antagonists, calcium-channel blockers, and α-blockers. The major objective is to achieve satisfactory control of BP and overall cardiovascular risk. In many patients, this requires a combination of antihypertensive medications to achieve therapeutic targets. Overall, the major drug groups have similar efficacy in ↓ BP in most groups of patients (African patients excluded) with mild to moderate hypertension.

β-blockers are no longer preferred as first-line therapy as, according to a recently published update by NICE (www.nice.org.uk), they raise a patient's risk of developing diabetes.

Target BP

Target BP is <130/85mmHg, but some patients, especially the elderly, might not achieve or tolerate these levels. The achievement of target levels in patients with diabetes mellitus is particularly important.

The optimal outcome is to attain target levels of BP using only one preparation and once-daily dosing. If the initial drug chosen does not achieve target levels, one worthwhile strategy is to consider ↑ the dose or changing to an acceptable substitute until monotherapy is successful or clearly fails. If possible, allow at least 1 month before changing therapy to allow steady-state effects to occur at each dose level. Alternatively, use an appropriate drug in combination.

Further reading

NICE (2006). *Clinical Guideline CG34. Hypertension: Management of Hypertension in Adults: in Primary Care.* ℘ http://guidance.nice.org.uk/CG127

1 NICE (2006). *Clinical Guideline CG34. Hypertension: Management of Hypertension in Adults: in Primary Care.* ℘ http://guidance.nice.org.uk/CG127
2 British Hypertension Society: ℘ http://www.bhsoc.org

Table 17.2 Guidance on selecting antihypertensive therapy with concomitant disease

Drug	Compelling indications	Possible indications	Compelling contraindications	Possible contraindications
Hypertensive patients aged ≥55 years or Black patients of all ages: first-choice initial therapy should be either a calcium-channel blocker or a thiazide-type diuretic (Black patients—does not include patients of mixed race or Asian patients)				
Low-dose thiazides		Diabetes mellitus	Gout	Dyslipidaemia
Thiazide-like drugs	Heart failure			Symptomatic orthostatic hypertension
	Elderly patients			
	Systolic hypertension			
Calcium-channel blockers	Angina	PVD	Heart block	Congestive heart failure
	Elderly patients			
	Systolic hypertension			
Hypertensive patients aged <55 years: first-choice initial therapy should be an ACE inhibitor (or an angiotensin receptor blocker if an ACE inhibitor is not tolerated)				
ACE inhibitor	Heart failure		Pregnancy	
	Left ventricular dysfunction		Hyperkalemia	
	Acute myocardial infarct		Bilateral renal artery stenosis	
	Diabetes mellitus			
Angiotensin II receptor blockers	ACE inhibitor cough	Heart failure	Pregnancy	
	Type 2 diabetes		Hyperkalaemia	
			Bilateral renal artery stenosis	

If initial therapy was with a calcium-channel blocker or thiazide-type diuretic and a second drug is required, add an ACE inhibitor (or an angiotensin receptor blocker if an ACE inhibitor is not tolerated). If initial therapy was with an ACE inhibitor, add a calcium-channel blocker or a thiazide-type diuretic

Triple therapy: ACE inhibitor, thiazide-type diuretic, calcium-channel blocker

If a fourth drug is required, one of the following should be considered: • a higher dose of a thiazide-type diuretic or the addition of another diuretic (careful monitoring is recommended) or • β-blockers or • selective α-blockers

β-blockers	Angina	Pregnancy	Asthma and COPD	Dyslipidaemia
	Acute myocardial infarct	Diabetes mellitus	Heart block	Athletes and physically active patients
	Tachyarrhythmias			PVD
	Heart failure			
α-blockers	Prostatic hypertrophy	Glucose intolerance	Orthostatic hypotension	
		Dyslipidaemia		

Understanding anticoagulation

After injury, three separate mechanisms are activated to ↓/halt bleeding: vasoconstriction, gap plugging by platelets, and the coagulation cascade. These mechanisms can be activated inappropriately and predispose patients to stroke.

The endothethial surface cells of blood vessels are involved in the balance between clotting and bleeding by secreting compounds such as von Willebrand factor, tissue plasminogen activator (t-PA), and prostaglandins (e.g. prostacyclin). The surface cells are also involved in the balance between fibrinolysis and fibrin formation.

Platelet response

- Adhesion
- Secretion
- Aggregation
- Propagation of procoagulant activity.

Regulation of coagulation and fibrinolysis

The coagulation factors consist of 12 plasma proteins that circulate in their inactive form. Coagulation of blood causes a cascading series of proteolytic reactions that result in an active protease which activates (in an enzymatic way) the next clotting factor until a fibrin clot is formed.

Coagulation factors

- Vitamin-K-dependent factors (II, VII, IX and X).
- Contact activation factors (XI, XII, prekallikrein, and high molecular weight kininogen).
- Thrombin-sensitive factors (V, VIII, XIII and fibrinogen).
- Clotting begins at either an intrinsic or an extrinsic pathway, with activation cascading to the common pathway.
- Tissue injury releases either of the following factors (see Fig. 17.1).
  - Tissue factor (extrinsic to blood), which activates the extrinsic pathway through factor VII.
  - Subendothelial membrane contact with factor XII initiates intrinsic pathway (intrinsic—all necessary coagulation factors are present in blood).

Fibrinolysis

Formation of a fibrin clot occurs as a result of the coagulation system. The fibrinolytic system opposes coagulation, dissolving the developing clot and restoring blood flow. The process starts by the release of t-PA from endothelial cells. In response to thrombin or venous stasis, t-PA is incorporated into the forming clot by binding to fibrin. t-PA converts inactive plasminogen into plasmin, which digests fibrin and dissolves the clot.

Laboratory tests

Bleeding time

Bleeding time measures the length of time to the cessation of bleeding following a standardized skin cut.

Factors that prolong bleeding time include the following:

- thrombocytopenia.
- platelet dysfunction.
- aspirin/NSAIDs.
- SSRIs.

Prothrombin time (PT)

Thromboplastin is added to test the extrinsic system. PT is expressed as a ratio compared with control (INR) and has a normal range or 0.9–1.2. The INR is prolonged by warfarin, vitamin K deficiency, and liver disease.

Thrombin time

Thrombin is added to plasma to convert fibrinogen to fibrin (normal range, 10–15s). The thrombin time is ↑ by heparin therapy, disseminated intravascular coagulation (DIC), and fibrinogen deficiency.

Kaolin cephalin clotting time (KCCT) APTT = PTT (partial thromboplastin time)

Kaolin activates the intrinsic system (normal range, 26–34s). KCCT is prolonged by heparin therapy or haemophilia.

Fig. 17.1 The intrinsic and extrinsic pathways of blood coagulation. Reproduced with permission from Longmore M, Wilkinson IB, and Rajagopalan S (2004). *Oxford Handbook of Clinical Medicine* (6th edn). Oxford: Oxford University Press.

Clinical use of anticoagulants

Prevention of venous thromboembolism (VTE)

VTE is the collective term for deep vein thrombosis (DVT) and pulmonary embolism (PE). VTE is a common complication of hospital admission, causing an estimated 25 000 deaths in the UK each year. All patients must be assessed for their risk of VTE on admission to hospital, 24h after admission and again whenever the clinical situation changes. Each risk assessment needs to be documented in the patient's medical notes. The risk of developing VTE during hospitalization, immobilization at home, or in a nursing home depends on factors related to the individual patient and the features of any predisposing medical illness or surgical procedure performed. Patients must also be assessed for their risk of bleeding (Tables 17.3 and 17.4).

Types of thromboprophylaxis

Pharmacological and non-pharmacological methods of prophylaxis are both effective in preventing VTE, and their use in combination is additive.

Pharmacological prophylaxis

- Unfractionated heparin (UFH) was the first pharmacological agent to be used for thromboprophylaxis. Because of its presentation as a high-strength heparin product (25 000units/mL), it is generally reserved for second- or third-line choice for those patients unable to use low molecular weight heparin (LMWH) or fondaparinux.
- LMWH has been shown to be clearly superior to UFH in preventing DVT in patients undergoing orthopaedic surgery and should be used in that situation. Its efficacy in other high- and moderate-risk situations is at least that of UFH, and it is considered a reasonable alternative first-line choice.
- Fondaparinux is a selective anti-Xa inhibitor which, unlike UFH and LMWH, has no antithrombin activity. Fondaparinux is more effective at DVT prevention than LMWH in patients undergoing hip and knee arthroplasty and hip fracture surgery, and is a suitable option for those procedures. Fondaparinux is also a treatment option for many patients who have a history of heparin-induced thrombocytopenia (HIT), although it is not licensed for all patient groups—check product literature.
- Aspirin has only a weak effect in preventing venous thrombosis and should not be considered adequate as sole prophylaxis.
- DVT prophylaxis should continue until the patient is fully ambulant and fit for hospital discharge. In particularly high-risk clinical situations, including hip and knee arthroplasty and oncology surgery, prolonged prophylaxis of 28 days duration should be strongly considered.
- In situations where the slightest risk of local bleeding is unacceptable (e.g. after neurosurgery, ophthalmic surgery, some plastic surgery, head injury, or haemorrhagic stroke), anticoagulant therapy should be avoided and mechanical preventive methods should be used.

Table 17.3 Risk factors for VTE

Medical patients	Surgical patients and patients with trauma
• If mobility significantly reduced for ˜3 days **or** • If expected to have ongoing reduced mobility relative to normal state plus any VTE risk factor	• If total anaesthetic + surgical time >90 min **or** • If surgery involves pelvis or lower limb and total anaesthetic + surgical time >60min **or** • If acute surgical admission with inflammatory or intra-abdominal condition **or** • If expected to have significant reduction in mobility **or** • If any VTE risk factor present

VTE risk factors

- Active cancer or cancer treatment
- Age >60 years
- Critical care admission
- Dehydration
- Known thrombophilias
- Obesity (BMI >30kg/m^2)
- One or more significant medical comorbidities (e.g. heart disease, metabolic, endocrine, or respiratory pathologies, acute infectious diseases, inflammatory conditions)
- Personal history or first-degree relative with a history of VTE
- Use of HRT
- Use of oestrogen-containing contraceptive therapy
- Varicose veins with phlebitis

Table 17.4 Risk factors for bleeding

All patients who have any of the following

- Active bleeding
- Acquired bleeding disorders (such as acute liver failure)
- Concurrent use of anticoagulants known to increase the risk of bleeding (such as warfarin with INR >2.0)
- Lumbar puncture/epidural/spinal anaesthesia within the previous 4h or expected within the next 12h
- Acute stroke
- Thrombocytopenia (platelets <75 x 10^9/L)
- Uncontrolled systolic hypertension (˜230/120mmHg)
- Untreated inherited bleeding disorders (such as haemophilia or von Willebrand's disease)
- Neurosurgery, spinal surgery, or eye surgery
- Other procedures with high bleeding risk

Mechanical prophylaxis

Methods of mechanical prophylaxis include graduated compression stockings providing 16–20mmHg pressure at the ankle, sequential pneumatic compression devices, and pneumatic foot compression. These should be applied the evening before surgery and continued until the patient is fully ambulant.

Prophylaxis treatment

The type of prophylaxis recommended depends on the patient's risk category. However, in all patients it is advisable to avoid dehydration and to commence mobilization as soon as possible.

Effective regimens for prophylaxis include the following.

- UFH 5000units SC every 8–12h.
- Enoxaparin 40mg or dalteparin 5000units SC daily, or other LMWH (commencing ≥6h postoperatively in surgical patients) for high- and moderate-risk surgical and medical patients.
- Enoxaparin 20mg or dalteparin 2500units SC daily, commencing ≥6h postoperatively, for low-risk surgical patients (or for patients with a very low body weight or if significant renal impairment is present).
- Fondaparinux 2.5mg SC daily (commencing ≥6h postoperatively in surgical patients).

Treatment of acute DVT

The aim of treatment for established venous thrombosis is to prevent thrombus extension, pulmonary embolism, the post-thrombotic syndrome and recurrent VTE. The type of therapy employed depends on the anatomical extent of the thrombus (Table 17.5).

Anticoagulation

Before anticoagulant therapy is instituted, blood should be collected for determination of APTT, PT, and platelet count. A thrombophilia screen should be considered if there is a family history of VTE, recurrent VTE, and possibly if there is spontaneous VTE. This should include activated protein C resistance, fasting plasma homocysteine, prothrombin, protein C, protein S, antithrombin III, lupus anticoagulant, blood count, and anticardiolipin antibody tests. More specialized testing is occasionally indicated.

LMWH has been shown to be at least as effective and safe as an IV UFH infusion in the initial management of DVT. LMWH has the advantages of not requiring routine laboratory monitoring and enabling management in a hospital out-patient or general practice setting in selected cases, and is now the treatment of choice.

Any of the following regimens are recommended:

- Enoxaparin 1.5mg/kg body weight SC daily (up to a maximum dose of 150mg daily).
- Dalteparin once-daily dose graduated to weight (see *BNF*) or 100units/kg body weight SC twice daily (for patients at higher risk of bleeding or obese patients).
- Tinzaparin 175units/kg body weight SC daily.

- In the presence of renal impairment LMWH requires factor Xa monitoring and possible dose adjustment (calculated creatinine clearance ≤30mL/min).
  - Oral anticoagulation can be commenced as soon as the diagnosis is confirmed.
  - A normal loading dose of warfarin is 15–30mg, divided between 3 days (it is vital to follow local protocol as determination of the first INR will differ for different loading regimes).
- The INR should be monitored daily and the dose adjusted according to the INR until a therapeutic level is achieved. The initial dose of warfarin should be ↓ in the elderly.
- LMWH should be given for a minimum of 5 days or until the INR has been >2 on two consecutive days, whichever is the longer.
- An infusion of UFH or treatment-dose fondaparinux are suitable alternatives for patients who cannot be treated with LMWH.
- Warfarin should not be commenced alone (i.e. without a LMWH) because this is associated with a high rate of DVT recurrence.
- The duration of anticoagulation depends on the risk of both recurrent VTE and bleeding.
- Graduated compression stockings ↓ the incidence and severity of the post-thrombotic syndrome and should be used in all cases. Stockings should provide 30–40mmHg pressure at the ankle and extend to the level of the knee. Graduated compression stockings should be worn for 18 months and indefinitely if the post-thrombotic syndrome is present. This important therapy is often overlooked. Patients should be encouraged to mobilize as soon as possible.

Table 17.5 Overview of the treatment of deep vein thrombosis

Extent of DVT	Therapy
Proximal veins (the popliteal or more proximal veins	Anticoagulation and graduated compression stockings
Distal veins	Anticoagulation or ultrasound surveillance programme and graduated compression stockings

Warfarin dosing

Loading dose

A normal loading dose of warfarin is 15–30mg, divided over 3 days—see Table 17.6 for a suggested loading regime. The individual response is unpredictable and factors that particularly influence first doses should be considered.

- Age and weight—consider ↓ loading dose if patient >60 years old or weight <60kg.
- Pathophysiological changes—consider ↓ loading dose in the following conditions:
  - liver disease
  - cardiac failure
  - nutritional deficiency.
- Drug interactions—check *BNF* (Appendix 1). Remember over-the-counter medicines and complementary therapies.

Maintenance dose

The response to the loading dose can be used to predict the maintenance dose. Aim for an INR of 2–4, depending on the indication (Table 17.7). If the loading regime has been followed and INRs are determined at the correct intervals, the dose for Day 4 in Table 17.6 is a good predictor of maintenance dose in the majority of patients. For those patients who are particularly sensitive or resistant to the effects of warfarin, your local anticoagulation service can be contacted for advice.

Monitoring therapy

It is important to take account of trends rather than single results. If a patient has an unusual individual result, consider whether recent changes in behaviour (e.g. diet, alcohol consumption) could have affected it. If so, these changes should be 'corrected' rather than correcting the warfarin dose.

Factors that can affect response to warfarin include the following.
- Compliance—including timing of dose.
- Changes in kinetic parameters—e.g. weight change and fluid balance.
- Diseases—e.g. infection, congestive cardiac failure, malabsorption, liver disease, renal impairment, and GI disturbances.
- Changes in social behaviour—e.g. smoking and, alcohol.
- Diet (green vegetables contain significant amounts of vitamin K).
- Stress.
- Drug interactions—consult *BNF* (Appendix 1) or Stockley.[1]

---

1 Baxter K (ed) (2010). *Stockley's Drug Interactions* (9th edn). London: Pharmaceutical Press.

Table 17.6 Suggested loading regime for warfarin

Days 1 and 2	Day 3		Day4	
	INR	Dose (mg)	INR	Dose
Give 5mg each evening if baseline INR is ≤1.3 (PT <17s)	<1.5	10	<1.6	10
	1.5–2.0	5	1.6–1.7	7
	2.1–2.5	3	1.8–1.9	6
	2.6–3.0	1	2.0–2.3	5
	>3.0	0	2.4–2.7	4
			2.8–3.0	3
			3.1–3.5	2
			3.6–4.0	1
			>4.0	0

Table 17.7 INR targets and durations for anticoagulant therapy

Indication	Target INR (range)	Duration
Antiphospholipid syndrome syndrome (arterial thrombosis)	3.5 (3.0–4.0)	Consider long term
Antiphospholipid syndrome (venous thrombosis)	2.5 (2.0–3.0)	Consider long term
Arterial thromboembolism	3.5 (3.0–4.0)	Discuss with haematologist
AF	2.5 (2.0–3.0)	Long term
Calf DVT	2.5 (2.0–3.0)	3 months
Cardiomyopathy	2.5 (2.0–3.0)	Long term
Cardioversion	2.5 (2.0–3.0)	3 weeks before and 4 weeks after
Mechanical prosthetic heart valve (MHV)	3.5 (3.0–4.0)	Long term
Mural thrombosis	2.5 (2.0–3.0)	3 months
Proximal DVT	2.5 (2.0–3.0)	6 months
Pulmonary embolus	2.5 (2.0–3.0)	6 months
Recurrence of VTE (if no longer on oral anticoagulants)	2.5 (2.0–3.0)	Consider long term
Recurrence of VTE (while on oral anticoagulants)	3.5 (3.0–4.0)	Consider long term

Counselling patients treated with warfarin

After the decision had been made to initiate anticoagulation therapy, the ward pharmacist should counsel the patient about the risks associated with warfarin.

Counselling

All patients, whether initiated within the hospital setting or in the community should ideally be given written information on anticoagulants. The following points should be covered.

- Dose—how much, how often, and how long?
- The colour of tablets corresponds to strength. (Imperative to check the patient's understanding on how to work out which tablet(s) to take to allow for the correct dose. This can be done by getting them to explain what they would take for a selection of doses.)
- Missed doses—what to do?
- Importance of compliance.
- How warfarin works—might need to be simplistic for certain patients (i.e. makes the blood take longer than usual to clot; ↓ the risk of clot extending).
- Need for blood tests.
- Importance of telling or reminding healthcare professionals (dentist, community pharmacist, and practice nurse) about their warfarin treatment.
- Signs of overdose/underdose and what to do.
- Recognition of drug interactions, including over-the-counter medicines and herbal preparations.
- Alcohol and diet.
- Pregnancy (if appropriate).
- Record detail of dose and INR result.
- Follow-up and duration of therapy, including arrangements for further monitoring (e.g. need to attend GP practice or out-patient clinic).

Patients should be informed that the dose of warfarin might need to be changed from time to time, and that monitoring their blood is necessary for as long as the therapy is administered. The therapeutic range is narrow and varies according to the indication. It is measured as the ratio to the standard PT.

Each patient should have an explanation of intended duration of therapy, indication for therapy, concurrent medical problems, other medication that must be continued, and target coagulation laboratory values for the patient's condition. This information also needs to be communicated to the patient's primary care team.

Thereafter, there should be a mechanism to ensure that the patient's therapy is monitored in terms of efficacy and risk during the duration of anticoagulation therapy.

Ideally, discharged patients should be reviewed within 48h of discharge (for new patients), but certainly no later than 1wk (new AF patients or existing stable patients). Each condition requires a specific range of

INR values. Therefore adjusting the oral anticoagulant loading dose and maintenance doses is very necessary. Some patients could be particularly sensitive to warfarin—e.g. the elderly, those with high-risk factors, such as liver disease, heart failure, or diabetes mellitus, those who regularly consume alcohol, those on drug therapy that is known to ↑ or ↓ the effect of oral anticoagulation, and those with poor compliance. Knowledge of concomitant medical problems and medication is essential for the safe management of anticoagulation.

Reversing the effects of warfarin (or other vitamin K antagonists)

Because of the unpredictable nature of warfarin dosing, or when an anti-coagulated patient needs to go for an invasive procedure, it may be necessary to reverse the anticoagulant effects of warfarin.

Reversal of over-anticoagulation

In all cases of over anticoagulation proceed as follows.
- Identify the precipitating cause.
- Establish whether it is temporary (e.g. other medications) or permanent (e.g. liver failure).
- Review the need for ongoing anticoagulation.
- If the patient is to continue with anticoagulation therapy, the degree of reversal must be decided. For example, patients with metallic heart valves will need to continue their anticoagulation after the event, so complete reversal may not be indicated (except in the case of severe bleeding).

The risk of bleeding on warfarin increases significantly when the INR is ≥5.0. Therapeutic decisions regarding reversal depend on the INR level and the degree of bleeding.

Major/life-threatening bleeding requiring immediate/ complete reversal

This relates to patients with intracranial or rapid-onset neurological signs, intra-ocular (not conjunctival) bleeds, compartment syndrome, peri-cardial bleeds, or active bleeding and shock. These patients need urgent assessment of clotting.

Patients on warfarin may be haemorrhagic for reasons other than the effect of the anticoagulant, such as DIC or factor VIII inhibitor. An urgent full blood count should be requested as well as APTT and INR.
- Stop warfarin and reverse anticoagulation with prothrombin complex concentrate (PCC) *and* IV phytomenadione (vitamin K)
- Anticoagulation can be effectively reversed with approximately 50units/kg of PCC (maximum 3000units) *and* 5–10mg phytomenadione
- As soon as PCC has been given, another clotting screen should be performed to assess the degree of correction of INR. If not corrected, advice should be sought from a haematologist
- All patients with bleeding should be evaluated to see if there is a local anatomical reason for bleeding.

Minor bleeding

INR ≥5.0

- Omit warfarin.
- Give IV phytomenadione 0.5-1mg (or 5–10mg if anticoagulation is to be stopped).

INR <5.0

- A clinical decision needs to be made as to whether lowering the INR is required. If this is the case, consider giving IV phytomenadione 0.5–1mg and modifying the warfarin dose.

No bleeding

INR 5.0–7.9

- Omit warfarin.
- Restart at a lower dose when INR <5.0.

INR 8.0–12.0

- Omit warfarin.
- Give 1–5mg oral phytomenadione.

INR >12.0

- Omit warfarin.
- Give 5mg oral phytomenadione.

Product details

Phytomenadione

- For administration guidelines, see local or national injectables monographs.
- Oral phytomenadione will work within 16–24h of administration; IV phytomenadione will work within 6–8h.

Prothrombin complex concentrate

- Examples of PCCs are Beriplex® and Octaplex®.
- PCCs are derived from human plasma which has been virally inactivated, and they contain coagulation factors II, VII, IX and X.
- The dose should be rounded to the nearest complete vial.
- Doses stated are based on factor IX content.
- Administration of PCC more rapidly than is stated in the product literature is a clinical decision based on risk versus benefit.

Safe medication practice

- Fresh frozen plasma (FFP) is not recommended for warfarin reversal. In non-urgent situations, phytomenadione is sufficient, and in urgent situations PCC is more effective
- Anticoagulated patients should not be given IM injections
- Oral phytomenadione should generally be measured in multiples of 1mg so that doses can be accurately measured using the oral syringes provided with the licensed preparation
- The effects of PCC will wear off relatively quickly, so IV phytomenadione must be given as well if the reversal is to be sustained.

Out-patient anticoagulation clinics

Anticoagulation management is a good example of an area in which patient care is undertaken by a multidisciplinary team of physicians, nurses, and pharmacists. Although warfarin is an effective anticoagulant, its use is complicated in clinical practice by its narrow therapeutic index, with a relatively small margin between safety and toxicity, dietary fluctuations in vitamin K, the effects of certain disease states, and physiological, genetic, and patient-specific factors (e.g. compliance with therapy).

The major implications of long-term therapy with anticoagulants are a tendency to bleeding, haemorrhage, and other factors, such as interaction between warfarin and other drugs, which make it difficult to maintain anticoagulant control in the therapeutic range.

The anticoagulation clinic provides ongoing monitoring of the INR and continual recommendations for warfarin dose adjustment, including management of drug interactions involving warfarin and out-of-range INRs. The goal is to provide follow-up and dose adjustment adequate to maintain the INR within designated therapeutic ranges specific to the conditions for which the anticoagulation is indicated.

Hospital-based clinics

Oral anticoagulation monitoring has traditionally taken place in secondary care because of the need for laboratory testing. The need for frequent monitoring and close patient follow-up introduced the need for coordinated warfarin management by means of an organized system of clinical follow-up. Anticoagulation clinics have historically fulfilled this role. The patients attend the hospital for venepuncture; blood is then sent to the laboratory for testing. The pharmacist, doctor, or nurse is informed of the results and can then discuss dosage adjustment and arrange a further appointment for blood test and review. The healthcare professional also discusses whether any changes in the patient's diet or recent change in alcohol consumption, for example, might have been the reason for the INR being outside the patient's therapeutic range.

GP-surgery-based clinics

The development of reliable near-patient testing systems for INR estimation has facilitated the ability to manage patients within primary care. With the introduction of finger-prick testing services, there is no longer a reliance on the hospital pathology laboratory for INR measurement. The GP discusses compliance with patients and recommends dose and the follow-up date for INR recheck.

Outreach DVT service

In some cases, coordination between primary and secondary care is established. Patients attend their local surgery for blood sampling, the samples for laboratory analysis are collected, and subsequent dosing and patient management are undertaken within the secondary-care anti-coagulation clinic.

Domiciliary service

This service is only suitable for patients who are on the telephone and whose anticoagulation is reasonably well controlled. The patient's GP sends a district nurse to the patient's home to collect blood samples.

Future of services

- The emergence of novel anticoagulant therapies might have dramatic implications not only for patient management, but also for anti-coagulation clinics. Oral direct thrombin inhibitors (DTIs) and direct factor Xa inhibitors show promise as future agents to improve the field of oral anticoagulation management.
- Dabigatran (oral DTI) and rivaroxaban (oral direct factor Xa inhibitor) are in the most advanced phases of clinical development.
- Both of the aforementioned newer agents are currently licensed for thromboprophylaxis post elective hip or knee arthroplasty, and both are seeking marketing authorization for many other indications including stroke prevention in AF and secondary prevention of VTE following standard treatment.
- In theory, both agents have several advantages over warfarin. They have a wider therapeutic index, a predictable dose–response profile (i.e. they do not require dosing adjustments and monitoring), they are not metabolized through known hepatic microsomal enzymes and they seem to lack CYP450-related drug and food interactions. These advantages make them easier and more convenient to administer than warfarin therapy.
- The introduction of the newer agents could lead to a significant drop in the volume of warfarin patients referred to anticoagulation clinics for monitoring. However, because they are relatively expensive compared with warfarin (including the costs associated with ongoing monitoring of warfarin therapy) and clinicians have limited clinical experience of its use (especially with respect to bleeding complications), anticoagulation services will remain a necessary service for the foreseeable future.

Further reading

NICE (2010) Clinical Guideline CG92. Venous Thromboembolism—Reducing the Risk. http://guidance.nice.org.uk/CG92/NICEGuidance/pdf/English.
National Patient Safety Agency (2007). *Safety Alert 18. Actions That Can Make Anticoagulation Therapy Safer*. London: NPSA.
Baglin TP *et al.* (2006). Guidelines on oral anticoagulation (warfarin): third edition – 2005 update. *British Journal of Haematology* **132**: 277–85.
Baglin TP *et al.* (2006). Guidelines on the use and monitoring of heparin. *British Journal of Haematology* **133**: 19–34.
BJH Guideline on Treatment of VTE (due late 2010).
NICE Guidelines on Treatment of VTE (due late 2011/early 2012).

Acute coronary syndrome

- These syndromes are attributable to myocardial ischaemia secondary to coronary obstruction. The syndromes cover a spectrum of conditions ranging from unstable angina to STEMI.
- Unstable angina is a syndrome of chest pain caused by myocardial ischaemia; MI is heart muscle damage caused by prolonged ischaemia. The two conditions share the same pathophysiology, similar symptoms, and the same early management.
- The syndrome depends on the extent of thrombosis, distal platelet and thrombus embolization, and resultant myocardial necrosis.
- The acute coronary syndromes are differentiated according to the extent and duration of chest pain, electrocardiogram (ECG) changes, and biochemical markers.
- Acute coronary syndromes are differentiated into syndromes associated with the following.
  - ST-segment elevation on the ECG (ST-segment elevation MI (STEMI))
  - Without ST-segment elevation (non-ST-segment elevation MI (NSTEMI)), which is associated with ST-segment depression, T-wave inversion, or no changes on the ECG.
- NSTEMI is differentiated from unstable angina by biochemical evidence of myocardial necrosis. The diagnosis of myocardial necrosis is indicated by an ↑ troponin I level. Troponin I is detectible in serum 3–6h after an MI (peaks at 12–24h; elevated for 14 days). If troponin is normal >6h after the onset of pain and the ECG is normal, the risk of MI is small.
- Unstable angina and NSTEMI represent a continuum, and their management is similar.
- Patients presenting with pain at rest or severe exacerbation of stable angina are differentiated into high, low, or intermediate risk, depending on various factors.
- Patients with unstable angina are classified according to the highest-risk category of which they exhibit at least one feature.
- High-risk features.
  - Prolonged (>10min) ongoing chest pain/discomfort.
  - ST-segment elevation or depression (>0.5mm) or deep T-wave inversion in three or more ECG leads.
  - ↑ serum markers of myocardial injury (especially cardiac troponin I or T) (Fig. 17.2).
  - Diabetes mellitus.
  - Associated syncope.
  - Associated heart failure, mitral regurgitation, or gallop rhythm.
  - Associated haemodynamic instability (SBP <90mmHg, cool peripheries, and diaphoresis).
- Intermediate-risk features.
  - Prolonged, but resolved, chest pain/discomfort.
  - Nocturnal pain.
  - Age >65 years.
  - History of MI or revascularization.

- ECG normal or pathological Q-waves.
- No significant (<0.5mm) ST-segment deviation, or minor T-wave inversion in <3 ECG leads.
- Low-risk features.
  - ↑ angina frequency or severity.
  - Angina provoked at a lower threshold.
  - New-onset angina >2 weeks before presentation.
  - Normal ECG and negative serum troponin.
  - No high-risk or intermediate-risk features.

Fig. 17.2 Enzyme changes following acute MI. Reproduced with permission from Longmore M, Wilkinson IB, Rajagopalan S (2004). *Oxford Handbook of Clinical Medicine*, 6th edn. Oxford: Oxford University Press.

ST-segment elevation myocardial infarction (STEMI)

- If the thrombus that occurs on a ruptured plaque completely occludes the coronary artery so that there is no flow beyond it, the result is severe transmural myocardial ischaemia with ST-segment elevation on the ECG.
- This can cause sudden death from ventricular fibrillation.
- If the coronary occlusion is not relieved, MI develops progressively over the next 6–12h.
- The aim of emergency treatment of STEMI is as follows:
  - prevent and treat cardiac arrest
  - relieve pain
  - reperfuse the myocardium urgently to minimize infarct size.
- In STEMI it is important to reopen the artery and re-establish flow as soon as possible. This can be achieved by the administration of thrombolytic therapy or primary percutaneous coronary intervention (PCI).
- Thrombolytic therapy consists of a combination of a fibrinolytic agent, an antiplatelet agent, and antithrombin therapy.
- Reperfusion therapy should be delivered as soon as feasible. Current standards indicate that if thrombolytic therapy is chosen, it should be given within 30min of arrival in hospital.
- If primary PCI is the selected therapy, the aim should be to have the artery reopened within 60min of arrival at hospital.
- Early risk assessment allows categorization in terms of prognosis and choice of treatment. Initial indicators of high risk are ECG evidence of a large infarct, clinical and radiographic evidence of circulatory congestion, hypotension and shock, and serious arrhythmias.

STEMI: prehospital management

- The patient should be advised to call the ambulance directly, rest until it arrives, and immediately take aspirin 300mg (chewed or dissolved before swallowing), if available.
- The patient should also be advised to take a short-acting nitrate, if available.
  - GTN spray 400micrograms sublingually. Repeat after 5min if pain persists (up to a maximum of two metered doses).
  - GTN tablet 500micrograms sublingually. Repeat every 3–5min (up to a maximum dose of 1500micrograms, three tablets).
  - administer supplemental oxygen.
- If a doctor is present, add the following for pain relief, if required.
  - Morphine 2.5–5mg IV. Repeat as necessary.

STEMI: immediate and early hospital management

- An ECG should be performed immediately. If on the basis of clinical assessment and ECG, a diagnosis or presumptive diagnosis of STEMI can be made, give the following treatment.
  - Aspirin 300mg chewed or dissolved before swallowing (if aspirin has not been given) plus O_2 therapy.
- Patients known to have severe obstructive airway disease could underventilate with O_2 therapy and retain CO_2, becoming drowsy.
- For chest pain, use the following treatment:
  - GTN 500micrograms sublingually. Repeat after 5min if pain persists, provided that SBP >95mmHg.
- For persisting chest pain, add the following treatment.
  - Morphine 2.5–5mg IV (repeat as necessary) plus reperfusion therapy.

STEMI: reperfusion therapy

Patient selection for reperfusion therapy

Reperfusion therapy is indicated in the following circumstances.

- Ischaemic/infarction symptoms >20min. This includes not only chest pain, but also other symptoms of MI such as chest discomfort or pressure, shortness of breath, pulmonary oedema, sweating, dizziness, and light-headedness.
- Patient's symptoms commenced within 12h.
- ST-segement elevation or left bundle branch block on the ECG.
- No contraindications to reperfusion therapy.

Percutaneous coronary intervention (PCI)

PCI is the therapy of choice if it is available in a timely manner. Adjuvant therapy for PCI includes aspirin/clopidogrel and heparin. Some patients need a glycoprotein IIb/IIIa inhibitor. The timing of delivery of the agents is determined by the individual interventionalist.

Fibrinolytic therapy

Fibrinolytic therapy is indicated in the following situation: prolonged ischaemic chest pain that has begun within the previous 12h in the presence of significant ST-segment elevation or left bundle branch block (presumed new).

The decision whether or not to give fibrinolysis requires analysis of risk versus benefit. Patients likely to gain most benefit from fibrinolytic therapy present early with large MI, usually anterior, especially if there is any evidence of heart failure. Those with small MI, often inferior, benefit less. After 24h, the chances of benefit are very small and there is ↑ risk of cardiac rupture.

Contraindications to fibrinolytic therapy can be absolute or relative.

Absolute contraindications

- Risk of bleeding:
  - active bleeding
  - recent (<1 month) major surgery or trauma.

- Risk of intracranial haemorrhage:
  - any history of haemorrhagic stroke or history: ischaemic stroke within the past 2–6 months
  - anatomical abnormalities, intracerebral neoplasms, and arteriovenous malformation.

Relative contraindications
- Risk of bleeding:
  - previous use of anticoagulants or INR >2.0
  - non-compressible vascular punctures
  - prolonged cardiopulmonary resuscitation (>10min)
- Risk of intracranial haemorrhage:
  - previous stroke at any time
  - previous transient ischaemic attack (TIA).
- Other:
  - pregnancy
  - severe hypertension that cannot be controlled (>180mmHg SBP and/or >110mmHg DBP).

Patients with absolute contraindications should be transferred for a PCI. With relative contraindication, the risks and benefits of treatment must be weighed up.

Use one of the following thrombolytic agents.
- Alteplase 15mg bolus IV, followed by an IV infusion of 0.75mg/kg body weight over a period of 30min (up to a maximum of 50mg); then 0.5mg/kg body weight over a period of 60min up to 35mg (the total dose should not exceed 100mg).
- Reteplase 10IU bolus IV, followed by 10IU 30min later.
- Streptokinase 1.5 million IU by IV infusion over a period of 20–30min. If SBP <80mmHg, the infusion rate should be halved. If SBP <70mmHg, stop the infusion until BP >70mmHg and then restart at half the previous rate.
- Tenecteplase 500micrograms/kg body weight over a period of 30s (up to a maximum dose of 50 mg).

The plasminogen activators alteplase, reteplase, and tenecteplase are superior to streptokinase but considerably more expensive. Thus streptokinase is the drug of choice. Because antibodies are produced against streptokinase, there is ↑ risk of allergic reactions if the patient is re-treated within 1 year. Prolonged exposure of antibodies to streptokinase can ↓ the effectiveness of subsequent treatment, and streptokinase should not be used again beyond 4 days of the first administration.

The bolus agents reteplase (double bolus) and tenecteplase (single bolus) have major advantages in terms of convenience and can be used in the pre-hospital setting, usually by suitably trained paramedic staff.

Recurrence of chest pain with ST-segment elevation is evidence of re-occlusion, and therefore further thombolysis or urgent angioplasty might be indicated. Hypotension can occur, particularly with streptokinase, and should be treated by raising the foot of the bed and adjusting the infusion rate.

Allergic reactions are common with streptokinase and include bronchospasm, periorbital swelling, angio-oedema, urticaria, itching, flushing, nausea, headache, and musculoskeletal pain. Delayed hypersensitivity reactions, such as vasculitis and interstitial nephritis, have also been observed. Anaphylactic shock is rare.

For mild or moderate allergic reactions and fever, use promethazine 25mg IV and/or hydrocortisone 100mg IV. For severe allergic reactions, immediately discontinue streptokinase and give adrenaline 1:10 000 solution, 1mL IV, over a period of 5min.

Antithrombin therapy

- There is still debate about the use of IV heparin with streptokinase.
- However, there seems to be a small, but significant, benefit. IV UFH is usually given routinely in conjunction with alteplase, reteplase, or tenecteplase. Use UFH 60IU/kg body weight initially (up to a maximum of 4000IU), followed by 12IU/kg body weight adjusted according to the APTT.
- The initial APTT should be taken in 3h and adjusted according to local protocol.
- LMWH has been used in conjunction with fibrinolytic agents. It seems to ↓ reinfarction, but at the cost of ↑ bleeding. It is currently under-going assessment in a large clinical trial. LMWH is not formally approved for use in combination with fibrinolytic agents. Particular care is needed in patients >75 years old; excess bleeding, including intra-cranial haemorrhage, has been reported.
- Occasionally, bleeding can occur following treatment with fibrinolytic therapy and heparin. Intracranial haemorrhages are devastating and life-threatening. Systemic bleeding and GI bleeding can occur, in which case the following treatments are advised:
  - Reverse heparin with protamine. Protamine dosage depends on the level of anticoagulation. Use 1mg of protamine for every 100IU of UFH or 1mg of protamine sulphate for every 100IU (anti-Xa) of dalteparin. The usual maximum dose is 50mg given by slow IV injection (rate not exceeding 5mg/min).
  - Replace fibrinogen using cryoprecipitate (two bags) or fresh frozen plasma (as required).
  - Give blood, as necessary.

Other therapy

- An IV β-blocker should be considered for patients with persistent pain and tachycardia that is not related to heart failure, those with hypertension, and those with a large MI:
  - atenolol 5–10mg IV infusion at a rate of 1mg/min or metoprolol 5–15mg IV infusion at a rate of 1–2mg/min.
- Titrate doses to the maximum dose of the recommended range, provided that SBP does not fall below 95mmHg and heart rate does not fall below 55bpm.
- β-blockers are contraindicated in patients with a significant history of bronchospasm or symptomatic bradycardia.

- The routine use of magnesium in the management of patients with acute MI is not recommended. Electrolyte abnormalities should be corrected appropriately.

Subsequent management of STEMI

On the basis of the probable contribution to clinical decision-making, further investigation should be considered. Many patients will undergo coronary angiography. Provided that there are no contraindications, continue with following treatment regimen:

- aspirin 75–300mg oral daily or (if intolerant of aspirin) clopidogrel 75mg oral daily.

β-blocker therapy

- β-blockers offer prognostic benefit following MI, especially in high-risk patients such as those with significant left ventricular dysfunction and/or ongoing ischaemia, and should be commenced during hospital admission unless contraindicated. Any of the following regimens is recommended:
  - atenolol 25–100mg oral daily
  - metoprolol 25–100mg oral twice daily
  - timolol 5–10mg twice daily
  - propranolol 40–80mg four times daily.
- Titrate doses to the maximum dose in the recommended range, provided that SBP does not fall below 95mmHg and heart rate does not fall below 55bpm.
- The benefit of β-blocker therapy persists long term, and it should be continued indefinitely in high-risk patients.
- The usual contraindications to the use of β-blockers apply. Patients with significant left ventricular dysfunction should be observed closely for the development of congestive heart failure.

ACE inhibitor therapy

- ACE inhibitors improve outcome after acute MI. Start ACE inhibitor therapy within 24–48h of acute MI in patients with previous MI, diabetes mellitus, hypertension, anterior location of infarct on ECG, elevated heart rate (>80bpm), and clinical or radiographic evidence of left ventricular failure or significant dysfunction (ejection fraction <45%).
- ACE inhibitors should be continued long term in patients with a low ejection fraction.
- Contraindications to early ACE inhibitor use include haemodynamic instability and hypotension (SBP <100mmHg). Complications of early ACE inhibitor therapy include persistent hypotension and renal dysfunction.

- BP should be closely monitored, and renal function and plasma electrolytes should be monitored on alternate days while the patient is in hospital. If the maintenance dose has not been achieved at discharge, the dose must be ↑ more slowly as an out-patient (e.g. weekly), with renal function and plasma electrolytes determined before each increase in dose.
- Angiotensin II receptor antagonists should be reserved (for this indication) for patients who develop a persistent cough with ACE inhibitor therapy.

Statin therapy
Statin therapy reduces premature death, MI, and other adverse outcomes, such as stroke and revascularization post-MI. Statin therapy should be continued, or initiated, during hospital admission, no matter what the underlying cholesterol level.

Calcium-channel blocker therapy
The use of calcium-channel blockers should be reserved for patients who have post-MI angina and a contraindication to a β-blocker.

Drug treatment in acute coronary syndromes

Drug treatment of high-risk unstable angina/NSTEMI

- Initial therapy for high-risk patients is hospitalization, with subsequent ECG monitoring and platelet inhibition, antithrombin therapy, use of a β-blocker and, potentially, glycoprotein IIb/IIIa inhibitors, and revascularization.
- For pain relief in patients requiring hospital admission, give GTN 10micrograms/min by IV infusion; ↑ by 10micrograms/min every 3min until pain is controlled provided that SBP >95mmHg (dose range for GTN is 10–200micrograms/min).
- Normally, IV GTN is required for only a short period; prolonged infusion rapidly induces tolerance.
- For patients in whom there is a contraindication to β-blockers, a non-dihydropyridine calcium-channel blocker can be substituted. For example, use one of the following regimens:
  - diltiazem 30–120mg oral, three times daily
  - diltiazem controlled release 180–360mg oral, daily
  - verapamil 40–120mg oral, twice to three times daily
  - verapamil sustained release 160–480mg oral, daily.
- For patients in whom angina has not been controlled with a β-blocker alone, a dihydropyridine calcium-channel blocker can be added— e.g. nifedipine sustained release or amlodipine.
- When the pain is nocturnal, long-acting nitrates might best be given at night rather than during the day.
- Isosorbide mononitrate 20–120mg oral, daily in divided doses.
- Avoid nitrates if the patient has used sildenafil (Viagra®) in the previous 24h or tadalafil (Cialis®) in the previous 5 days.
- Pain nearly always settles promptly.
- After initial assessment and management, patients gradually return to the same risk as patients with stable angina.
- Patients who have undergone revascularization procedures involving a coronary stent must be on aspirin and clopidogrel for at least 1 month, and for those receiving drug-eluting stents, this should be for a minimum of 3 months.

Platelet inhibition
Aspirin 75–300mg oral, daily, and clopidogrel 75mg oral, daily (initial loading dose of 300mg).

Antithrombin therapy
- UFH or LMWH should be given in addition to aspirin. One of the following regimens is advised.
  - enoxaparin 1mg/kg body weight SC, twice daily
  - dalteparin, 120units/kg body weight SC, twice daily (up to a maximum of 10 000units).
  - UFH 5000units bolus IV, followed by 1000units/h by IV infusion and then dose adjustment according to the APTT.

- UFH or LMWH should be administered for a minimum of 3days and possibly longer, depending on the clinical response.
- The advantages of LMWH are that it can be given subcutaneously and it has a more predictable effect, so constant monitoring is not required. However, the fact that its effect cannot easily be reversed is a disadvantage for the high-risk patient who might require urgent intervention. Care should be taken in the elderly and in those with impaired renal function, in whom the dose should be decreased in accordance with the drug's SPC or with renal dosing guidelines.
- For patients on IV UFH, the APTT should be checked initially every 6h, with a target range of 60–80s, and should be checked daily after therapy has been stabilized.

β-blocker

- All patients without contraindications to β-blockade should be commenced on a β-blocker. Either of the following regimens is recommended:
  - atenolol 25–100mg oral, once daily
  - metoprolol 25–100mg oral, twice daily.

Glycoprotein IIb/IIIa inhibitors

These agents prevent the binding of fibrinogen, thereby blocking platelet aggregation.

- Some glycoprotein IIb/IIIa inhibitors are beneficial in ↓ MI and death in patients with NSTEMI or high-risk unstable angina. They are of particular benefit in patients who have an elevated troponin level and/or who are undergoing PCI. They are recommended for patients who are at high risk and have abnormal ECGs or a positive troponin test.
- Treatment with glycoprotein IIb/IIIa inhibitors occurs in two different clinical situations.
  - Patients might be treated in the coronary care unit (with tirofiban only) for a number of hours (up to 9h) before undergoing investigation and PCI, if appropriate.
  - Patients might be treated (with abciximab only) at the time of the procedure.

Tirofiban (non-peptide antagonist of glycoprotein IIb/IIIc receptors)

- Approved for use in combination with heparin for patients with unstable angina who are being treated medically and for those undergoing PCI.
- When administered IV, more than 90% of platelet aggregation is inhibited.
- A loading dose of tirofiban 400ng/kg body weight/min is administered over 30min, followed by a maintenance infusion of 100ng/kg body weight/min for up to 108h.

Abciximab (chimeric human–murine monoclonal antibody)
- Approved for use in elective/urgent/emergent PCI.
- Binds to receptor with high affinity and reduces platelet aggregation by 80%. Persists for up to 48h after end of infusion.
- Loading dose of abciximab 250micrograms/kg body weight bolus before the intervention, followed by a maintenance infusion dose of 125ng/kg body weight/min (up to a maximum of 10micrograms/min) administered over the 12h following the PCI.

Eptifibatide
- Antagonist of the platelet glycoprotein IIb/IIIc receptor, which reversibly prevents von Willebrand factor, fibrinogen, and other adhesion ligands from binding to the receptor.
- Prevention of early MI in patients with unstable angina or NSTEMI with last episode of chest pain within 24h.
  - Unstable angina—180micrograms/kg IV bolus, followed by continuous infusion until discharge or surgery.
  - PCI—135micrograms/kg IV bolus administered before PCI, followed by a continuous infusion of 0.5micrograms/kg/min.

Prasugrel
Used in combination with aspirin for the prevention of atherothrombotic events in patients with acute coronary syndromes undergoing PCI only when immediate primary PCI is necessary for STEMI, or stent thrombosis occurred during treatment with clopidogrel, or the patient has diabetes mellitus.
- 60mg as a single dose, then 10mg daily in patients >60kg, or 5mg daily in patients <60kg or aged >75 years.

Revascularization
Revascularization should be considered in all patients who are at high risk. Clinical trials have demonstrated the benefit of an early invasive strategy.

Drug treatment of intermediate-risk unstable angina/ NSTEMI

Patients who are deemed to be at intermediate risk are admitted for monitoring and reassessment of clinical status, ECG, and biochemical markers. They are then reclassified, depending on the results of these investigations, into high or low risk. If it is thought probable that the patient has coronary artery disease, treatment while undergoing assessment should include aspirin (or clopidogrel) and heparin.

Drug treatment of low-risk unstable angina/NSTEMI

Patients who are low risk need cardiac assessment to rule out coronary disease. This involves stress testing, which could be exercise testing with an ECG, stress echocardiography, or nuclear stress study. Patients proved to have coronary disease should proceed to further investigation and management. Patients should be treated with platelet inhibitors (usually aspirin) while being assessed.

Cardiopulmonary resuscitation

Cardiac arrest in adults: what the pharmacist needs to know

The management of cardiopulmonary arrest can be divided into two categories: basic and advanced life support. Note that this advice applies to **adults only.**

Basic life support

Basic life support is the 'first-responder' phase of the chain of survival. It can be carried out by anyone who has the relevant knowledge or training (Fig. 17.3).

Shout for help. Ask someone to call the arrest team and to bring the defibrillator. Note the time.

Before approaching the patient, the first responder should always check that it is safe to do so. The patient should then be assessed (e.g. check consciousness by calling the patient's name or shaking (if no response) to confirm that an arrest has occurred. This is done by checking the airway, breathing, and circulation (ABC).

- Airway
  - Tilt head (if no spine injury) and lift chin/jaw thrust. Clear the mouth. If this does not restore breathing then:
- Breathing
  - Pinch the patient's nose shut and give two breaths (each inflation should be 2s long), ideally using the Ambu system. Otherwise give mouth-to-mouth resuscitation (unless poisoning is suspected).
- Chest compressions
- Check for pulse, taking no longer than 10s. If no pulse found, then:
  - Give 30 compressions to 2 breaths (30:2). Cardiopulmonary resuscitation (CPR) should not be interrupted, except to give shocks or intubate. Use the heel of the hand with the other hand placed on top and straight elbows. in the middle of the lower half of the sternum, which should be depressed by ~5cm. Compressions should be fairly fast (~100/min). Chest compressions work to promote the forward flow of blood. (Allow the chest to recoil completely between each compression.)
  - Do not start chest compressions if you do not think that you can continue until the cardiac arrest team arrives, as compressions may lead to asystole whereas prior to compressions there may have been some (although inefficient) activity. Alternatively the person providing chest compressions should change about every 2min.

The most common cause of cardiac arrest is an arrhythmia—ventricular fibrillation. Ventricular fibrillation is known as a 'shockable rhythm' because it responds to defibrillation.

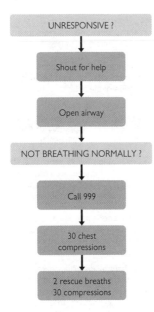

UNRESPONSIVE ?

↓

Shout for help

↓

Open airway

↓

NOT BREATHING NORMALLY ?

↓

Call 999

↓

30 chest
compressions

↓

2 rescue breaths
30 compressions

Managing the airway

- You open the airway by tilting the head and lifting the chin—but only do this if there is no question of spinal trauma.
- Use a close-fitting mask if available, held in place by thumbs pressing downwards either side of the mouthpiece; palms against cheeks.

Chest compressions

- Cardiopulmonary resuscitation (CPR) involves compressive force over the lower sternum with the heal of the hands placed one on top of the other, directing the weight of your body through your vertical, straight, arms.
- Depth of compression: ~4cm.
- Rate of compressions: 100/min.

Fig. 17.3 UK adult basic life support algorithm. Reproduced with permission from the Resuscitation Council (UK).

Advanced life support

Advanced life support starts when medical personnel arrive, and is nominally provided by the cardiac arrest team (Fig. 17.4).

- Basic life support maintained.
- The patient's airway is secured and O_2 is administered.
- IV access is obtained (in hospital, blood is taken for urgent blood gas analysis and determination of electrolyte levels).

The patient is attached to the cardiac monitor on the defibrillator to allow diagnosis of the arrhythmia. Further management depends on whether or not the type of arrhythmia present responds to defibrillation. In addition to ventricular fibrillation, pulseless ventricular tachycardia responds to defibrillation.

Treat ventricular fibrillation/pulseless ventricular tachycardia (VF/VT) with a single shock, followed by immediate resumption of CPR (30 compressions to 2 ventilations). Do not reassess the rhythm or feel for a pulse. After 2min of CPR, check the rhythm and give another shock (if indicated).

- The recommended initial energy for biphasic defibrillators is 150–200J. Give second and subsequent shocks at 150–360J.
- The recommended energy when using a monophasic defibrillator is 360J for both the initial and subsequent shocks.

Asystole and electromechanical disturbance cannot be corrected using defibrillation. Asystole is the absence of any heart rhythm. Electromechanical disturbance (also known as pulseless electrical activity) is the presence of organized electrical activity that fails to result in mechanical contraction of the heart.

Pharmaceutical aspects of cardiopulmonary resuscitation

Basic CPR and early defibrillation are the only interventions proved to benefit survival in cardiac arrest. However, drugs have a role and should always be considered.

In hospital, an 'arrest box', containing a variety of drugs, is usually kept with the arrest trolley. Drugs in the arrest box commonly tend to be pre-assembled syringes.

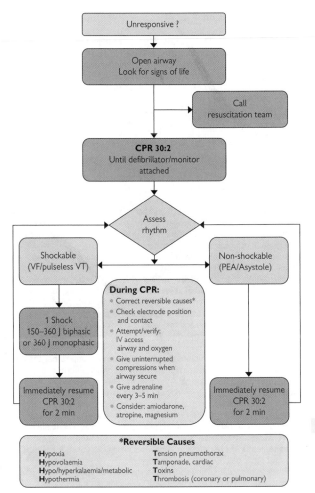

Fig. 17.4 UK adult advanced life support algorithm. Reproduced with permission from the Resuscitation Council (UK).

Drug administration

- *Adrenaline*
  - When treating VF/VT cardiac arrest, current guidelines recommend the administration of 1mg of adrenaline IV (i.e. 10mL of 1 in 10 000 pre-filled syringe) is given after the third shock once chest compressions have restarted and then every 3–5min during resuscitation. IV doses >1mg are no longer considered to be of benefit and should not be used.
  - For IV administration, a flush of 20mL of sodium chloride 0.9% solution should be administered after each drug dose to enhance its passage from the peripheral circulation to the central circulation. Alternatively, the dose can be given in tandem with a fast-flowing IV fluid.
  - If IV access is unattainable, giving drugs via a tracheal tube is no longer recommended. Drugs should be given by the intraosseous (IO) route (tibial and humeral sites preferred).
- *Atropine* was often used in the management of asystole or bradycardia to block any excessive vagal activity that might be contributing to a ↓ in heart rate. Atropine is no longer recommended for asystole and slow pulseless electrical activity (<60/min). Smaller doses (0.5–1mg IV) can be given in bradycardia, up to a maximum total of 3mg.
- *Amiodarone* is the anti-arrhythmic of choice in resistant ventricular fibrillation or pulseless ventricular tachycardia. If VF/VT persists after three shocks, a dose of 300mg in 20mL glucose 5% solution is given as a slow bolus over a period of at least 3min before delivery of the fourth shock. Remember that amiodarone is incompatible with normal saline, and bags of glucose 5% solution should be available to enable prompt setting up of the infusion and for flushing after dose(s). A further 150mg can be given, followed by an infusion of 1mg/min for 6h, and then 0.5mg/min for 6h. It is recommended that, if possible, amiodarone is administered using a volumetric control infusion pump rather than drip-counting technique because of the drug's affect on drip size. If amiodarone is not available, lidocaine 1mg/kg can be used as an alternative, but do not give lidocaine if amiodarone has already been given. Do not exceed a total dose of 3mg/kg during the first hour.
- *Magnesium sulphate* is the agent of choice in torsades de pointes, a type of arrhythmia that is often drug-induced. It can also be useful in resistant arrhythmias, especially if they are associated with hypo-magnesaemia (more common in patients taking diuretics). A bolus of 8mmol (4mL of a 50% w/v) is usually given.
- *Sodium bicarbonate* Giving sodium bicarbonate routinely during cardiac arrest and CPR is not recommended. Give sodium bicarbonate (50mmol) if cardiac arrest is associated with hyperkalaemia or tricyclic antidepressant overdose. Repeat the dose according to the clinical condition of the patient and the results of repeated blood gas analysis. Should only be administered after arterial blood gas analysis where pH has fallen below 7.1. A 50mmol dose (50mL of the 8.4%solution) would normally be given as a slow IV bolus.

- *Oxygen* Once return of spontaneous circulation is achieved and oxygen saturation of arterial blood can be monitored (by pulse oximetry and/or arterial blood gas analysis), inspired oxygen should be titrated to achieve SaO$_2$ of 94–98%.
- *Calcium chloride* 10mL of the 10% preparation (equivalent to 6.8mmol of calcium ions) is administered in suspected or actual calcium-channel blocker overdose or in magnesium-induced heart block. Calcium can slow the heart rate and precipitate arrhythmias. ▶ Do not give calcium solutions and sodium bicarbonate simultaneously by the same route.

Resuscitation is generally stopped after 20min if there is refractory asystole or electromechanical dissociation.

After successful resuscitation, perform the following:
- 12-lead ECG, CXR, U&Es, glucose, blood gases, FBC, creatinine kinase/troponin levels.
- Transfer to coronary care unit.
- Monitor vital signs.
- Communicate to relatives.

Suggested contents of the adult emergency drug box used in pre-arrest and arrest situations
- 5x adrenaline 1:10 000 solution, 1mg in 10mL pre-filled syringe (pre-assembled syringe).
- 1x atropine 3mg in 10mL pre-filled syringe (pre-assembled syringe).
- 1x amiodarone 300mg in 10mL pre-filled syringe (pre-assembled syringe).
- 1x 5% glucose, 50mL to flush amiodarone.

Suggested contents of back-up emergency box, containing the following drugs
- 6x adenosine, 6mg in 2mL vial.
- 5x adrenaline 1:1000 solution, 1mg in 1mL ampoule.
- 2x amiodarone 150mg in 3mL ampoule.
- 6x atropine 500mg in pre-filled syringe (pre-assembled syringe).
- 1x calcium chloride 6.8mmol in 10mL (10%) pre-filled syringe (pre-assembled syringe).
- 1x 50% glucose solution in 50mL vial.
- 1x magnesium sulphate 10mmol in 5mL (50% solution) pre-filled syringe (pre-assembled syringe).
- 1x sodium bicarbonate 8.4% in 50mL pre-filled syringe (pre-assembled syringe).

It is envisaged that back-up emergency boxes are normally issued to the wards and departments with manual defibrillators.

Therapy-related issues: respiratory system

Asthma management in adults: British Thoracic Society
    and SIGN guidelines *390*
Inhaler techniques *392*

Asthma management in adults: British Thoracic Society and SIGN guidelines

Aims
- Minimize symptoms during the day and night.
- Minimize need for reliever medication.
- No exacerbations.
- No limitation on physical activity.
- Achieve best possible pulmonary function.

Treatment
- Initiate treatment at the level most appropriate to the severity of asthma (Table 18.1).
- Step up treatment as necessary.
- Before initiating new therapy re-check compliance and inhaler technique, and eliminate trigger factors.
  - If trials of add-on therapies are ineffective, stop.
  - If trials of ↑ steroids are ineffective, return to original dose.
- Step down treatment levels if control is good:
- Review regularly while treatment is stepped down.

Table 18.1 Management of chronic asthma in adults

Level	Reliever therapy	Additional therapies	Further advice/therapy considerations
Step 1			
Mild Intermittent asthma	Inhaled short-acting β_2-agonist PRN		Review patients with high usage of reliever (>10 puffs/day is a marker of poorly controlled asthma)
Step 2			
Regular preventer therapy	Inhaled short-acting β_2-agonist PRN	Add inhaled steroid (200–800 micrograms daily)	Start at a dose appropriate to the severity and titrate to lowest effective dose. Usual dose is 400micrograms/daily
			Initially, divide dose twice daily; use once daily if good response is established

Table 18.1 (Contd.)

Level	Reliever therapy	Additional therapies	Further advice/therapy considerations
Step 3			
Add-on therapy	Inhaled short-acting β_2-agonist PRN	Add inhaled steroid (200–800 micrograms daily)	Good response to LABA—continue
			Improvement with LABA but poor response—continue and ↑ inhaled steroid to 800micrograms daily
		Add inhaled long-acting β_2-agonist (LABA)	If control is still inadequate, go to step 4
			No response to LABA—discontinue LABA and ↑ inhaled steroid dose to 800micrograms daily. If control still inadequate, trial other therapies—e.g. leukotriene receptor antagonists, theophylline, and slow-release oral β_2-agonists
			If control still inadequate, go to step 4
Step 4			
Persistent poor control	Inhaled short-acting β_2-agonist PRN	Add inhaled steroid (800micrograms daily)	Consider trials of ↑ inhaled steroids, up to 2000micrograms daily. Consider trials of fourth drug—e.g. leukotriene receptor antagonists, theophylline, and slow-release oral β_2 agonists
		Inhaled LABA (unless discontinued because of poor response)	
Step 5			
Continuous or frequent use of oral steroids	Inhaled short-acting β_2-agonist PRN	High-dose inhaled steroid (2000 micrograms daily)	Consider other treatments to minimize use of oral steroids
			Refer to a specialist
		Use oral steroids at lowest dose for adequate control	

Inhaler techniques

Metered-dose inhalers

The checklist steps for using a pressurized MDI are as follows.

- Sit or stand upright.
- Remove cap and shake the inhaler vigorously.
- Breathe out slowly and completely.
- Hold the inhaler in the upright position.
- Insert mouthpiece into mouth, between closed lips.
- Depress the canister once . . .
- . . . and at this time, begin slow, deep inhalation.
- Remove inhaler, with lips closed.
- Hold breath for 10–15s.
- Wait for 20–30s before starting the second puff.

Emphasize that coordination of the commencement of breathing with the release of medicament is very important and can require practice to maximize benefit.

The pharmacist may need to consider the use of a spacer or Haleraid® device for specific patients.

Points for the pharmacist/technician

- Demonstrate the correct method of use with a placebo inhaler, and ask the patient to show you how they use it. Most patients are on long-term therapy and many might have developed bad habits.
- The degree of benefit can be demonstrated to the patient by determining peak expiratory flow rates before dosing and 30min afterwards.
- Patients with anything other than mild occasional attacks derive considerable benefit from learning about their disease and how to manage it. They should measure peak expiratory flow rates regularly and keep a diary of the results.

Advice to the patient

- Keep the device clean and replace the mouthpiece cap after use.
- The plastic housing can be cleaned with warm mild detergent solution. Ensure that it is dried before use.

Dry-powder inhalers

Several devices are now available to deliver the medicament in a dry-powder inhaler. Because the medicines are dry powder, they must be inhaled fast enough so that the medicine is released. The basic technique for using a dry-powder medication is as follows.

- Exhale.
- Put the mouthpiece in your mouth.
- Breathe in quickly and deeply.

Diskhaler®

A Diskhaler® is a dry-powder inhaler that holds small pouches (or blisters), each containing a dose of medication, on a disk. The Diskhaler® punctures each blister so that its medication can be inhaled.

The basic technique for using the Diskhaler® is as follows.

- Remove the cover and check that the device and mouthpiece are clean.
- If a new medication disk is needed, pull the corners of the white cartridge out as far as they will go and then press the ridges on the sides inwards to remove the cartridge.
- Place the medication disk with its numbers facing upwards on the white rotating wheel. Then slide the cartridge all the way back in.
- Pull the cartridge all the way out, and then push it all the way in until the highest number on the medication disk can be seen in the indicator window.
- With the cartridge fully inserted and the device kept flat, raise the lid as far as it will go to pierce both sides of the medication blister.
- Move the Diskhaler® away from your mouth and breathe out.
- Place the mouthpiece between teeth and lips, making sure that you do not cover the air holes on the mouthpiece. Inhale quickly and deeply. Do not breathe out.
- Move the Diskhaler® away from your mouth and continue holding your breath for 10s.
- Breathe out slowly.
- If you need another dose, pull the cartridge out all the way and then push it back in all the way. This will move the next blister into place. Repeat procedure.
- After you have finished using the Diskhaler®, put the mouthpiece cap back on.

Turbohaler®

The basic technique for using the Turbohaler® dry-powder inhaler is as follows.

- Remove the cap from the Turbohaler® by unscrewing it.
- Hold the Turbohaler® with the mouthpiece up.
- Turn the bottom of the Turbohaler® all the way to the right and back to the left. You will hear it click.
- Hold the Turbohaler® away from your mouth and gently breathe out.
- Seal your lips around the mouthpiece.
- Inhale rapidly and deeply. Continue to take a full deep breath.
- Resume normal breathing.
- Repeat procedure if more than one puff is prescribed.
- Keep the Turbohaler® cap on when not in use.

Other points to tell patients include the following.

- When the red dot appears at the top of the window, there are 20 doses left. Plan to get a new Turbohaler® when you see the red dot.
- When the red dot is at the bottom of the window, the Turbohaler® is empty. Start using a new Turbohaler®.

Accuhaler®

The basic technique for using the Accuhaler® dry-powder inhaler is as follows.

- Open the Accuhaler® by holding the outer case in one hand and putting the thumb of the other hand on the thumb grip. Push your thumb away as far as it will go until a click is heard.
- Prime the dose by sliding the lever at the right of the mouthpiece away from you until a click is heard. Every time the lever is pushed back, a blister is opened and the powder is made available for inhaling. This is shown by the counter.
- Hold the Accuhaler® away from your mouth and breathe out as far as comfortable. Remember—never breathe into the Accuhaler®.
- Put the mouthpiece to your lips, and breathe in quickly and deeply.
- Remove the Accuhaler® from your mouth. Hold your breath for about 10s or for as long as is comfortable.
- Close the Accuhaler® by sliding the thumb grip back towards you. It should click shut.

Therapy-related issues: central nervous system

Pain: a definition *396*
Assessment of pain *398*
Acute pain: incidence *401*
Acute pain *402*
Treating cancer pain *404*
Equianalgesic doses for opioids *406*
Compatibility of drugs in pain and palliative care *407*
Chronic pain *408*

Pain: a definition

The International Association for the Study of Pain defines pain as *'an unpleasant sensory and emotional experience associated with actual or potential tissue damage, or described in terms of such damage'*.

Pain is always subjective. Each individual learns the application of the word through experiences related to injury in early life. Accordingly, pain is that experience we associate with actual or potential tissue damage. It is unquestionably a sensation in a part or parts of the body, but it is always unpleasant and therefore is also an emotional experience.

Many people report pain in the absence of tissue damage or any likely pathophysiological cause. Usually this happens for psychological reasons. There is usually no way to distinguish their experience from that caused by tissue damage if we take the subjective report. If they regard their experience as pain and if they report it in the same way as pain caused by tissue damage, it should be accepted as pain. This definition avoids tying pain to the stimulus.[1] In view of this, pharmacists should be wary of expressing opinions about whether a particular patient is in pain or not.

Types of pain

Nociceptive pain

'Nociceptive pain' is pain that occurs when nociceptors (pain receptors) are stimulated. This is normal pain in response to injury of the body. The purpose of this type of pain is to discourage the use of injured body parts, which could potentially extend the injury further. This pain normally responds to conventional analgesics, such as paracetamol, NSAIDs, and opioids (Fig. 19.1).

Neuropathic pain

'Neuropathic pain' is pain initiated or caused by a primary lesion or dysfunction in the nervous system. The pain is often triggered by an injury, but this injury might or might not involve actual damage to the nervous system. It seems to have no physiological purpose. The pain frequently has burning, lancinating (stabbing), or electric-shock qualities. Persistent allodynia, pain resulting from a non-painful stimulus such as a light touch, is also a common characteristic of neuropathic pain. The pain can persist for months or years beyond the apparent healing of any damaged tissues. This pain might not respond to standard analgesics but might respond to unconventional analgesic treatments, such as antidepressants, anticonvulsants, and various other therapies, such as clonidine or capsaicin. (Fig. 19.1).

---

1 International Association for the Study of Pain. ✍ http://www.iasp-pain.org

Fig. 19.1 Treating pain—methods available.

Assessment of pain

There are good validated scales for assessing pain. These are usually derived from assessment of both pain intensity and pain relief when analgesics are used. Both visual analogue scales (VASs), a line moving from 'no pain' to 'worst possible pain', and categorical scales, using words such as 'none', 'slight', 'moderate' or 'severe', are employed, often together. They can be useful to monitor progress in patients who are suffering from pain.

Categorical scales

Categorical scales use words to describe the magnitude of the pain. The patient picks the most appropriate word; most research groups use four words (none, mild, moderate, and severe). Scales to measure pain relief were developed later. The most common is the five-category scale (none, slight, moderate, good, and complete).

For analysis, numbers are given to the verbal categories (for pain intensity, none = 0, mild = 1, moderate = 2, and severe = 3, and for relief, none = 0, slight = 1, moderate = 2, good or lots = 3, and complete = 4).

The main advantages of categorical scales are that they are quick and simple. However, the small number of descriptors could force the scorer to choose a particular category when none describes the pain satisfactorily.

Visual analogue scales

VASs, lines with the left end labelled 'no relief of pain' and the right end labelled 'complete relief of pain', seem to overcome this limitation (Fig. 19.2). The standard VAS is 100mm long. Patients mark the line at the point that corresponds to their pain. The scores are obtained by measuring the distance between the 'no relief' end and the patient's mark, usually in millimetres. The main advantages of VASs are that they are simple and quick to score, avoid imprecise descriptive terms, and provide many points from which to choose. More concentration and coordination are needed, which can be difficult postoperatively or with neurological dis-orders.

Pain relief scales are perceived as more convenient than pain intensity scales, probably because patients have the same baseline relief (zero), whereas they could start with different baseline intensities (usually moderate or severe). They are based on the same approach of a 100mm scale but are asked to rate the amount of relief from 0 to 100mm. Relief scale results are then easier to compare. They can also be more sensitive than intensity scales. A theoretical drawback of relief scales is that the patient has to remember what the pain was like to begin with.

Global subjective efficacy ratings, or simply 'global scales', are designed to measure overall treatment performance. Patients are asked questions such as 'How effective do you think the treatment was?' and answer using a labelled numerical or categorical scale. Although these judgements probably include adverse effects, they can be the most sensitive way to discriminate between treatments.

Judgement of pain by the patient, rather than by a carer, is the ideal. Carers tend to overestimate the pain relief compared with the patient's version (Fig. 19.2).

Instructions

It is important that the use of the scale is explained to each patient. Patients are instructed to place a mark on the line to report the intensity or quality of the sensation experienced. Instructions should be written above the scale, e.g. INSTRUCTION: Put a mark on the line at the point that best describes HOW MUCH PAIN YOU ARE HAVING RIGHT NOW. Notice that what is measured is 'the perception right now', not a comparison such as: 'What is your pain compared with what you had before?'

Fig. 19.3 can be completed to show changes in pain intensity and/or pain relief across time. This can be valuable when introducing changes to analgesia and provides an ongoing assessment of progress.

A range of pain assessment tools including those in a range of languages and some for children, can be found at the Partners Against pain website.[1]

An example of a chart for patients with chronic pain is presented in Fig. 19.3. Patients are asked to assess their pain on a weekly basis and to bring their charts when attending clinics.

(Low end)		(High end)
No pain		Worst
at all		possible
		pain
–> –> –>	100mm	<– <– <–

Fig. 19.2 Example of a VAS for pain intensity.

---

1 ⅏ http://www.partnersagainstpain.com

Fig. 19.3 Oxford chronic pain record chart.

Acute pain: incidence

Acute pain is common. A survey of >3000 patients newly discharged from hospital revealed the results shown in Table 19.1.
- Not all of the patients in the survey had undergone surgery, so this is not just a problem for surgical wards.
- Pain can be a problem after operations, dental procedures, and wound dressings. Some types of surgery have a less painful recovery than others, so analgesia must be tailored.
- The need for pain relief in medical settings such as MI, sickle cell crisis, musculoskeletal disease, and renal colic must be considered along with the needs of cancer, trauma, burns and obstetric patients.

Table 19.1 Responses to questions on pain by 3163 in-patients[*]

	Proportion of patients (%)
Pain was present all or most of the time	33
Pain was severe or moderate	87
Pain was worse than expected	17
Had to ask for drugs	42
Drugs did not arrive immediately	41
Pain was present all or most of the time	33

[*] http://www.medicine.ox.ac.uk/bandolier/painres/Painresstuff/whypain.html

Acute pain

NSAIDs and non-opioids

Effective relief can be achieved with oral non-opioids and NSAIDs. It is clear from the NNT chart (Fig. 19.4) that NSAIDs are superior to paracetamol and to paracetamol combined with codeine. Combining paracetamol with an NSAID can enhance pain relief for a number of patients in the acute phase post surgery. The current vogue of supplying separate paracetamol and codeine is to be discouraged (as a cost-saving exercise) because it leads to confusion in some patients, and there have been cases of (inadvertent) codeine overdosing leading to hospitalization.

There is wisdom in the saying that if patients can swallow, they should receive medicines by mouth. There is no evidence that NSAIDs given rectally or by injection work better or faster than the same oral dose. They do not ↓ the risk of GI damage either. Gastric upset and bleeding are important adverse effects. Ibuprofen is probably the safest in this respect; however, long-term NSAID treatment should be covered with a gastric-protecting agent such as a PPI. Beware also of using NSAIDs in patients with pre-existing kidney problems; an NSAID can precipitate acute renal failure, requiring dialysis.

The belief that NSAIDs should not be used after orthopaedic surgery because they inhibit healing is a myth.

Opioids

- These are first-line treatment for acute pain. Intermittent doses might provide effective relief, but patient-controlled analgesia is the preferred method. There are many stories of adequate doses being withheld because of misconceptions, fear, and ignorance.
- Dependence is not a problem in acute pain, and respiratory depression is only a problem if the patient is either not in pain or given doses larger than those needed to treat the pain.
- The key principle is to titrate the analgesic until either pain relief is obtained or unacceptable side effects are experienced.
- There is no evidence that one opioid is better than another, although pethidine (meperidine) should be avoided because of its toxic metabolites, which can accumulate, acting as a CNS irritant and eventually inducing convulsions, particularly if underlying renal failure is present. There is no evidence for the view that pethidine (meperidine) is best for renal colic pains.
- The metabolite of morphine (morphine-6-glucuronide) can accumulate in renal disease, with the effect of prolonging the action of morphine. Provided that the dose is titrated carefully, this should not be a problem.
- It makes good sense to select one opioid for the treatment of acute pain, so that everyone is familiar with its profile. In most settings, morphine does the job.

Regional anaesthesia

- Regional anaesthesia works by interrupting pain transmission from a localized area. The risk of neurological damage is the main concern.
- Pharmacists should be aware of the compatibility issues surrounding medicines for epidural or intrathecal use, in addition to careful monitoring of the doses used. Preservative-free morphine should be used as a rule (because of the potential neurotoxicity of preservatives), unless patients are in the terminal phase of illness.

Topical agents

- Topical agents can be useful in treating acute injuries, such as strains, sprains and soft tissue trauma. There is limited evidence for the benefits of rubifacients, which work by producing a counter-irritation to relieve musculoskeletal pains. The NNT is ~2, but this is based on three small trials (with 180 participants).
- There is good systematic review evidence to show that topical NSAIDs are effective in acute pain. The NNT for pain relief is 2–4 based on 37 placebo-controlled trials with a range of NSAIDs. Ketoprofen, felbinac, ibuprofen, and piroxicam are superior to placebo, but indometacin and benzydamine are no better than placebo. Adverse events for NSAIDs were no different than placebo.

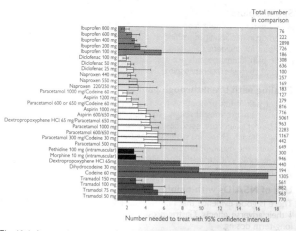

Fig. 19.4 Acute pain treatments: league table of the NNT.

Treating cancer pain

Since the introduction of the WHO three-step ladder (Fig. 19.5), potent opioids (usually morphine) have been the analgesics of choice for managing cancer pain.

Morphine is still considered the benchmark by the European Association for Palliative Care mainly because it is available in a number of different dose forms, it has extensive clinical experience, and it has an ability to provide analgesia. However, it is not always ideal, with wide individual variation in dose needs and active metabolites that can accumulate, particularly in renal failure. There is no maximum dose for morphine, but a systematic review showed that mean daily doses range from 25 to 300mg and, in unusual cases, can reach 2000mg daily. The adverse effects of morphine are not tolerated in ~4% of patients.

Drugs such as hydromorphone and oxycodone can be substituted, but these offer no real advantages. Transdermal fentanyl has become popular in recent years and can offer less constipation and daytime drowsiness.

Methadone can produce similar analgesia to morphine and has similar side effects, but it has a narrower dose range. It is the safest in renal failure; it also has a long and unpredictable half-life and its potency is often underestimated.

Spinal opioids

A few patients benefit from spinal opioids if they are unable to tolerate oral morphine. Spinal morphine in combination with a local anaesthetic is helpful for incident pain, and the addition of clonidine can help neuropathic pain. Spinal opioids are associated with greater risks, especially of epidural abscesses, cerebrospinal fluid leaks, and catheter problems.

Dealing with breakthrough pain

Cancer pain often presents as a continuous pain, with intermittent more serious pain breaking through. This can arise in up to 80% of patients with cancer pain. Four episodes daily is about the average, with each pain lasting ~30min. There are several dose strategies to manage breakthrough pain, with the usual 4h dose every 1–2h as needed (as an instant-release formulation). With transmucosal fentanyl, there seems to be little relationship between the rescue dose and the daily dose.

Use of NSAIDs with opioids

There is good evidence that NSAIDs can ↓ the total dose of opioids and ↓ their adverse effects. Gastric protective agents are needed for chronic long-term dosing.

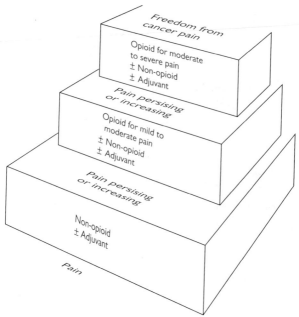

Fig. 19.5 WHO analgesic ladder.

Equianalgesic doses for opioids

Calculating equivalent doses is not an exact science, so care is needed. The literature contains much conflicting information, so key points are listed in the next section together with some external sources for suggested conversion factors.

Key points to consider when converting patients from one opioid to another

- Ratios for acute pain might not be the same as those for chronic pain.
- Ratio tables are for guidance only—they can be useful, but there can be wide variation between individuals. Therefore the dose needs to be started cautiously and titrated to effect.
- Monitor pain and pain relief—use of pain-assessment tools and adverse-effect monitoring should be considered.
- Tolerance to one opioid might not be carried over to another—this can lead to greater potency than expected. This can be anticipated by ↓ the equianalgesic dose by a further 30–50% and providing further analgesic rescue in the early stages.
- Be careful if treating patients with renal impairment—certain metabolites accumulate in renal impairment, so caution is needed. Fentanyl probably does not produce active metabolites in renal impairment, but caution is still advised.

Further reading

There is an opioid conversion software program for use on a handheld computer (and now a desktop version) at the Johns Hopkins Center for Cancer Pain Research. You can download the program free. Free registration is required. ℘ http://www.hopweb.org

Department of Anesthesiology and Critical Care Medicine at Johns Hopkins Medical Center has a useful website with additional suggested resources. ℘ http://www.hopkinsmedicine.org/anesthesiology/index.shtml

Pereira J et al. (2001). Equianalgesic dose ratios for opioids. Journal of Pain and Symptom, Management **22**: 672–87.

Regnard C (1998). Conversion ratios for transdermal fentanyl. European Journal of Palliative Care **5**: 204.

Compatibility of drugs in pain and palliative care

There are a number of mixtures in common use, including opioids combined with drugs such as baclofen, midazolam, or local anaesthetics.

It is common to differentiate between chemical and physical compatibilities. Ideally, information for the former would be available for all mixtures, but in practice this is often hard to find. Some information is available in the peer-reviewed pharmacy literature and a search of international pharmaceutical abstracts can be helpful.

Time and temperature are two key components affecting chemical reactions, so it is wise not to leave mixtures sitting in syringe drivers for many hours in a warm room. An ↑ number of drugs mixed together and the greater the concentration will ↑ the risk of incompatibility.

The majority of recommendations are desired from on physical compatibility, i.e. drugs are mixed and no obvious colour change or precipitation occurs, even when examined microscopically. Additionally, no change in pharmacological effect is seen when the drugs are administered.

Further reading

There are several useful sources for information on common opioid mixtures, as follows.

Trissel L (2005). *Handbook of Injectable Drugs* (13th edn). Bethesda, MD: American Society of Health System Pharmacists.

Dickman A et al. (2005). *The Syringe Driver: Continuous Subcutaneous Infusions in Palliative Care.* Oxford: Oxford University Press.

Twycross R, Wilcock A (2002). *Palliative Care Formulary.* Abingdon: Radcliffe Medical Press.

Trissell LA (2005). *Trissel's Stability of Compounded Formulations* (3rd edn). Washington, DC: American Pharmacists' Association.

Chronic pain

Overview

- Chronic pain is a major under-treated illness. The Pain in Europe study interviewed >46 000 people and it makes grim reading.
- Chronic pain is a widespread problem in Europe, affecting 1 in 5 adults. More than one-third of European households contain a pain sufferer. Two-thirds of chronic pain sufferers experience moderate pain, whereas one-third experience severe pain. The most common pain is back pain, and the most common cause of this is arthritis.
- People with chronic pain have been suffering on average for 7 years, with one-fifth of sufferers reporting a >20 year history. One-third of sufferers have pain all the time. Adequate pain control took >2 years to achieve in >50% of sufferers. Pain has a huge social impact. One in five sufferers have lost their job as a result of their pain. A similar number have been diagnosed with depression as a result of their pain. Generally, patients are satisfied with their care, but only 23% of sufferers have seen a pain management specialist and only 1 in 10 have been evaluated using pain scales.
- In terms of treatment, two-thirds of sufferers report that their pain control is inadequate at times, and one-third of sufferers believe that their doctor does not know how to control their pain.

What about the UK?

Almost 1 in 7 people in the UK suffer from chronic pain (~7.8 million people).

One-third of UK households are affected by chronic pain. 50% of chronic pain sufferers report the following:

- feel tired all the time
- feel helpless
- feel older than they really are
- do not remember what it feels like not to be in pain.

In addition, the following statistics here been reported.

- One in five sufferers say the pain is sometimes so bad that they want to die.
- Two-thirds of sufferers are *always* willing to try new treatments, but almost as many sufferers are worried about potential side effects of pain medication.
- Pain sufferers are proactive, with 80% of chronic pain sufferers treating their pain in some way, mainly with prescription medications.
- More than 1 in 5 (22%) sufferers have tried, and then stopped taking, prescription pain medication.
- Weak opioids are the most used class (50%) of pain medication.
- Other commonly prescribed drugs are paracetamol (38%) and NSAIDs (23%).
- The mean number of tablets taken every day is 5.7.

Despite this, much can be done to alleviate the suffering of patients with of chronic pain. The approach to treatment is the same as for acute pain, i.e. to titrate with analgesics until either pain relief or unacceptable side effects occur. In addition, there is a wide range of medicines other than analgesics that can provide relief.

Analgesics

In treating chronic pain, it is important to start with the simplest and most obvious treatments first, rather than move directly to unconventional analgesics. NSAIDs and/or paracetamol should be tried early. The combination of NSAIDs and paracetamol can be effective and can ↓ the dose of NSAID needed. The addition of a weak opioid can help in chronic pain. Patients on long-term NSAIDs should be given gastric protection and informed of the reasons for this. Approximately 1 in 120 patients who take an NSAID for >2 months without gastric protection develop a bleeding ulcer, and ~1 in 1200 patients die of a bleeding ulcer.

If simple analgesics are insufficient, there are other choices including so-called 'unconventional analgesics', such as antidepressants and anticonvulsant drugs. A strong opioid can be justified for some patients, provided that adequate steps are taken to screen patients before initiating treatment.

Non-pharmacological interventions can also help. Weight loss in overweight patients who suffer with arthritis can have a real benefit. Transcutaneous electronic nerve stimulation (TENS) can also be a useful addition. Radiotherapy can be effective in dealing with painful bony metastases. In specialist clinics, nerve blocks and epidural injections can also be helpful. A list of unconventional analgesics that can be effective in chronic neuropathic pain follows. It is usual to start at low doses and titrate the dose upwards until pain relief, unacceptable adverse effects, or the maximum dose is reached:

- Amitriptyline 50–150mg at night, or similar tricyclic antidepressants.
- Carbamazepine 100mg three times daily initially, ↑ slowly up to a maximum of 1200mg daily.
- Gabapentin, doses up to 3.6g daily
- Clonazepam 0.5mg twice daily, increasing to 1mg three times daily.
- Baclofen 5mg three times daily, increasing to 10mg three times daily.
- Pyridoxine 100mg up to five times daily.
- Capsaicin cream.
- Other anticonvulsants, such as pregabalin, lamotrigine, phenytoin, and sodium valproate.
- SSRIs can also be beneficial, but evidence for their use is very limited.

Antidepressant drugs for neuropathic pain

- Neuropathic pain refers to a group of painful disorders characterized by pain caused by dysfunction or disease of the nervous system at a peripheral or central level, or both. It is a complex entity, with many symptoms and signs that fluctuate in number and intensity over time. The three common components of neuropathic pain are steady and neuralgic pain paroxysmal spontaneous attacks and hypersensitivity.

- This type of pain can be very disabling, severe, and intractable, causing distress and suffering for individuals, including dysaesthesia and paraesthesia. Sensory deficits, such as partial or complex loss of sensation, are also commonly seen.
- The clinical impression is that both antidepressants and anticonvulsants are useful for neuropathic pain, but there are unanswered questions, including the following.
  - Which drug class should be the first-line choice?
  - Is one antidepressant drug superior to another?
  - Is there any difference in response to antidepressants in different neuropathic syndromes?
- The mechanisms of action of antidepressant drugs in the treatment of neuropathic pain are uncertain. Analgesia is often achieved at lower dosage and faster (usually within a few days) than the onset of any antidepressant effect, which can take up to 6wks. In addition, there is no correlation between the effect of antidepressants on mood and pain. Furthermore, antidepressants produce analgesia in patients with and without depression.
- Two main groups of antidepressants are in common use: the older tricyclic antidepressants, such as amitriptyline, imipramine, and many others, and a newer group of SSRIs. The clinical impression was that tricyclic antidepressants are more effective in treating neuropathic pain. However, SSRIs are gaining acceptance for pain relief.
- Tricyclic antidepressants exhibit more significant adverse effects which limit clinical use, particularly in the elderly. The most serious adverse effects of tricyclic antidepressants occur within the cardiovascular system:
  - postural hypotension
  - heart block.
  - arrhythmias.
- The most common adverse effects are:
  - sedation
  - anticholinergic effects (e.g. dry mouth, constipation, and urinary retention).
- SSRIs are better tolerated. They are free from cardiovascular side effects, are less sedative, and have fewer anticholinergic effects than tricyclic antidepressants.

Therapy-related issues: infections

Basic microbiology 412
Modes of action of antibacterials 416
Selection and use of antimicrobials 418
Antimicrobial prophylaxis 428
Optimizing antimicrobial use 430
Antimicrobial prescribing guidelines 432
Antimicrobial resistance 436
Infection control 440

Basic microbiology

Micro-organisms are classified in many ways. The most important classifications are as follows.

- Category—e.g. viruses, bacteria, and protozoa.
- Genus—i.e. the 'family' that the micro-organism belongs to, such as
  Staphylococcus.
- Species—i.e. the specific name, such as *aureus*.

To name a micro-organism correctly, both the genus and the species name
must be used—e.g. *Staphylococcus aureus, Haemophilus influenzae*.

Identifying micro-organisms

To diagnose and treat an infection correctly, the micro-organism must be
identified. This is usually done by examining samples of faeces, blood, and
sputum in various ways.

Microscopy

The sample is examined under the microscope. Sometimes the organism
can easily be seen and identified—e.g. some helminths (worms) and their
ova (eggs).

Dyes are used to stain cells so that they can be seen more easily.
Differential staining uses the fact that cells with different properties stain
differently and therefore can be distinguished. Bacteria are divided into
two groups according to whether they stain with the Gram stain. The
difference between Gram-positive and Gram-negative bacteria is in the
permeability of the cell wall when treated with a purple dye followed by
a decolorizing agent. Gram-positive cells retain the stain, whereas Gram-
negative cells lose the purple stain and appear colourless, until stained
with a pink counterstain (Fig. 20.1).

Mycobacteria have waxy cell walls and do not readily take up the Gram
stain. A different staining technique is used, and then the sample is tested
to see if it withstands decolorization with acid and alcohol. Mycobacteria
retain the stain and thus are known as acid-fast bacilli (AFB), whereas
other bacteria lose the stain.

Examination of stained films allows the shape of the cells to be seen,
which can aid identification.

Bacteria are classified as follows:

- Cocci (spherical, rounded)—e.g. streptococci.
- Bacilli (straight rod)—e.g. *Pseudomonas* species.
- Spirochaetes (spiral rod)—e.g. *Treponema* species.
- Vibrios (curved, comma-shaped)—e.g. *Vibrio cholerae*.

Culture

Bacteria and fungi can be grown on the surface of solid, nutrient media.
Colonies of many thousands of the micro-organism can be produced from
a single cell. Colonies of different species often have characteristic appear-
ances, which aids identification. For most species, it takes 12–48h for a
colony to develop that is visible to the naked eye. Some organisms (e.g.
mycobacteria) multiply much more slowly and can take several weeks to
develop.

Samples can be grown in an environment from which O_2 has been excluded. Bacteria that grow in the absence of O_2 are known as 'anaerobes' and bacteria that need O_2 to grow are 'aerobes'. Bacteria are often described as a combination of their Gram-staining, shape, and anaerobic/aerobic characteristics. This helps to narrow the range of bacteria under consideration before lengthier tests identify the individual organism (Table 20.1). Other tests that can be used to identify the organism include the following.

• Detection of microbial antigen.
• Detection of microbial products—e.g. toxin produced by *Clostridium difficile*.
• Using gene probes.
• Polymerase chain reaction.

Discussion of these tests is beyond the scope of this topic. For further information the reader is referred to microbiology texts.

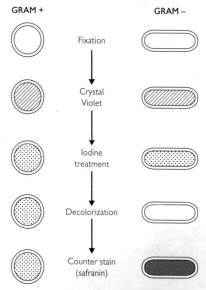

Fig. 20.1 Gram-staining procedure.

Table 20.1 Examples of pathogens from various types of bacteria

Gram-positive cocci	Gram-negative cocci
Staphylococci	Neisseria
Coagulase +ve, e.g. *Staph.aureus*	*N.meningitidis* (meningitis, septicaemia)
Coagulase –ve, e.g. *Staph.epidermidis*	*N.gonorrheae* (gonorrhoea)
Streptococci*	Moraxella
B-haemolytic streptococci	*M.catarrhalis* (pneumonia)
Strep.pyogenes (Lancefield group A)	**Gram-negative bacilli (rods)**
α-haemolytic streptococci	Enterobacteriaceae
Strep. mitior	*Escherichia coli*
Strep.pneumoniae (pneumococcus)	*Shigella species*
Strep. sanguis	*Salmonella species*
Enterococci (non-haemolytic)†	*Citrobacter freundii, C. koser*
E.mutans, E. faecalis	*Klebsiella pneumoniae, K.oxytoca*
Anaerobic streptococci	*Enterobacter aerogenes, E.cloacae*
Gram-positive bacilli (rods)	*Serratia morascens*
Aerobes	*Proteus mirabilis/vulgaris*
Bacillus anthracis (anthrax)	*Morganella morganii*
Corynebacterium diphtheriae	*Providencia species*
Listeria monocytogenes	*Yersinia Y.enterocolitica*
Nocardia species	*Y.pestis, Y.paratuberculosis*
Anaerobes	*Pseudomonas aeruginosa*
Clostridium	*Haemophilus influenzae*
C.botulinum (botulism)	*Brucella species*
C.perfringens (gas gangrene)	*Bordetella pertussis*
C.tetani (tetanus)	*Pasterurella multocida*
C.difficile (diarrhoea)	*Vibrio cholerae*
Actinomyces	*Camphylobacter jejuni*
A.israeli, A.naeslundii	
A.odontolyticus, A.viscosus	

Table 20.1 (Contd.)

Obligate intracellular bacteria	Anaerobes
Chlamydia	*Bacteroides* (wound infections)
C.trachomatis	*Fusobacterium*
C.psittaci	*Helicobacter pylori*
C.pneumoniae	**Mycobacteria**
Coxiella burnetii	*Mycobacterium tuberculosis*
Bartonella, Ehrlichia	*M.bovis*
Rickettsia (typhus)	*M.leprae* (leprosy)
Legionella pneumophilia	**'Atypical' mycobacteria**
Mycoplasma pneumoniae	*M.avium intracellulare*
	M.scrofulaceum, M.kansasii
	M.marinum, M.malmoense
	M.ulcerans, M.xenopi, M.gordonae
	M.fortuitum, M.chelonae, M.flaverscens
	M.smegmatis-phlei
	Spirochaetes
	Treponema (syphilis. yaws, pinta)
	Leptospira (Weil's dis., canicola fever)
	Borrelia (relapsing fever; Lyme disease)

*Streps are classified according to haemolytic pattern: (α–β or non-haemolytic) or by Lancefield antigen (A–G), or by species (e.g. Strep. pyogenes). There is crossover among these groups; this table is a generalization for the chief pathogens.

†Clinically, epidemiologically and in terms of treatment, enterococci behave unlike other streps.

Reproduced with permission from Longmore M et al. (2004). *Oxford Handbook of Clinical Medicine*, 6th edn. Oxford: Oxford University Press.

Modes of action of antibacterials

To avoid unwanted toxic effects on human cells, most antibacterials have a mode of action that affects bacterial but not mammalian cells.

There are many possible sites of action of antimicrobial agents. However, the most common mechanisms are as follows:
- inhibition of cell wall synthesis
- alteration of the cell membrane (usually antifungals)
- inhibition of protein synthesis
- inhibition of nucleic acid synthesis.

Inhibition of cell wall synthesis
- Mammalian cells do not have a cell wall (only a cell membrane) so this mode of action does not affect mammalian cells.
- Penicillins, cephalosporins, and other β-lactam antibacterials interfere with the synthesis of a substance called peptidoglycan. Peptidoglycan is an essential component of bacterial cell walls. If synthesis of peptidoglycan is inhibited, it is unable to support the cell wall and thus the bacteria lose their structure and eventually lyse (disintegrate) and die.
- Isoniazid also acts on the cell wall. It inhibits enzymes that are essential for synthesis of mycolic acids and the mycobacterial cell wall. The mode of action of ethambutol is not clear, but it might be the same as that of isoniazid.

Inhibition of protein synthesis
- The mechanism of protein synthesis is similar in bacterial and mammalian cells, but there are differences in ribosome structure (involved in protein synthesis) and other target sites, which ↓ the risk of toxicity to mammalian cells.
- Tetracyclines, aminoglycosides, macrolides, and chloramphenicol all work by inhibiting synthesis of proteins essential to the growth and reproduction of bacteria.
- Tetracyclines, macrolides, and chloramphenicol interfere with the binding of new amino acids onto peptide chains.
- Aminoglycosides prevent initiation of protein synthesis and cause non-functional proteins to be created.

Inhibition of nucleic acid synthesis
- Sulphonamides are structural analogues of para-amino benzoic acid (PABA). PABA is an essential precursor in bacterial synthesis of folic acid, which is necessary for the synthesis of nucleic acids. Mammalian cells are not affected as they use exogenous folic acid.
- Trimethoprim is an inhibitor of dihydrofolic acid reductase, an enzyme that reduces dihydrofolic acid to tetrahydrofolic acid. This is one of the stages in bacterial synthesis of purines and thus DNA. Trimethoprim inhibits dihydrofolic acid reductase 50 000 times more efficiently in bacterial cells than in mammalian cells.
- Sulphonamides and trimethoprim produce sequential blocking of folate metabolism and therefore are synergistic.

- Bacteria use an enzyme called DNA gyrase to make the DNA into a small enough package to fit into the cell. This is called supercoiling. The quinolones inhibit DNA gyrase and supercoiling.
- Rifampicin inhibits bacterial RNA synthesis by binding to RNA polymerase. Mammalian RNA polymerase is not affected.
- Nitro-imidazoles (e.g. metronidazole) cause the DNA strand to break (cleavage).

Selection and use of antimicrobials

To treat or not to treat

The presence of micro-organisms does not necessarily mean that there is infection. The human body hosts a wide range of micro-organisms (mostly bacteria), but these rarely cause infection in an immuno-competent host. These organisms are known as 'commensals' and some have an important role in host defences. For example, *Clostridium difficile* is a pathogen that is normally suppressed by normal bowel flora. Eradication of the bowel flora (e.g. by broad-spectrum antibacterials) allows overgrowth of *C.difficile*, leading to diarrhoea and, sometimes, pseudo-membraneous colitis. Indiscriminate drug therapy can thus ↑ the risk of other infection.

Some organisms might be commensals in one part of the body and pathogens in another—e.g. *Escherichia coli* is part of the normal bowel flora but if it gets into the bladder it can cause urinary tract infection.

Some pathogenic organisms can reside on the host without causing infection. This is known as 'colonization', and signs and symptoms of infection are absent. A skin or nasal swab positive for meticillin-resistant *Staphylococcus aureus* (MRSA) does not usually require treatment except where elimination of MRSA carriage is required—e.g. prior to surgery.

Some infections are self-limiting and resolve without treatment. Many common viral infections resolve without treatment, and in any case most do not have specific antiviral drugs.

Choice of therapy

If infection is confirmed or is strongly suspected, appropriate therapy must be selected. Ideally, the pathogen is identified before antimicrobial therapy is started. However, identification of an organism by the laboratory usually takes a minimum of 24h and antimicrobial sensitivity tests can take a further 24h. For some slow-growing organisms, such as mycobacteria, culture and sensitivity results can take several weeks. Thus, in most cases, therapy will be started using 'best guess' (empirical) antimicrobials and tailored after culture and sensitivity results are known (Table 20.2).

Whenever possible, samples for culture and sensitivity tests should be taken before starting antimicrobial therapy so that growth is not inhibited. However, this delay might not be possible in very sick patients—e.g. those with suspected bacterial meningitis.

Factors that should be taken into account when selecting an antimicrobial are described as follows:

Clinical

- Does the patient have an infection that needs treating?
- Diagnosis/likely source of infection.
- Anatomical site of infection.
- Severity or potential severity of infection (and possible consequences—e.g. loss of prosthetic joint).
- Patient's underlying condition (if any) and vulnerability to infection— e.g. neutropenic patients more susceptible to sepsis.
- Patient-specific factors, e.g. allergies and renal function.

- Does the infection require empirical therapy or can antimicrobials be delayed until culture and sensitivity results are available?
- Foreign material, necrotic tissue, and abscesses are relatively impervious to antimicrobials. Abscesses should be drained and necrotic tissue debrided. If possible, foreign material should be removed.

Microbiology

- What are the pathogens?
  - Identified by microscopy or culture.
  - Presumed, according to epidemiology and knowledge of probable infecting organisms for the site of infection.
- Sensitivity of organisms to antimicrobial agents (Table 20.3):
  - national and local resistance patterns
  - culture and sensitivity data.

Pharmaceutical

- Evidence of clinical efficacy:
  - against the organism.
  - at the site of infection.
- Bactericidal versus bacteriostatic agents:
  - Bactericidal drugs generally give more rapid resolution of infection.
  - Bacteriostatic drugs rely on phagocytes to eliminate the organisms and therefore are not suitable for infection in which phagocytes are impaired (e.g. granulocytopenia) or do not penetrate the site of infection (e.g. infective endocarditis).
- Spectrum of activity.
  - Narrow-spectrum antimicrobials are preferred if the organism has been identified.
  - Broad-spectrum antimicrobials might be required in empirical therapy or mixed infection.
  - Indiscriminate use of broad-spectrum antimicrobials ↑ the risk of development of drug resistance and super-infection, e.g. *C.difficile*.
- Appropriate route of administration.
  - Topical antimicrobials should be avoided, except where specifically indicated—e.g. eye or ear infection or metronidazole gel for fungating tumours.
  - Oral therapy is preferred and most antimicrobials have good bioavailability.
  - IV therapy might be necessary in the following circumstances:
    — if the infection is serious
    — if the drug has poor oral bioavailability
    — if the patient is unconscious or unable to take oral drugs (e.g. perioperatively).
- Possible side effects or drug interactions.
- Pharmacokinetics:
  - tissue penetration—will the antimicrobial reach the site of infection?
  - clearance in liver/kidney impairment.
- Dose and frequency must be sufficient to give adequate blood levels but avoid unacceptable toxicity. Serum levels four to eight times the minimum inhibitory concentration (MIC) are considered adequate.

- Duration of treatment:
  - not too long—e.g. uncomplicated urinary tract infection only requires 3–5 days therapy.
  - not too short—e.g. bone infection might require therapy for several weeks or months.
- Local policies/restrictions on antimicrobial use.
- Cost.

Combined antimicrobial therapy

Combined antimicrobial therapy may be prescribed for certain indications.

- To give a broad spectrum of activity in empirical therapy, especially in high-risk situations such as neutropenic sepsis.
- To treat mixed infection if one drug does not cover all possible pathogens.
- To achieve a synergistic effect, thus ↑ efficacy but ↓ the dose required of each drug (and thus ↓ the risk of side effects)—e.g. penicillin and gentamicin in the treatment of streptococcal endocarditis. Relatively low doses of gentamicin are used, ↓ the risk of nephrotoxicity.
- To ↓ the probability of the emergence of drug resistance—e.g. treatment of TB requires a minimum of two drugs and antiretroviral therapy requires a minimum of three drugs.
- To restore or extend the spectrum of activity by including an enzyme inhibitor—e.g. co-amoxiclav.

Penicillin and cephalosporin hypersensitivity

Up to 10% of people are allergic to penicillins and up to 7% of these people are also allergic to cephalosporins. This can range from mild rash to fever to a serious anaphylactic reaction. Penicillins and cephalosporins should never be used again in a patient who has had a severe hypersensitivity reaction. If a patient has had a severe hypersensitivity reaction to penicillins, it is advisable to avoid cephalosporins unless there is no alternative. If the penicillin allergy is relatively mild (e.g. rash) cephalosporins can be prescribed cautiously.

Some patients state that they have had an allergic reaction when they have really only had nausea or a headache. This is not drug allergy and therefore it is safe to use penicillins and cephalosporins in these patients.

Ampicillin and amoxicillin can cause rashes in patients who have had glandular fever or leukaemia, or who are HIV positive. This is not a true allergic reaction and penicillins can be used again in these patients.

Monitoring therapy

It is essential to monitor and review antimicrobial therapy regularly, both to ensure that treatment is working and to avoid inappropriate continuation of therapy (Fig. 20.2) The pharmacist should monitor the following parameters.

- Temperature should ↓ to normal (36.8°C). (Note: drug hypersensitivity is a possible cause of persistent pyrexia.)
- Pulse, BP, and respiratory rate revert to normal.
- Raised white cell count decreases.
- Raised C-reactive protein decreases (normal <8).
- Symptoms such as local inflammation, pain, malaise, GI upset, headache, and confusion resolve.

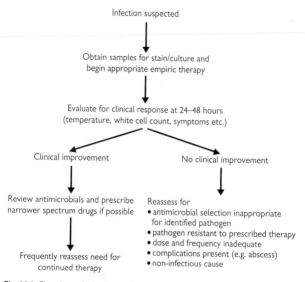

Fig. 20.2 Flowchart of selection and use of antimicrobials.

Reasons for treatment failure

- Wrong antimicrobial.
- Drug resistance.
- The isolated organism is not the cause of the disease.
- Treatment started too late.
- The wrong dose, duration, or route of administration.
- Lack of patient compliance.
- Difficulty getting the drug to the site of infection.
- ↓ immunity of the patient.

Further reading

Wickens H, Wade P (2005). How pharmacists can promote the sensible use of antimicrobials. *Pharmaceutical Journal* **274**: 427–30.

Wickens H, Wade P (2005). The right drug for the right bug. *Pharmaceutical Journal* **274**: 365–8.

Table 20.2 In vitro activity of antibacterials

✓ = usually sensitive   ? = variable sensitivity   X = usually resistant or inappropriate therapy

Note: These are generalizations. There are major differences between countries, areas and hospitals. Check local Public Health or Microbiology laboratories for local sensitivity patterns. Antibacterials may not be licensed to treat the bacteria for which they are active.

	Gram positives								Anaerobes			Gram negatives									Atypicals		
	Staphylococcus aureus MSSA	*Staphylococcus aureus* MRSA	*Staphylococcus epidermidis*	Haemolytic streptococci (Strep A, C, G and Strep B)	*Enterococcus faecalis*	*Enterococcus faecium*	*Streptococcus pneumoniae*	*Listeria monocytogenes*	*Clostridium perfringens*	*Clostridium difficile*	*Bacteroides fragilis*	*Neisseria meningitidis*	*Neisseria gonorrhoeae*	*Haemophilus influenzae*	*Escherichia coli*	*Klebsiella* spp	*Proteus mirabilis*	*Proteus vulgaris*	*Pseudomonas aeruginosa*	*Moraxella catarrhalis*	*Legionella* spp	*Mycoplasma pneumoniae*	*Chlamydia* spp
Penicillins																							
Phenoxymethylpenicillin	×	×	×	✓	✓	?	✓	×	✓	×	×	✓	?	×	×	×	×	×	×	×	×	×	×
Benzylpenicillin	×	×	×	✓	✓	?	✓	✓	✓	×	×	✓	?	×	×	×	×	×	×	×	×	×	×
Ampicillin/Amoxicillin	×	×	×	✓	✓	?	✓	✓	✓	×	×	✓	?	?	?	×	?	×	×	✓	×	×	×
Co-amoxiclav	✓	×	?	✓	✓	?	✓	×	✓	×	✓	✓	?	✓	✓	?	✓	✓	×	✓	×	×	×
Flucloxacillin	✓	×	?	✓	×	×	✓	×	×	×	×	×	×	×	×	×	×	×	×	×	×	×	×
Pip+tazobactam (Tazocin®)	✓	×	?	✓	✓	?	?	×	✓	×	✓	✓	?	?	✓	✓	✓	✓	?	✓	×	×	×
Cephalosporins																							
Cefradine / Cefalexin	✓	×	?	✓	×	×	✓	×	×	×	×	×	×	?	✓	?	✓	×	×	✓	×	×	×
Cefotaxime	✓	×	?	✓	×	×	✓	×	×	×	×	✓	✓	✓	✓	✓	✓	✓	×	✓	×	×	×
Cefuroxime	✓	×	?	✓	×	×	✓	×	×	×	×	✓	?	?	✓	✓	✓	×	×	✓	×	×	×
Ceftriaxone	✓	×	?	✓	×	×	✓	×	×	×	×	✓	✓	✓	✓	✓	✓	✓	×	✓	×	×	×
Ceftazidime	?	×	?	✓	×	×	?	×	×	×	×	✓	?	✓	✓	✓	✓	✓	✓	✓	×	×	×

	Gram positives								Anaerobes			Gram negatives										Atypicals	
	Staphylococcus aureus MSSA	*Staphylococcus aureus* MRSA	*Staphylococcus epidermidis*	Haemolytic streptococci (Strep A, C, G and Strep B)	*Enterococcus faecalis*	*Enterococcus faecium*	*Streptococcus pneumoniae*	*Listeria monocytogenes*	*Clostridium perfringens*	*Clostridium difficile*	*Bacteroides fragilis*	*Neisseria meningitidis*	*Neisseria gonorrhoeae*	*Haemophilus influenzae*	*Escherichia coli*	*Klebsiella* spp	*Proteus mirabilis*	*Proteus vulgaris*	*Pseudomonas aeruginosa*	*Moraxella catarrhalis*	*Legionella* spp	*Mycoplasma pneumoniae*	*Chlamydia* spp
Carbapenems																							
Ertapenem	✓	✗	✓	✓	?	✗	✓	?	✓	✗	✓	✓	✓	✓	✓	✓	✓	✓	✗	✓	✗	✗	✗
Meropenem/ Imipenem	✓	✗	✓	✓	?	?	✓	?	✓	✗	✓	✓	✓	✓	✓	✓	✓	✓	✓	✓	✗	✗	✗
Macrolides/ Lincosamides																							
Azithromycin	✓	✗	✗	✓	✗	✗	✓	?	✓	✗	✗	✓	?	✓	✗	✗	✗	✗	✗	✓	✓	✓	✓
Erythromycin	✓	?	?	✓	✗	✗	✓	✗	✓	✗	✗	✓	?	?	✗	✗	✗	✗	✗	✓	✓	✓	✓
Clarithromycin	✓	?	?	✓	✗	✗	✓	?	✓	✗	✗	✓	?	✓	✗	✗	✗	✗	✗	✓	✓	✓	✓
Clindamycin	✓	✗	✗	✓	✗	✗	✓	✗	✓	✗	✓	✗	✗	✗	✗	✗	✗	✗	✗	✗	✗	✗	✗
Aminoglycosides																							
Amikacin	✓	✓	?	✗	✓	✗	✗	✓	✗	✗	✗	✗	✗	✓	✓	✓	✓	✓	✓	✓	✓	✗	✗
Gentamicin	✓	✓	?	✗	✓	✓	✗	✓	✗	✗	✗	✗	✗	✓	✓	✓	✓	✓	✓	✓	✓	✗	✗
Diaminopyrimidines and sulphonamides																							
Co-trimoxazole	✓	?	?	?	✗	✗	?	✗	✗	✗	✗	✓	?	?	✓	✓	✓	✓	✗	✓	✓	✗	✗
Trimethoprim	?	?	?	?	✓	✗	?	✗	✗	✗	✗	✗	✗	?	✓	✓	✓	✓	✗	✓	✗	✗	✗
Quinolones																							
Ciprofloxacin	✓	✗	✓	✗	✓	✗	✗	✗	✗	✗	✗	✓	✓	✓	✓	✓	✓	✓	✓	✓	✓	✓	✓
Levofloxacin	✓	?	?	?	✓	?	✓	✗	✗	✗	?	✓	✓	✓	✓	✓	✓	✓	?	✓	✓	✓	✓
Moxifloxacin	✓	✗	✓	✓	✓	?	✓	✗	✓	✗	?	✓	✓	✓	✓	✓	✓	✓	?	✓	✓	✓	✓

(continued)

Table 20.2 (Contd.)

	Gram positives								Anaerobes			Gram negatives									Atypicals		
	Staphylococcus aureus MSSA	Staphylococcus aureus MRSA	Staphylococcus epidermidis	Haemolytic streptococci (Strep A, C, G and Strep B)	Enterococcus faecalis	Enterococcus faecium	Streptococcus pneumoniae	Listeria monocytogenes	Clostridium perfringens	Clostridium difficile	Bacteroides fragilis	Neisseria meningitidis	Neisseria gonorrhoeae	Haemophilus influenzae	Escherichia coli	Klebsiella spp	Proteus mirabilis	Proteus vulgaris	Pseudomonas aeruginosa	Moraxella catarrhalis	Legionella spp	Mycoplasma pneumoniae	Chlamydia spp
Glycopeptides																							
Vancomycin (IV)	✓	✓	✓	✓	✓	?	✓	✓	✓	✓²	×	×	×	×	×	×	×	×	×	×	×	×	×
Teicoplanin	✓	✓	?	✓	✓	?	✓	✓	✓	×	×	×	×	×	×	×	×	×	×	×	×	×	×
Nitroimidazoles																							
Metronidazole	×	×	×	×	×	×	×	×	✓	✓	✓	×	×	×	×	×	×	×	×	×	×	×	×
Oxazolidinones																							
Linezolid	✓	✓	✓	✓	✓	✓	✓	✓	✓	?	?	×	×	×	×	×	×	×	×	×	×	×	×
Tetracyclines																							
Doxycycline	✓	?	×	✓	?	?	✓	✓	✓	×	?	✓	✓	?	✓	?	?	?	×	✓	✓	✓	✓
Miscellaneous																							
Chloramphenicol	?	×	×	✓	×	?	✓	✓	?	×	✓	✓	✓	✓	✓	✓	?	?	×	✓	×	✓	✓
Quinupristin / dalfopristin (Synercid®)	✓	✓	✓	✓	×	✓	✓	×	✓	?	✓	×	×	?	×	×	×	×	×	✓	✓	✓	✓

[1] Sensitive if used synergistically with penicillins/glycopeptides.
[2] IV vancomycin ineffective for *Clostridium difficile*.

Table 20.3 Diseases, potential causative bacteria and typical treatment choices*

Specific condition	Potential bacterial pathogens	Typical empirical treatment
Meningitis	*Streptococcus pneumoniae*, *Neisseria meningitidis*, *Haemophilus influenzae*. Group B streptococcus (seen in neonates). Less commonly, *Escherichia coli* and *Listeria monocytogenes*. Other Gram negative bacteria and *Staphylococcus* spp usually associated with neurosurgery	Cefotaxime and ceftriaxone provide broad cover and good central nervous system penetration. Ampicillin or amoxicillin is required to cover *Listeria* spp (elderly and neonates). Causative agents can also be mycobacterial, viral or, rarely, fungal and these will require appropriate therapy.
Brain abscess	*S.aureus*, anaerobic streptococci, *Bacteroides* spp. Gram negatives, such as *Escherichia*, *Proteus*, *Klebsiella* spp	Cefotaxime or ceftriaxone, meropenem if broader cover required (avoid imipenem due to CNS side effects). The condition can occasionally be fungal or parasitic.
Otitis media	*Strep. pneumoniae*, *H.influenzae*, *Moraxella catarrhalis*, *S.aureus*, mixed anaerobes	Antibacterial therapy not always necessary. Amoxicillin or co- amoxiclav. Can also be viral (e.g. influenza, respiratory syncitial virus, enteroviruses).
Otitis externa	*Pseudomonas aeruginosa* ("swimmer's ear"), *S.aureus* (pustule)	Topical gentamicin. Less commonly fungal (*Candida albicans*, *Aspergillus* spp).
Upper respiratory tract infections		
Pharyngitis/tonsillitis	*Strep. pyogenes* (group A)	Phenoymethylpenicillin but note that 50% of sore throats are viral in origin.
Epiglottitis	*H.influenzae*, *Strep. pyogenes* (group A)	Ceftriaxone or cefotaxime.
Sinusitis	*Strep. pneumoniae*, *H.influenzae*, mixed anaerobes, *S.aureus*, *M. catarrhalis*	Co-amoxiclav. Sinusitis may be viral (e.g. rhinovirus, influenza) or occasionally, fungal.

(continued)

Table 20.3 (Contd.)

Specific condition	Potential bacterial pathogens	Typical empirical treatment
Lower respiratory tract infections‡		
Community-acquired	Strep. pneumoniae, H.influenzae, M. catarrhalis, atypical organisms (Mycoplasma pneumoniae, Chlamydia pneumoniae and, rarely, Legionella pneumophila).	Amoxicillin oral or ceftriaxone intravenous (depending on severity) ± macrolide if atypical organisms are suspected or clarithromycin ± rifampicin for Legionella.
Hospital-acquired	E.coli, Ps. aeruginosa, and other gram negative organisms, methicillin-resistant S.aureus (MRSA)	Broad spectrum antibacterials are required until a definitive diagnosis is made e.g. meropenem/imipenem/piperacillin + tazobactam (Tazocin®), vancomycin + quinolone if MRSA suspected. Infection can be viral. Fungal infection is more likely in immunocompromised patients.
Endocarditis	Enterococcus spp. Viridans group streptococci, S.aureus, coagulase-negative staphylococci.	Benzylpenicillin and gentamicin (synergistic action) or flucloxacillin and gentamicin if staphylococci are suspected (often seen in injecting drug users).
Gastrointestinal infections	E.coli, Shigella spp, Campylobacter jejuni, Salmonella spp, S aureus, Bacillus cereus (toxin mediated)	Gastrointestinal infections are generally self-limiting and often viral. Fluid replacement may be all that is required. Expert advice should be sought if antibacterials are considered necessary. In severe disease, ciprofloxacin is used for Salmonella spp and erythromycin for Campylobacter.
Urinary tract infections	E.coli, enterococci, Klebsiella spp. Enterobacter spp. Pseudomonas spp (UTI)/Pyelonephritis Proteus spp	For UTI use amoxicillin, cefradine/cefalexin, trimethoprim or nitrofurantoin depending on local resistance patterns. For uncomplicated UTI in a young woman, three days treatment should be sufficient. A longer course may be required in men. Recurrent or complicated UTIs require further investigation, consideration of resistant organisms and use of second-line agents. Co-amoxiclav or ceftriaxone (± single dose of gentamicin) are often used for pyelonephritis.

Skin and soft tissue infection (cellulitis)	S.aureus, Strep. pyogenes (group A)	Penicillin +/- flucloxacillin (oral or intravenously depending on severity). Always check (and treat) for co-existing athlete's foot which can be an entry point for organisms.
Septic arthritis	S.aureus, Strep. pneumoniae, occasionally Gram negatives guided by culture results.	Flucloxacillin or ceftriaxone empirically, but therapy should be guided by culture results
Osteomyelitis	S.aureus, Strep. pneumoniae, coagulase negative staphylococci (usually associated with implanted material). Many other organisms infrequently cause disease.	Flucloxacillin or ceftriaxone empirically, but therapy should be guided by culture results. Infections involving prostheses will require longer therapy.
Sepsis		
Neutropenic	S aureus (MRSA), Strep. viridans, coagulase-negative staphylococci, E.coli, Klebsiella spp, Ps aeruginosa or Pneumocystis jiroveci (carinii) pneumonia (PCP).	Meropenem/imipenem/piperacillin+tazobactam plus gentamicin. Vancomycin if staphylococcus species (including MRSA) suspected. Co-trimoxazole for PCP. If fever persists consider fungal or viral infections
Non-neutropenic	S.aureus (MRSA), Streptococcus. spp. E.coli, Pseudomonas spp.	Therapy depends on source of infection. Empirically – flucloxacillin/ ceftriazone +/– gentamicin. Vancomycin if MRSA suspected. Meropenem/imipenem/piperacillin + tazobactam initially in septic shock

*Pathogens/therapy may differ in children and neonates—seek specialist advice.
†Patients with MRSA or high risk of MRSA, add vancomycin or teicoplanin.
‡See also British Thoracic Society Guidelines for the management of community acquired pneumonia in adults. Thorax (2001) **56** (suppl 4) 1–64 www.brit-thoracic.org.uk.
Adapted with permission from Wickens H and Wade P (2005) The right drug for the right bug. The Pharmaceutical Journal, **274** 365–8.

Antimicrobial prophylaxis

Indiscriminate and prolonged courses of antimicrobials should be avoided, but in some situations short- or long-term antimicrobial prophylaxis might be appropriate to prevent infection (and thus further courses of antimicrobials).

Surgical prophylaxis

Antibacterial drugs are given to ↓ the risk of the following.
- Wound infection after potentially contaminated surgery—e.g. GI or genitourinary surgery and trauma.
- Losing implanted material—e.g. joint prosthesis.

It is important that there are adequate concentrations of antibacterials in the blood at the time of incision ('knife-to-skin time') and throughout surgery. Thus it is important to administer antibacterials at an appropriate time (usually 30–60min) before surgery starts and repeat doses of short-acting antibacterials if surgery is delayed or prolonged. It is rarely necessary to continue antibacterials after wound closure. More prolonged therapy is effectively treatment rather than prophylaxis.

The choice of antibacterial depends on the type of surgery and local bacterial sensitivities. Vancomycin or teicoplanin should be used for patients with proven or suspected MRSA colonization.[1] Drugs are usually administered by IV infusion to ensure adequate levels at the critical time.

Medical prophylaxis

Medical prophylaxis is appropriate for specific infections and for high-risk patients, as follows.
- Contacts of sick patients—e.g. meningitis and TB.
- Immunosuppressed patients—e.g. organ-transplant recipients, HIV-positive patients, and splenectomy patients.
- Malaria.
- Post-exposure prophylaxis, following exposure to HIV or hepatitis B.

Further reading

Prophylaxis regimens can be found in the *British National Formulary* and on www.sign.ac.uk.
Rahman MH, Anson J (2004). Peri-operative antibacterial prophylaxis. *Pharmaceutical Journal* **272**: 743–5.

1 Gemmell CG *et al.* (2006).Guidelines for the prophylaxis and treatment of methicillin-resistant *Staphylococcus aureus* (MRSA) in the UK. *Journal of Antimicrobial Chemotheraphy* **57**: 589–608.

Optimizing antimicrobial use

↓ antimicrobial use might not actually ↓ the rate of resistance, but it might limit the rate at which new resistance emerges. Pharmacists have an important role in optimizing antimicrobial use—often known as 'antimicrobial stewardship'. In the UK, the Department of Health has specifically promoted the role of pharmacists in monitoring and optimizing antimicrobial use. In many hospitals, specialist antimicrobial pharmacists work alongside microbiologists and infectious diseases doctors to promote good antimicrobial stewardship through education, audit, and production of prescribing policies. However, all pharmacists, whether in hospitals or the community, have a role in ensuring 'prudent use' of antimicrobials.

Strategies for antimicrobial stewardship

- Use of non-antimicrobial treatment as appropriate, e.g. draining abscesses and removing infected invasive devices such as catheters.
- Improved systems for resistance testing and better communication of resistance data in the hospital and community settings to enable better-directed therapy.
  - Avoid continued use of ineffective drugs.
  - Enable switching from broad-spectrum to narrower-spectrum antimicrobials.
- Faster diagnosis of infection to ↓ the amount of unnecessary empirical therapy.
- Ensuring that empirical therapy considers the following adjustments, as necessary.
  - Therapy is stopped if infection is ruled out.
  - Therapy is changed, as necessary, when culture results are available.
- Production of antimicrobial prescribing policies and promoting adherence to guidelines.
- Ensuring choice, dose, and duration of therapy, including the following.
  - Monitoring serum levels and adjusting doses for antimicrobials that require TDM.
  - Ensuring that kinetic factors are taken into account—e.g. nitrofurantoin is not excreted into the urine in adequate concentrations to be effective in patients with renal impairment.
- Avoiding unnecessary/overlong use of broad-spectrum antimicrobials.
- Appropriate use of antimicrobials for surgical prophylaxis, including avoiding prolonged courses.
- Use of combination therapy if there is a high risk of resistance emerging—e.g. rifampicin should never be used alone for TB or other infections.
- Avoiding co-prescribing of antimicrobials that have the same or an overlapping spectrum of activity—e.g. co-amoxiclav and metronidazole.
- Considering rotational use of antimicrobials (cycling) in some circumstances.
- Educating patients to take antimicrobials correctly and that some infections do not require antimicrobial therapy.

Points to consider when reviewing a prescription for an antimicrobial

- Is it the right choice for the infection (or appropriate empirical therapy)?
- Does it comply with local policies/restrictive practices?
- Could a narrower-spectrum antimicrobial be used?
- Should it be used in combination with another antimicrobial?
- Is more than one antimicrobial with an overlapping spectrum of activity being used, and if so, why?
- Will the antimicrobial be distributed to the target (infected) organ?
- Is the dose correct taking into account the following?
  - Renal impairment.
  - Severity of infection.
  - Patient weight.
- Is TDM and subsequent dose adjustment required?
- Is the route of administration appropriate?
- Is the duration of therapy appropriate?
- Does the patient understand the dosing instructions and importance of completing the course?

Further reading

Wicken H, Wade P (2005). Understanding antibiotic resistance. *Pharmaceutical Journal* **274**: 501–4.
European Surveillance of Antimicrobials. ℘ http://www.ua.ac.be/esac
Department of Health. *The Path of Least Resistance*. London: Department of Health. ℘ http://www.dh.gov.uk/prod_consum_dh/groups/dh_digitalassets/@dh/@en/documents/digitalasset/dh_4120729.pdf
Patient information sheets on:
- *C.difficile*: ℘ http://www.dh.gov.uk/assetroot/04/11/34/79/04115884.pdf
- MRSA: ℘ http://www.dh.gov.uk/assetroot/04/11/58/84/04113479.pdf

Get Smart for Healthcare (advice for clinicians, fact sheets, and posters). ℘ http://www.cdc.gov/getsmart/healthcare/resources/factsheets/hc_providers.html

Antimicrobial prescribing guidelines

Antimicrobials are the second most frequently prescribed class of drugs, after analgesics. In England, about 50 million prescriptions for antimicrobials are dispensed each year. Approximately 80% of antimicrobial prescribing is in the community, and although the emergence of 'superbugs' is less of a problem than in hospitals, resistance and cost are still an issue. Education of patients and GPs to reduce pressure to prescribe has contributed to a reduction in antimicrobial usage in the community. The remaining 20% of antimicrobial prescribing is in hospitals. However, this class represents some of the more expensive drugs used in secondary care and antimicrobial resistance in the hospital setting is an increasing problem, notably with MRSA.

Both WHO and the UK Department of Health have emphasized the need for 'prudent use' of antimicrobials. WHO defines this as: '*the cost-effective use of antimicrobials which maximises their clinical therapeutic effect, while minimising both drug-related toxicity and the development of antimicrobial resistance*'.

A good antimicrobial prescribing policy or guidelines will contribute to prudent (and thus cost-effective) use of antimicrobials.

Type and format of guidance

Antimicrobial prescribing guidelines come in many formats. Before starting to write guidelines, both the format and the intent must be decided:
• advisory or mandatory
• policy, guidelines, restricted list
• educational.

It has been shown that prescribers prefer an educational approach and this may have the best long-term impact. However, it may be necessary to give mandatory advice on the use of certain high-cost/sensitive drugs.

The format must be easily accessible to prescribers at the time of prescribing. Computer-based guidelines offer the opportunity to provide additional educational material and may be linked to a computerized prescribing package. This may be the best approach in the community where most GP practices use electronic prescribing. However, few hospitals in the UK use electronic prescribing and most doctors will not have a computer at the bedside. Thus most hospital guidelines are presented as a booklet, card, or Filofax insert which can be kept in the pocket. An ideal format is a pocket-size ready reference linked to more detailed electronic guidelines.

The amount of detail will be determined by the presentation. As a minimum the recommended drug and an alternative (if needed) due to allergy, (adult) dose, route, and duration should be included. More detailed policies might also include side effects, contraindications, use in children, in the elderly, and in pregnancy, etc.

Style and layout must be clear and easy to follow. In lengthier guidelines an index or contents list should be provided. Use plain English throughout and avoid Latin abbreviations such as 'tds' (if space permits). Note that different countries use different abbreviations, which may cause confusion for visiting staff—e.g. the US abbreviation 'qd' means once a day but may be misinterpreted as the UK 'qds' or four times a day. During the drafting process it is advisable to 'pilot' the guidelines to ensure that potential users interpret them in the way intended.

Hard-copy guidelines should be robust, using card (laminated if possible) rather than paper and good-quality printing.

Target audience

This should be identified. Are restrictions just applicable to junior doctors or to senior medical staff as well? Write the guidelines as if they are aimed at a doctor who has newly joined the hospital/GP practice and who needs to find what to prescribe in a situation quickly and easily.

Authors

Hospital antimicrobial guidelines are usually produced as a collaboration between microbiology and pharmacy. To ensure local ownership, consultants in the relevant specialities should be invited to contribute or comment— e.g. surgeons for surgical prophylaxis. In the community, guidelines may be produced by a committee of GPs from one or more practices, usually with the assistance of the prescribing adviser. Ideally, local primary and secondary care policies should be linked.

Content

Guidelines should:
- be evidence based and recommendations referenced as appropriate
- advise on when **not** to prescribe, as this is as valid as advice on when and what antimicrobial to prescribe
- discourage unnecessary use of the parenteral route
- include contact numbers for microbiology, pharmacy medicines information service
- be cross-referenced to other relevant hospital/practice guidelines.

Cost may be included but may become outdated before the guidelines are due for revision. As a minimum, the following areas should be covered.
- Surgical prophylaxis.
- Meningitis prophylaxis.
- Empirical treatment (first and second choice) for:
  - meningitis
  - urinary tract infection
  - lower respiratory tract infection
  - sepsis.

Other areas which should be included are as follows.
- Prophylaxis in asplenic patients.
- Empirical treatment for:
  - GI infection
  - MRSA
  - upper respiratory tract infection
  - skin infection.

A suggested list of recommended areas to cover is provided at ✍ http://www.jac.oxfordjournals.org/content/60/suppl_1/i87.full

Updating

The guidelines should state the issue date and frequency of review. As a minimum, guidelines should be reviewed and updated as necessary every 2 years.

Monitoring and audit

Adherence to the guidelines should be monitored. For example, a specific area such as vascular surgery prophylaxis can be audited. If there is significant non-adherence, the reasons should be established and addressed.

Antimicrobial resistance

Resistance is an almost inevitable consequence of antimicrobial use. As bacteria, viruses, or other micro-organisms reproduce, mutations can spontaneously occur. These mutations might provide some protection against the action of certain antimicrobials. 'Survival of the fittest' means that when these micro-organisms are exposed to antimicrobials, the fully sensitive ones are suppressed but resistant ones survive, reproduce, and become the dominant strain. Most attention has been focused on bacterial resistance, but the principles discussed here apply to all micro-organisms.

Mechanisms of resistance

- Change in cell wall permeability, thus ↓ drug access to intracellular target sites. The relatively simple cell wall of Gram-positive bacteria makes them inherently more permeable and therefore this resistance mechanism is more common in Gram-negative than Gram-positive bacteria.
- Enzyme degradation of the drug—the best known is breakdown of the β-lactam ring of penicillins, cephalosporins, and carbapenems by β-lactamases.
- Efflux pumps actively remove the drug from the cell.
- Mutation at the target site.
  - Alteration of penicillin-binding proteins leads to resistance to β-lactam antibiotics.
  - Changes in the structure of the enzyme reverse transcriptase leads to resistance to reverse transcriptase inhibitors.

Some organisms can develop multiple resistance mechanisms—e.g. *Pseudomonas aeruginosa* manifests resistance to carbapenems through production of β-lactamase, ↑ in efflux pumps, and changes to the bacterial cell wall.

Implications of antimicrobial resistance

Antimicrobial resistance leads to ↑ in the following.

- Morbidity:
  - patients might be sicker for longer
  - hospital stays are ↑
  - alternative antimicrobials might be more toxic
  - residential placements might be difficult
  - isolation and institutionalization.
- Mortality.
- Cost.
  - Newer, potentially more expensive antimicrobials might have to be used.
  - Extended hospital stay.
  - More nursing time.
  - ↑ use of disposables (e.g. aprons and gloves).
  - In some cases, equipment might have to be discarded.

New strains of resistant bacteria are appearing at an alarming rate. Within the hospital environment, MRSA has been a problem for many years but the emergence of vancomycin-resistant MRSA (VRSA) and community-acquired MRSA (C-MRSA) is of significant concern. Other increasingly problematic resistant organisms are as follows:

- vancomycin-resistant enterococci (VRE)
- extended-spectrum β-lactamases (ESBLs)
- *Acinetobacter baumanii.*

At present, agents to treat these resistant organisms are available, but they tend to be expensive, with a higher risk of side effects. However, the production of new drugs is not keeping up with development of new resistant bacteria, and the possibility of resistant species emerging for which there is no antibacterial therapy available is very real.

Measuring resistance

In vitro resistance tests generally require the organism to be cultured in the presence of antimicrobials.

Disk diffusion

Disk diffusion involves culturing bacteria on an agar plate that has had samples (impregnated disks) of an antibacterial placed on it. If there is no growth around the antibacterial, the bacteria are sensitive to the antibacterial, but if the bacteria grow around the sample, this means that they are resistant. Partial growth represents intermediate susceptibility.

E-test

The E-test is based on similar principles to disk diffusion, but here an impregnated strip containing a single antibacterial at ↑ concentrations is placed on the agar plate. Bacterial growth is inhibited around the strip after it reaches a certain concentration. This is equivalent to the MIC.

These tests can be problematic for slow-growing bacteria, such as mycobacteria, and for organisms that are difficult to culture, such as viruses. Newer tests involve amplifying and examining the genetic material of the organism to look for mutations that are known to be associated with resistance. This technique is used for HIV-resistance testing.

Risk factors for antimicrobial resistance

Excessive and inappropriate antimicrobial use results in selective pressures that facilitate the emergence of resistant micro-organisms. It is estimated that up to 50% of antimicrobial use is inappropriate. Unnecessary antimicrobial use contributes to resistance without any clinical gain. This includes the following.

- Use of antimicrobials for infections that are trivial or self-limiting.
- Use of antibacterials to treat infection of viral origin—e.g. the common cold.
- Over-long antimicrobial prophylaxis or treatment courses.

Even appropriate antimicrobial therapy is ↑ worldwide, in addition to ↑ use of broad-spectrum antibacterials and prolonged courses. This is due to the following reasons.

- ↑ numbers of severely ill hospital patients.
- More frequent use of invasive devices and procedures.
- Presence of more severely immunocompromised patients in hospitals and the community. ↑ opportunity for dissemination of infection ↑ the possibility of spread of resistant organisms between patients. This is facilitated by the following.
  - Overcrowding in hospital and community healthcare facilities.
  - ↑ hospital throughput.
  - Poor cleaning and disinfection of rooms, equipment, and hands.

Strategies to ↓ or contain antimicrobial resistance

Three main strategies are required to ↓ or contain antimicrobial resistance.
- Prevention of infection through the following mechanisms:
  - vaccines.
  - prophylaxis.
  - ↓ use of invasive devices.
  - good hygiene.
- ↓ dissemination of antimicrobial-resistant organisms (see 📖 p.440, 'Infection control').
- Limiting or modifying antimicrobial use.

Further reading

Standing Medical Advisory Committee, Subgroup on Antimicrobial Resistance (1998). *The Path of Least Resistance.* ℅ http://www.dh.gov.uk/prod_consum_dh/groups/dh_digitalassets/@dh/@en/documents/digitalasset/dh_4120729.pdf

Infection control

Infection control is important in hospital and community residential facilities for the following reasons.
- To prevent cross-transmission of infection.
- To prevent the spread of resistant micro-organisms.

Special attention should be paid to infection control in areas where patients are most vulnerable:
- intensive care units
- neonatal units
- burns wards
- vascular wards
- units treating immunocompromised patients.

Special attention should also be paid to infection control where procedures or devices make patients more vulnerable:
- urinary catheters
- intravascular devices
- surgical procedures
- respiratory care equipment
- enteral or parenteral feeding.

Infection control should be an integral part of the culture of any institution. This requires the following considerations.
- There is an infection control lead clinician or nurse.
- There are written procedures for infection control.
- Staff (including temporary staff and locums) receive education and training on infection control procedures.
- There are adequate supplies and facilities—e.g. availability of aprons and gloves.
- There is documentation of additional infection control requirements, as necessary, for individual patients.
- Healthcare staff are immunized, as needed, for hepatitis B, TB, chickenpox, and influenza.
- There are written procedures for managing occupational exposure to blood-borne viruses, and staff are made aware of these procedures.

Universal precautions

Strict attention to hygiene is essential. All body fluids and contaminated equipment, including linen, from all patients should be handled as if infected. This is known as 'universal precautions' and includes taking appropriate measures to ensure the following.
- Prevent contamination—e.g. wearing apron and gloves and bagging dirty linen.
- Dispose of waste safely—e.g. use of clinical waste bins and sharps boxes.
- Protect staff against occupational exposure to blood-borne viruses—e.g. hepatitis B and C, and HIV.

Isolation of patients

It might be necessary to nurse patients in isolation in the following circumstances.

- They are a potential source of infection—e.g. MRSA, *C.difficile* diarrhoea, and TB.
- They are particularly vulnerable to infection ('reverse barrier nursing')—e.g. severely neutropenic patients.

Isolation procedures include the following.

- Nursing patients in a side room or, if more than one patient has the same infection, in a cordoned-off area.
- Wearing protective clothing when in contact with the patient. This includes staff who might be in contact with the patient elsewhere in the hospital (e.g. hospital porters).
- Ensuring that equipment is disinfected immediately after use.
- Ensuring that aprons, gloves, and other disposables are disposed of safely (usually bagged within the room).
- Ensuring that visitors take appropriate measures to prevent cross-contamination—e.g. handwashing and wearing protective clothing for particularly vulnerable patients.

Handwashing or decontamination

Hand hygiene is an essential part of infection control. It is effective for prevention of cross-contamination, but unfortunately compliance is often poor—particularly if staff are overworked and stressed.

Education of all staff (clinical and non-clinical) on hand hygiene is essential, in addition to ensuring adequate facilities for washing or decontamination. The usual procedures include the following.

- Staff 'bare below the elbows' in clinical areas (i.e. wearing short or rolled-up sleeves, no wrist watches or bracelets, no rings except wedding rings) in order to facilitate hand hygiene.
- Hands must be decontaminated before and after any episode of patient contact, including handling patients' possessions at the bedside–e.g. when checking patients' own drugs.
- Visibly soiled or potentially grossly contaminated hands should be washed with soap and water; otherwise alcohol gel can be used (with the exception of potential exposure to *C.difficile* as the spores are resistant to alcohol).
- Attention should be paid to ensuring the whole of the hand is decontaminated, including the following:
  - wrists
  - thumbs
  - between the fingers
  - backs of hands.

Pharmacists and infection control

To avoid contamination of medicines, in addition to presenting a professional appearance, a high standard of cleanliness should be maintained in pharmacy shops and dispensaries. Special attention should be paid to ensuring that the following areas are kept clean and tidy.

- Dispensing benches, especially areas where extemporaneous dispensing is carried out.
- Drug refrigerators.
- Toilets.
- Storage areas (often neglected).

Pharmacy staff should have access to handwashing facilities with soap and hot water. Aprons, gloves, and (as appropriate) masks should be used when preparing extemporaneous preparations. Tablets and capsules should not be handled—use counting trays and tweezers or a spatula, and disinfect these frequently.

Note that the type of patient contact experienced in a community pharmacy is extremely unlikely to lead to transmission of infection, including MRSA and TB.

Pharmacists do not often have 'hands-on' contact with patients but they should still observe infection-control procedures. These include the following.

- Decontaminating hands on entering and leaving clinical areas, and before and after direct patient contact.
- Wearing gloves and an apron when in close or prolonged contact with high-risk patients—e.g. those with MRSA.
- Wearing gloves, as appropriate, for 'hands-on' patient contact—e.g. wound care.
- Checking that new staff, trainees and locums, or temporary staff, if necessary, have immunity to chickenpox, TB. and hepatitis B.

In the UK, NICE[1] has published guidelines on infection control in primary and community care (including antimicrobial treatment and prophylaxis) in the following areas:

- standard principles
- care of patients with long-term urinary catheters
- care during enteral feeding
- care of patients with central venous catheters.

1 NICE guidance: http://guidance.nice.org.uk/CG2/Guidance/pdf/English

Therapy-related issues: endocrine system

Diabetes mellitus *444*
Monitoring and control *449*
Thyroid disorders *450*

Diabetes mellitus

Diabetes mellitus (DM) affects approximately 4% of the UK population. In 2009, Diabetes UK reported that 2.6 million people in the UK have diabetes.

Type 2 diabetes accounts for 90% of all diabetes and is a result of insulin resistance and pancreatic β-cell dysfunction. Type 1 diabetes results from an absolute insulin deficiency secondary to autoimmune dysfunction.

Diabetes is the leading cause of kidney failure and the leading cause of blindness in 20–74-year-olds. Among diabetics, the risks for stroke, heart disease, and death from heart disease are 2–4 times higher than those of the non-diabetic population. Diabetes accounts for more than 60% of all non-traumatic lower limb amputations.

Diabetes is likely to reach epidemic proportions in the UK unless there are significant efforts to tackle lifestyle issues such as obesity and lack of exercise.

Oral therapy is used alone in the early stages and in combination with insulin to treat type 2 diabetes. Insulin is used as monotherapy in type 1 diabetes and in some type 2 patients.

Diagnosis

The main symptoms with which a patient with undiagnosed diabetes can present include:
- polydipsia
- polyuria
- nocturia
- extreme tiredness
- unexplained weight loss
- reduced wound-healing rates
- blurred vision
- genital itch/frequent episodes of thrush.

Together with these symptoms, a diagnosis of diabetes can be confirmed when any of the following results are noted in clinical tests.
- A random plasma glucose level ≥11mmol/L.
- A fasting plasma glucose ≥7mmol/L.
- A 2h plasma glucose concentration ≥11mmol/L after 75g glucose load in an oral glucose tolerance test.

NB: in practice, evidence of sugars in urine together with the symptoms stated is sufficient to instigate serious investigation.

Management

The management of diabetes involves lifestyle and pharmacological therapy. Pharmacological therapy includes insulin and oral hypoglycaemics. Adjustments to diet and increasing exercise remain the cornerstones for treatment of diabetes.

When glycosylated haemoglobin (HbA$_{1c}$) or blood glucose goals are not met by oral monotherapy, combination therapy is more effective than switching to another monotherapy. Switching or replacing drug therapy is not recommended.

Combination therapy allows for greater glucose lowering, addressing both major physiological defects of type 2 diabetes—insulin secretory failure and insulin resistance. It is important to keep in mind the percentage degree of HbA$_{1c}$-lowering achievable from monotherapy, combination, and triple therapy when making decisions to help patients reach HbA$_{1c}$ goals. Remember that statistical significance in trials needs to translate to clinical significance for patients.

Approximate HbA$_{1c}$-lowering values (not including insulin) are:
- monotherapy ~0.6–2.5%
- combination therapy ~2%
- triple therapy ~2%–2.5%.

HbA$_{1c}$-lowering value from insulin has no ceiling, but is limited by hypoglycaemia.

Insulin

Insulin is necessary for type 1 diabetics and for type 2 diabetics who are inadequately controlled or during periods of stress. Insulin is also used in gestational diabetics inadequately controlled by diet and exercise.

There are various types of insulin based on onset and duration of action (see Table 21.1) as well as premixed combination products.
- Generally mixing of insulins should be discouraged.
- Insulin glargine and detemir may not be mixed with any other insulins.

Table 21.1 Insulin types: human and insulin analogues

Insulin	Onset	Peak	Duration
Rapid-acting analogues (lispro, aspart, glulisine)	10–15min	1–2h	3–5h
Short-acting human regular (soluble)	30–60min	2–4h	5–8h
Intermediate-acting human (e.g. isophane)	1–2h	4–12h	10–16h
Protamine zinc is longer-acting			
Long-acting analogues			
Detemir[*]	3–8h	None	~24h
Glargine[*]	2–4h	None	Up to 24h

[*]Two or more injections may be required in some patients

- Insulin is stable for 28 days once opened (with the exception of detemir which is stable for 42 days) and can be stored in or out of the refrigerator, although generally pens in use are not stored in a refrigerator. Unopened refrigerated insulin is stable until the manufacturer's expiration date.
- The goal of any insulin regimen or combination is to target control, avoid hypoglycaemia, and be acceptable to the patient.
- Consider insulin therapy when HbA₁c >8% and the patient is already on combination or triple therapy and exhibits hyperglycaemia. Oral agents are often continued if a once- or twice-daily insulin regime is chosen.
- Although premixed insulin offers the advantage of decreased injections, it is difficult to adjust either insulin component successfully.
- Insulin dosage can be adjusted every 3–7 days on the basis of patient's self-monitoring of blood glucose. However, patients who have developed an understanding of the process will adjust more frequently to manage changes in lifestyle such as intensive exercise or a larger than normal meal.
- Insulin regimes are often tailored to fit preferences and lifestyle. Initiation of insulin therapy can be a challenging concept, and patients need time to adjust. There may be benefits in starting on a once- or twice-daily regime and moving to four times a day if control is difficult.

Insulin pens
- Insulin pens offer flexibility in patient schedules as they are more discreet and may offer an alternative to those who fear injections or have dexterity or visual impairments.
- Pens are either disposable or have replaceable cartridges.
- Pens hold 300 units (3mL) of insulin and come in boxes of five.
- The stability of insulin pen contents in use is usually 28 days, but this should be checked with the SPC as there are variations.

Oral agents
Second-generation sulfonylureas
- Mechanism: stimulate insulin release from binding to sulfonlyurea β-cell site.
- Target post-prandial glucose.
- Place in therapy: monotherapy, combination therapy, can be first line.
- Reduction in HbA₁c: 0.9–2.5%.
- Examples: gliclazide, glibenclamide.
- Risks: hypoglycaemia, weight gain.
- No additional benefit at doses >50% of maximum dose.

Biguanides
- Mechanism: decrease gluconeogenesis and increase peripheral utilization of glucose.
- Target fasting blood glucose.
- Place in therapy: considered first line, monotherapy, combination therapy.
- Reduction in HbA₁c: 1–1.3%.
- Available as metformin immediate release and metformin extended release (MR); no real advantage over standard formulation.

- Increase dose by 500mg/day weekly.
- Maximum effective dose is 2000mg/day.
- Lactic acidosis rare (<0.3%, but 50% fatal).
- Does not cause hypoglycaemia.
- Contraindicated with serum creatinine 133µmol/L in men and 124µmol/L in women.
- Use with caution in patients aged >80 years (should have normal renal clearance) and in those with hepatic dysfunction, alcoholism, unstable congestive heart failure (CHF), or dehydration.
- GI side effects (nausea, vomiting, diarrhoea) occur in up to 50% of patients; can give with food; start low and go slow.
- Improved lipid profile; weight neutral or weight loss.
- Decreased macrovascular events.

Meglitinides

- Mechanism: stimulate insulin release from binding to sulfonlyurea β-cell site.
- Target post-prandial glucose; short-acting.
- Place in therapy: monotherapy or combination therapy.
- Reduction in HbA_{1c}: 0.6–0.8%.
- Examples: repaglinide, nateglinide.
- Risks: hypoglycaemia; weight gain.
- The need for frequent dosing may adversely affect compliance.

Thiazolidinediones

- Mechanism: activate PPAR-G (peroxisome proliferator-activated receptor gamma), increasing peripheral insulin sensitivity in skeletal muscle cells.
- Target fasting blood glucose.
- Place in therapy: considered second line, but could be monotherapy in patients with lower HbA_{1c} range(6.5–8%), combination therapy.
- Reduction in HbA_{1c}: 1.5–1.6%.
- Example: pioglitazone.
- Oedema and weight gain occur more in combination with insulin.
- Contraindicated in NYHA Class III and IV heart failure; do not use in patients with underlying liver dysfunction.
- An increase in bone fracture rates has been reported in women.
- Delayed onset of action; may be 6–8wks (or as much as 12wks).
- Pioglitazone may have positive effects on lipids (↑HDL, ↓TG).
- In September 2010, following a Europe-wide review of available data on the risks and benefits of rosiglitazone, the UK Commission on Human Medicine (CHM) withdrew this product from clinical use in the UK because of increased risk of cardiovascular disorders including MI and cardiac failure.

α-glucosidase inhibitors

- Mechanism: slow carbohydrate absorption in gut.
- Target post-prandial glucose.
- Place in therapy: monotherapy or combination therapy.
- Reduction in HbA_{1c}: 0.6–1.3%.
- Example: acarbose.
- Must take with carbohydrate-containing meal.

- Decrease post-prandial glucose; must be taken with first bite of food.
- Start low and go slow to avoid GI intolerance.
- If hypoglycaemia occurs (risk if on insulin or sulfonylurea), must treat with glucose, not sucrose, as acarbose interferes with sucrose absorption.

Dipeptidyl peptidase inhibitors (DPP IV)

- Mechanism: slows inactivation of incretin hormone GLP-4, suppressing glucagon secretion and increasing glucose-dependent insulin release.
- Target post-prandial blood glucose.
- Place in therapy: monotherapy or combination therapy.
- Reduction in HbA_{1c}: 0.8%.
- Examples: sitagliptin, vildagliptin.
- Dosage adjustment necessary in renal dysfunction.
- Increase satiety.
- Delay gastric emptying.
- Weight neutral.

Newer antidiabetic treatments

Exenatide

- Glucagon-like peptide-1 (GLP-1) incretin mimetic; mimics incretin hormone given by injection.
- Mechanism: stimulates insulin secretion in response to glucose load; inhibits release of glucagon following a meal; increases satiety; slows absorption of nutrients through delayed gastric emptying.
- Place in therapy: adjunct therapy for use in combination with sulfonyl-ureas, metformin, or a combination of these.
- Reduction in HbA_{1c}: 0.8–0.9%.
- Common side effects include nausea and vomiting (dose-related).
- Recent reports of possible exenatide pancreatitis have arisen.
- Currently its use is not recommended in patients with a history of pancreatitis.

Biphasic insulin

A wide range of biphasic (mixed) insulins are available. Readers are referred to the *BNF* or relevant SPC for up-to-date information.

Monitoring and control

Monitoring

The place of blood glucose monitoring is well recognized in patients with diabetes who require insulin treatment. There are now a wide range of meters available, in addition to finger-pricking devices. It is important to be familiar with a range of machines. The list of those available can be found on the Diabetes UK website.[1] Most companies provide meters at low cost directly to patients, and this route is considerably cheaper than purchasing over the counter.

Recent developments have both ↓ the volume of blood required and ↓ the speed of analysis to 75s. Some can link to computer programs and estimate average levels according to chosen parameters.

Monitoring of patients with type 2 diabetes tends to be frowned upon by pharmaceutical advisers. However, there are good reasons for regular, if less frequent, monitoring, and it should be encouraged. A sensible pattern might be to monitor twice weekly to ensure that there are no major changes in glucose levels. It is also useful to monitor for lifestyle changes such as ↑ exercise, change of diet, fasting, and other influencing factors (e.g. mild illness).

Finger-pricking devices are often supplied with meters, which are not prescribable (the lancets are) but can be purchased from community pharmacies. Unfortunately, they all seem to be somewhat painful to use. Laser devices claim to be painless but are very expensive.

Control

Target glucose levels are usually set at 4–7mmol/L for fasting and <9mmol/L for post-prandial levels. In the UK, glucose is measured in units of mmol/L. Other countries use mg/100mL. The conversion is 1mmol/L equivalent to 18mg/100mL.

Regular monitoring of HbA_{1c} gives a good pattern of levels in the previous 3 months. The target level for HbA_{1c} should be <7%. However, some authorities set lower levels.

1 ॐ http://www.diabetes.org.uk/home.htm

Thyroid disorders

The thyroid gland is the only endocrine gland to store large quantities of pre-formed hormones. Found anterior to the trachea in the lower neck, it is the largest endocrine organ of the human body and regulates the body's metabolism through the release of thyroid hormones in response to thyroid-stimulating hormone (TSH) formed by the anterior pituitary gland. Cells are arranged within the gland in spherical follicles that surround a thyroid hormone store and release two hormones:

- thyroxine (T_4)—a pro-hormone that acts as a plasma reservoir
- tri-iodothyronine (T_3)—the active hormone

These hormones are derived from two molecules of iodine and the amino acid tyrosine, with T_3 containing three iodine atoms and T_4 containing four. The iodine required is acquired mainly from iodized salt, meat, and vegetables in the diet. The recommended daily intake of iodine is 150mg, though only a fraction of this amount is absorbed as the thyroid gland cells are the only cells in the body that can actively absorb and utilize plasma iodine. Iodine is then returned to the plasma by the breakdown of these hormones and excreted from the body mainly via the kidneys.

The T_3 and T_4 hormones released by the thyroid gland regulate the rate of metabolism in almost every cell in the body, oxygen consumption, and heat production. They also have a role in growth and development, as well as sensitizing the cardiovascular and nervous system to catecholamines.

Regulation of thyroid hormones

Hypothalamic thyrotrophin-releasing hormone (TRH) stimulates the release of TSH from the anterior pituitary gland which, in turn, acts on extracellular receptors on the surface of the thyroid follicular cells to stimulate the synthesis and secretion of T_3 and T_4. TSH also has long-term actions on the thyroid gland, increasing its size and vascularity to improve hormone synthesis.

Thyroid hormone release is inhibited by the presence of excess thyroid hormones in the bloodstream and glucocorticoids (e.g. cortisol) which act on the anterior pituitary to suppress TSH.

The active hormone T_3 affects almost every cell in the body. Peripheral tissues can regulate the amount of T_3 in circulation by increasing or decreasing the amount of T_3 synthesis. Most of the deiodination is carried out by the liver and kidney. T_4, a relatively inactive molecule, is converted to T_3 by deiodination. It is important to note the following.

- The majority of plasma T_3 is formed by deiodination of T_4 and not directly from the thyroid gland.
- The concentration of T_4 in circulation is much higher than that of T_3 by a ratio of 50:1.
- T_4 has a longer half life than T_3 (7 days versus 1 day).

Transport of the thyroid hormones

T_3 and T_4 hormones are carried in circulation bound to plasma proteins produced in the liver, thus protecting them from enzymatic attack. 70% is bound to thyroid-binding globulin (TBG) and 30% to albumin.

Only 0.1% of T_4 and 1% of T_3 are carried unbound. It is this free (unbound) fraction which is responsible for their hormonal activities.

Disorders of the thyroid gland

The thyroid gland is prone to a number of diseases that can alter its function and structure. As nearly all body tissues are affected by thyroid hormones, an alteration in their level of secretion affects the activity of virtually all body systems, giving rise to a wide range of presenting symptoms. The main categories of disease are:

• hyperthyroidism
• hypothyroidism
• goitre formation
• adenoma of the thyroid
• carcinoma of the thyroid.

Thyroid function tests

First-line diagnosis of primary hyper- and hypothyroidism is made from examination of serum TSH concentrations. However, this test alone is misleading in patients with secondary thyroid dysfunction.

Free hormone concentrations are unaffected by changes in binding protein concentration or affinity and usually correlate better with the metabolic state than do total hormone concentrations. Therefore serum T_3 and T_4 concentrations are measured using highly specific and sensitive radio-immunoassay.

As the presenting symptoms of thyroid disorders can be varied and non-specific, biochemical confirmation is necessary, but it is important to remember that these tests should never be used alone to diagnose and decide whether treatment is necessary as clinical features need to be taken into account. Indeed, abnormalities are noted in thyroid function tests during systemic illnesses. Therefore a diagnosis of hyper- or hypothyroidism should not be made in the presence of any recognized concurrent systemic illness, and the tests should be repeated once the illness has resolved to ensure an accurate representation of a patient's thyroid function. In instances where abnormal test results are detected in the absence of any signs or symptoms, close monitoring of the patient is required but no treatment.

Table 21.2 shows thyroid hormone concentrations seen with various thyroid abnormalities, and Table 21.3 shows the reference ranges against which variances are determined.

When interpreting the results of thyroid function tests, the effects of any drugs that the patient is taking should be borne in mind. Table 21.4 shows how the processes of the thyroid gland can be affected by certain medications.

Table 21.2 Thyroid hormone concentrations associated with various thyroid abnormalities

Condition	TSH	Free T_4	Free T_3
Primary hyperthyroidism	Undetectable	↑↑	↑
T_3 toxicosis	Undetectable	Normal	↑↑
Thyrotoxicosis	↓	↑	↑
Subclinical hyperthyroidism	↓	Normal	Normal
Secondary hyperthyroidism (TSHoma)	↑ or normal	↑	↑
Thyroid hormone resistance or consider adherence to treatment	↑ or normal	↑	↑
Primary hypothyroidism	↑	↓	↓ or normal
Secondary hypothyroidism	↓ or normal	↓	↓ or normal
Subclinical hypothyroidism	↑	Normal	Normal
Pituitary disease/sick euthyroidism	↓	↓	↓

Table 21.3 Typical reference ranges used in thyroid function tests

Test	Range
TS	0.4–4.5mU/L
Free T_3	3.5–7.8pmol/
Free T_4	9.0–25.0pmol/

Table 21.4 Influence of drugs on thyroid function tests

Metabolic process	Increased	Decreased
TSH secretion	Amiodarone (transiently: becomes normal after 2–3mo)	Glucocorticoids, dopamine agonists, phenytoin, dopamine
T_4 synthesis/release	Iodide	Iodide, lithium
Binding proteins	Oestrogen, clofibrate, diamorphine	Glucocorticoids, androgens, phenytoin, carbamazepine
T_4 metabolism	Anticonvulsants; rifampicin	
T_4/T_3 binding in serum		Salicylates, furosemide, glucocorticoids, mefenamic acid, amiodarone, β-blockers

Hyperthyroidism

Hyperthyroidism affects approximately 1% of the UK population and is six times more common in women. It is defined as overactivity of the thyroid gland leading to the release of excess T_3 and T_4 hormones which, when symptomatic, is called thyrotoxicosis. The two main causes in the UK, which account for more than 90% of cases, are as follows.

- Graves' disease—an autoimmune disease which is the most common cause of hyperthyroidism in the 20–50 age group. It is characterized by the presence of thyroid-stimulating antibodies in the blood which bind to TSH receptors in the thyroid and stimulate them to produce excess thyroid hormones in the same way as TSH stimulates the receptors.
- Solitary toxic nodule/toxic multinodular goitre (depending on the number of nodules).

Other causes are as follows.
- Solitary toxic adenoma.
- Thyroiditis due to viral infection, pregnancy, or some drugs such as amiodarone or interferon—usually transient.
- Exogenous iodine and iodine-containing drugs.
- Excessive T_3 and T_4 ingestion.

Clinical features

The presenting features in mild cases are often noted to mimic an anxiety state. The most common clinical features of hyperthyroidism are:
- weight loss (but normal appetite)
- sweating; heat intolerance
- increased rate and depth of respiration
- diarrhoea/increased frequency of defecation
- fatigue
- generalized muscle weakness and muscle tremor
- cardiac symptoms (palpitations, sinus tachycardia or atrial fibrillation, angina, heart failure).

Other symptoms include:
- agitation
- hyperkinesis
- insomnia
- oligomenorrhoea, infertility
- goitre
- eyelid retraction, lid lag.

Features specific to Graves' disease include periorbital oedema, proptosis, diplopia, opthalmoplegia, corneal ulceration, and loss of visual acuity, with pre-tibial myxoedema occurring in one-third of these patients. Untreated Graves' disease has a natural history of remission and relapse; 30–40% of patients only ever have a single episode of hyperthyroidism.

On rare occasions, patients with thyrotoxicosis present with a thyroid storm or crisis, which is considered a medical emergency as features include hyperpyrexia, dehydration, and cardiac failure.

Treatment of Graves' disease and nodular thyrotoxicosis

Anti-thyroid drugs

Carbimazole (the first choice of anti-thyroid drug in the UK) and propylthiouracil are both thionamides which inhibit thyroid peroxidase-catalysed iodination of T_4 residues and the coupling of iodotryosyl residues to reduce the synthesis of T_4 from iodine. These drugs are the first choice of therapy in younger patients with Graves' disease and are usually given for a period of 1–2 years, monitoring thyroid status during this time and after. A delay in effect of up to 4wks from initial administration is often seen because the pre-formed hormones are still being released from the thyroid gland when using this prescription.

Once thyroid function tests have revealed that the patient has reached a state of normal gland function (i.e. a euthyroid state), the prescribed dose can usually be reduced to a lower maintenance dose. The actual dose is determined by regular monitoring of thyroid function tests. 30–40% of patients treated with these drugs stay euthyroid for 10 years after discontinuation of therapy, with a further course of the same or alternative treatment given if the patient relapses.

NB: 5mg of carbimazole is roughly equivalent to 50mg of propylthiouracil, with propylthiouracil being the drug of choice during pregnancy and lactation because of its lower concentration in breastmilk and the possible association of carbimazole with aplasia cutis.

Two alternative treatment regimes are used.

Dose titration regime

As mentioned, the primary aim is to achieve a euthyroid state with high doses and then maintain euthyroidism with a low stable dose for approximately 18 months. The dose of thionamides is titrated according to the thyroid function tests performed every 4–8wks, aiming for a serum free T_4 in the normal range and a detectable TSH. A high serum TSH indicates a need for a dose reduction. TSH may remain suppressed for weeks or months.

The typical starting dose of carbimazole is 20–30mg daily and the treatment is continued for 18 months.

Block and replace regime

After achieving a euthyroid state on carbimazole alone, carbimazole at a dose of 40mg daily together with levothyroxine at a dose of 100micrograms daily can be prescribed. The main advantage of this regime is that fewer hospital visits are required and the duration of treatment is often reduced to 6 months. During treatment, free T_4 levels are measured 4wks after starting levothyroxine and the dose of levothyroxine is altered, if necessary, in increments of 25micrograms to maintain free T_4 in the normal range. Most patients do not require dose adjustments.

NB: relapses are common after either regime within the first year and are most likely in patients with large goitres and high T_4 levels at the time of diagnosis.

Side effects
Potential side effects of carbimazole and propylthiouracil are as follows.
- Pruritus and maculopapular rash—these can be treated with anti-histamines without discontinuing treatment
- Sensitivity reaction (e.g. arthralgia, jaundice, lymphadenopathy, vomiting, pyrexia.)—withdrawal from treatment is required in this instance. There is rarely cross-sensitivity between the two drugs. Therefore, once the patient has recovered, the other drug can be tried.
- Agranulocytosis—characterized by fever, systemic upset, mouth ulceration, and sore throat. This rare but serious side effect of both drugs is seen in 0.1–0.5% of patients and occurs very suddenly (usually within the first 3 months of therapy) in equal frequency with both anti-thyroid drugs. All patients prescribed with these drugs should be told to report these symptoms to their GP or hospital consultant and stop the drug immediately.

NB: one drug should not be substituted for the other after this reaction has been diagnosed.

Compliance with these drugs can be a problem as the patient may initially feel worse in terms of their presenting symptoms, with women often concerned about weight gain. Patients should be counselled that they will have adjusted to the change in metabolic rate after a few months, and a general improvement in symptoms will be seen.

β-blockers
β-blockers (e.g. propranolol at a dose of 20–80mg, three times a day), may provide effective temporary relief of cardiac symptoms, particularly palpitations and tremor as well as anxiety, while the anti-thyroid drugs (thionamides) take effect, but should be avoided in patients with asthma. However, it is important to consider that many of the symptoms of hyperthyroidism have a β_2 component, therefore contraindicating the use of cardioselective β-blockers.

Surgery
Thyroid surgery, a total or sub-total thyroidectomy, is rarely performed as a primary course of action as the thyroid overactivity needs to be controlled, usually with anti-thyroid drugs, prior to such a procedure to make the use of anaesthetic safe and reduce the risk of precipitating a dangerous hyperthyroid crisis or 'thyrotoxic storm'. To this end, β-blockers, usually propranolol at a dose of 20mg three times a day, can be prescribed to provide temporary symptomatic relief prior to surgery.

A recognized side effect of surgery is hypothyroidism, for which lifelong levothyroxine replacement will be needed.

Radioactive iodine
This is the primary choice of treatment for toxic nodular hyperthyroidism, if the goitre is not large, and for Graves' disease, especially if there is a relapse after medical treatment or subtotal thyroidectomy, with further doses given at 2–4 months to patients who have not responded.

Radioactive iodine-131 causes necrosis of the overactive gland with minimal local or systemic side effects to the patient and minimal radiation hazard. It is administered as a tasteless oral liquid after ensuring that anti-thyroid drugs have been stopped 1wk prior to commencement of this treatment. β-blockers can be maintained throughout. The thyroid gland may be tender for a few days after treatment.

The following precautions should be taken.

- Careful evaluation of the risks and benefits of this treatment option is needed as patients with thyroid eye disease are more likely to worsen with this therapy. However, worsening of eye symptoms may be prevented with a short course of corticosteroids.
- Although fertility is not affected by this treatment, it is advised that women should avoid becoming pregnant for 6 months following treatment and men should avoid fathering a child within 4 months of treatment. This treatment is contraindicated during pregnancy and it is advised not to breastfeed after therapy.

Treatment of thyroiditis

Many forms of thyroid inflammation (thyroiditis) are described as 'self limiting'. In instances where thyroiditis is painful or prolonged, anti-inflammatory agents or corticosteroids may be helpful, with patients suffering from severe symptoms of thyrotoxicosis finding potential benefit from β-blockers.

Subclinical hyperthyroidism

In cases of subclinical hyperthyroidism, the TSH level is suppressed but the free T_3 and T_4 levels are seen as being normal. This condition, regarded as a precursor of clinical hyperthyroidism, is currently the subject of debate as to whether or not it should be treated. Although treatment may be worthwhile in the elderly, particularly if the heart rhythm becomes abnormal or there is thinning of the bones, the decision of prescribed treatment is a matter for individual clinical assessment and evaluation.

Thyroid crisis

Thyroid crisis, or 'thyrotoxic storm', is a rare but life-threatening exacerbation of the manifestations of thyrotoxicosis and is associated with significant mortality. It is characterized by:

- severe hyperthyroidism associated with fever
- disproportionate tachycardia
- CNS dysfunction—especially confusion or severe irritability
- GI dysfunction—diarrhoea, vomiting, and jaundice

Treatment is needed immediately under intensive care, which is beyond the scope of this chapter.

Hypothyroidism

Hypothyroidism, defined as underactivity of the thyroid gland leading to deficient levels of serum T_3 and T_4, affects approximately 2% of the population in the UK and is 10 times more common in women than in men. When this becomes symptomatic, it is called myxoedema. The two main causes in the UK, which account for more than 90% of cases, are as follows.

- Autoimmune hypothyroidism (Hashimoto's thyroiditis), which typically affects middle-aged and elderly women, where the thyroid cells are destroyed by lymphocytes. It is usually accompanied by the presence of thyroid peroxidase (TPO) antibodies, which can be detected in the blood and therefore are a useful tool for diagnosis.
- Post surgery, radioactive iodine, and anti-thyroid drugs.

Other causes include:
- viral agents (De Quervain's thyroiditis)
- idiopathic atrophic hypothyroidism
- congenital factors
- dyshormonogenic hypothyroidism
- secondary to pituitary or hypothalamic disease
- iodine deficiency
- drugs—reversible cause mainly by amiodarone, lithium, and iodine.

Clinical features

The presentation of hypothyroidism is more gradual than that of hyperthyroidism, with many symptoms often being ignored. The onset may be insidious, with occasional symptoms noted. The clinical signs and symptoms reflect the diverse action that thyroid hormones have on the body, the most common being:
- lethargy
- cold intolerance
- dryness and coarsening of skin and hair and subcutaneous swelling (myxoedema)
- hoarseness
- weight gain
- hyperlipidaemia

Other clinical signs and symptoms include:
- anaemia—usually macrocytic
- depression, dementia, psychosis
- constipation
- bradycardia, angina, heart failure, pericardial effusion
- muscle stiffness
- carpal tunnel syndrome
- infertility, menorrhagia, galactorrhoea
- vitiligo.

Children with hypothyroidism may present with growth failure, delayed pubertal development, or deterioration in academic performance.

Goitre can occur in patients who are hypothyroid, particularly in the presence of Hashimoto's thyroiditis due to the accumulation of lymphocytes in the thyroid gland. However, in many recorded cases there is no goitre present and the thyroid is destroyed by the time diagnosis is confirmed.

Treatment

Thyroid hormone replacement, usually with T_4 (levothyroxine), is the treatment of choice for hypothyroidism, whereby the metabolic rate and demand for oxygen is increased. However, angina or MI may be precipitated if the latter occurs too quickly. Treatment with levothyroxine is preferable to replacement with T_3 for most patients because of its slower onset of action. T_3 is used occasionally where a more rapid response is indicated.

The required dose of levothyroxine ranges from 25 to 200micrograms daily. The initial dose is usually 50micrograms, increasing in increments of 50micrograms every 3–4wks. However, elderly patients and those with ischaemic heart disease are prescribed an initial dose of 25micrograms daily or on alternate days as indicated. The dose should be taken at least 30min before breakfast as food can reduce its absorption.

Although symptomatic improvement is often seen within 2–3wks, it may take up to 6wks before TSH levels respond fully. As a result, TSH levels should be checked after 6wks of commencement of levothyroxine therapy and adjusted accordingly by increments of 25–50micrograms.

Once TSH and T_4 levels return to normal and the patient is symptom free, the adequacy of continuing treatment should be assessed by conducting annual thyroid function tests.

Most patients prescribed with levothyroxine therapy require lifelong treatment. Dose requirements rarely change once the TSH and T_4 levels are stable, with the exceptions of a dose increase which may be necessary during pregnancy and a dose reduction which is sometimes indicated in the elderly. Advice is given to patients not to stop taking the treatment without consulting their doctor as the symptoms would recur. Patients in the UK issued with this prescription can obtain a medical exemption certificate from having to pay for this medication from the NHS Business Services Authority, having filled out a FP92A form available from GP surgeries.

NB: If undertreated, hypothyroidism can progress to a life-threatening myxoedema coma—a medical emergency with high mortality rate where T_3 (oral or injection) is the main treatment advised. However, this may be precipitated by infection, therapy with sedative drugs, or hypothermia, particularly in the elderly population.

Further reading

Turner HE, Wass JAH (2009). Thyroid. In: *Oxford Handbook of Endocrinology and Diabetes* (2nd edn), pp. 2–81. Oxford: Oxford University Press.

Association of Clinical Biochemistry, British Thyroid Association, British Thyroid Foundation (2006). *UK Guidelines for the Use of Thyroid Function Tests* (2006). Available at: ✍ http://www.btf-thyroid.org/images/stories/pdf/tft_guideline_final_version_july_2006.pdf (accessed 10 August 2010).

Toft AD (2002). Hyperthyroidism. In: Robinson S, Meeran K (eds), *Endocrine Specialist Handbook*, pp. 211–32. London: Martin Dunitz.

Lazarus JH, Obuobie K (2002). Graves' disease. In: Robinson S, Meeran K (eds), *Endocrine Specialist Handbook*, pp. 233–42. London: Martin Dunitz.

Wahid ST, Robinson ACJ (2002). Hypothyroidism. In: Robinson S, Meeran K (eds), *Endocrine Specialist Handbook*, pp. 243–55. London: Martin Dunitz.

Daniels GH, Dayan CM (2006). *Fast Facts: Thyroid Disorders*. Abingdon: Health Press.

British Thyroid Association: ✍ http://www.btf-thyroid.org

Therapy-related issues: obstetrics, gynaecology, and urinary tract disorders

Hormonal contraception 460

Hormonal contraception

Contraception has been an important part of human lives since the time of the early Egyptians. While methods have changed dramatically over the years, the purpose remains the same—to control fertility.

Most methods used today are female-driven and involve hormones. These methods are very effective in preventing pregnancy when taken or used as directed. Barrier methods rely on their availability at the time of intercourse and are more efficacious when used with spermicides.

Factors that need to be considered when selecting a method of contraception include the woman's potential ability to adhere to treatment, the age of the patient, medical history, personal history, and reversibility of the agent.

Failure rates for methods include the *perfect rate*, when the method is used perfectly all of the time, and the *typical rate*, which is more consistent with normal use.

Oral contraceptive pills

- Combination (COC)—containing an oestrogen and a progestogen. These are the most reliable in general use.
- Progestogen-only (POP)—these are a suitable alternative where oestrogens are contraindicated or not tolerated but they have a higher failure rate than COCs as good adherence is essential.
- The perfect-use failure rates for COCs and POPs are 0.1% and 0.5%, respectively.
- The typical failure rate is 5% for both pill types.
- Pharmacists should ensure that women are counselled on what to do if a pill is missed—because of either forgetting to take it or a GI upset (Box 22.1).

Transdermal patch

- Evra® contains ethinylestradiol and norelgestromin, a metabolite of norgestimate.
- The patch is changed weekly for 3wks, with the fourth week remaining hormone free.
- The failure rate is 1% for both perfect and typical use.
- Approximately 60% more oestrogen is absorbed into the bloodstream than with traditional 35micrograms pills. This places women at higher risk for thrombosis and myocardial infarctions.
- The patch is less effective in women weighing >90kg, and other methods should be considered.

If a patch change is forgotten in the first week, change the patch-change day and use alternative contraception for the first week of the new cycle. Patch changes forgotten in the second and third week do not need alternative contraception as long as the duration was <48h. Apply a new patch and keep the same day for the next patch-change day. If it was >48h, restart the entire cycle and use alternative contraception for the first week.

Box 22.1 Advice to women who have missed an OCP

A pill counts as missed
- If you have completely forgotten to take it
- If you vomit within 2h of taking a pill or have severe diarrhoea

Combined oral contraceptives

If you miss ONE pill (for 20micrograms pills) or ONE or TWO pills (for 30–35micrograms pills) anywhere in the pack
- Take a pill as soon as possible and continue to take the pills in the pack (even if it means taking two pills in 1 day).
- Use condoms or abstain from sex until you have taken pills for 7 days in a row.
- Emergency contraception is not required. Any pills missed in the last week of the previous pack should be taken into consideration when deciding on emergency contraception.

If you miss TWO or more pills (for 20micrograms pills) or THREE or more pills (for 30–35micrograms pills)
- Take the most recent pill as soon as possible and then continue taking pills daily at the usual time.
- Also use condoms or abstain from sex until pills have been taken for 7 days in a row.
- If pills are missed in week 1 (pills 1–7) and unprotected sex occurs in week 1 or the preceding pill-free interval (PFI), consider the use of emergency contraception.
- If pills are missed in week 2 (pills 8–14), no emergency contraception is needed.
- If pills are missed in week 3 (pills 15–21), finish the pills in your current pack and start a new pack the next day. If you miss out the PFI, no emergency contraception is needed.
- Remember: it is extending the pill-free interval that is risky.
- Take into account any pills missed in the last week of your previous pack when deciding about emergency contraception.

For every-day pill regimens
- If you miss any inactive pills, discard the missed pills and then continue taking the pills daily, one each day.

Progesterone-only pill
- Take it as soon as you remember and take the next pill at the usual time.
- If the pill was 3h late (12h for Cerazette®), use alternative contraception for the next 2 days.
- If you have unprotected sex before two further tablets are taken correctly, consider the use of emergency contraception.

Transvaginal ring

Nuvaring® contains ethinylestradiol and etonogestrel, a metabolite of desogestrel.

- The ring remains in place for 3wks and is removed for the fourth. A new ring is used each month. It can be removed for up to 3h.
- Side effects include increased vaginal discharge, irritation, or infection.
- The perfect-use failure rate is <0.3%, and the typical-use failure rate is 2%.
- The ring can be dislodged with bowel movements.
- If the ring is removed for <3h it should rinsed and reinserted—no alternative contraception is required. If it is removed for >3h:
  - During weeks 1 or 2 rinse and reinsert, and use alternative contraception for 7 days.
  - During week 3 insert a new ring or allow a withdrawal bleed and insert a new ring no later than 7 days after the old ring was removed. No alternative contraception is required provided that a new ring is inserted within 7 days.

Intrauterine

Mirena® contains levonorgestrel and releases the equivalent of three POPs per week.

- The device can remain in place for 5 years.
- Suitable for women taking drugs which are potent enzyme inducers (e.g. phenytoin).
- The failure rate is 0.1% for both perfect and typical use.

Injection

Depo-Provera®—medroxyprogesterone 150mg

- Given by IM injection every 3 months. First dose must be given within 5 days of the beginning of the cycle, or pregnancy must be ruled out if >5 days.
- Suitable for women taking drugs which are potent enzyme inducers (e.g. phenytoin).
- The failure rate is 0.3% for both perfect and typical use.
- Risk of reduction in bone mineral density and, rarely, osteoporosis. Avoid in adolescents or women with risk factors for osteoporosis unless other forms of contraception are unsuitable.

Noristerat®—norethisterone 200mg

- Given by deep IM within 5 days of the beginning of the cycle
- For short-term contraception only—may be repeated once only after 8wks.

Implantable

Nexplanon®—single-rod implant containing etonogestrel.

- Implanted within first 5 days of cycle
- Has a 3-year duration.
- Requires a specially trained professional for placement and removal.
- Failure rate is <0.1% for both perfect and typical use.

Risk of venous thromboembolism (VTE)

The risk of VTE is increased by oestrogen-containing hormonal contraception, though it is lower than the risk of VTE in pregnancy (Table 22.1). Progestogen-only methods appear not to be associated with increased risk of VTE (although evidence is limited). Factors which increase the risk are as follows.

- First year of use.
- Increasing age.
- Higher doses of oestrogen.
- Third-generation progestogen.
- Possible higher risk with transdermal patches than with COC.
- Presence of other risk factors (e.g. increased BMI).

Women should be counselled on the relative risks before starting hormonal contraception, and women on COC, transdermal patches, and the vaginal ring should be advised that they have an increased risk of VTE associated with long periods of immobility (e.g. long-haul travel). Women on oestrogen-containing contraception should be advised to stop their contraceptive 4wks before major elective surgery or any surgery involving immobilization of a lower limb. The contraceptive can be restarted at the beginning of the next cycle at least 2wks after mobility is restored. For non-elective surgery, where it has not been possible to stop the contraceptive in advance, VTE prophylaxis should be given.

Table 22.1 Risks of VTE associated with oestrogen containing contraception (cases per 100 000 women per year)

Healthy, non-pregnant, not using oestrogen-containing contraception	5–10
Using COC containing second-generation progestogen	15
Using COC containing third-generation progestogen	25
Pregnant women	60

Drug interactions

Enzyme-inducing drugs such as rifampicin (including 2 day course for meningitis prophylaxis), some anticonvulsants, St John's wort, and some antiretrovirals can significantly reduce the effectiveness of COCs, POPs, transdermal patches, and vaginal rings. Women should be counselled to use an alternative form of contraception while taking these drugs and until enzyme induction has completely resolved (4–8wks). Women on long-term therapy with enzyme-inducing drugs should use progestogen injection or an intrauterine device.

There is no evidence to support the theory that by reducing the bowel flora responsible for recycling enthinylestradiol from the large bowel, broad-spectrum antibacterials reduce the effectiveness of hormonal contraceptives. Women taking broad-spectrum antibacterials that are not enzyme inducers do not need to use alternative forms of contraception.

Counselling points

If a woman is using hormonal contraception for the first time or is switching from one form to another it is important that the pharmacist ensures that she is aware of the following points.

- Confirm that the risk of VTE has been explained when deciding on form of hormonal contraception—if not refer back to prescriber.
- When to take the first dose with respect to menstrual cycle and for how long alternative contraception should be continued after starting. This varies with the type of contraception—check SPC or *BNF*, Chapter 7
- What to do if a pill is missed, a patch is delayed or detached, or a vaginal ring is delayed, expelled, or broken.
- What to do if she vomits within 2h of taking pill.
- What to do if vomiting or diarrhoea last for >24h.
- Potential drug interactions, especially with respect to enzyme-inducing antibacterials and broad-spectrum antibacterials.
- Increased risk of VTE with long-haul travel if on oral contraception, patch, or vaginal ring.

Emergency hormonal contraception (EHC)

Two types of EHC are available in the UK.

- Levonorgestrel 1.5mg—single dose taken as soon as possible after unprotected intercourse and ideally within 72h. If a woman is on an enzyme-inducing drug, she should take two tablets (unlicensed dose).
- Ulipristal 30mg, a progesterone receptor modulator—single dose taken within 120h of unprotected intercourse. It is probable that enzyme inducers reduce the efficacy of ulipristal but there is no information at present on adjusting doses to compensate.

In the UK levonorgestrel 1.5mg tablets (Levonelle One Step®) can be sold as a P medicine to women aged >16. Pharmacists can supply EHC to women aged <16 on prescription or via a PGD.

Further reading

Biswas J *et al* (2008). Oral contraception. *Obstetrics, Gynaecology and Reproductive Medicine* **18**: 317–23 (🔗 http://cpd4gp.co.uk/PDF%20files/Contraception%20overview%20Dec%2008.pdf).

Guillebaud J (2007). *Contraception Today: A Pocketbook for Primary Care Practitioners* (6th edn). London: Informa Healthcare.

🔗 http://www.fsrh.org/pdfs/CEUguidanceEmergencyContraception11.pdf

Therapy-related issues: malignant disease and immunosuppression

Policy for the administration and handling of cytotoxic
    drugs 466
Clinical screening of chemotherapy prescriptions 470
Chemotherapy dosing 474
Antiemetics for the prophylaxis of chemotherapy-induced
    nausea and vomiting 478
Principles of extravasation 486
Extravasation of chemotherapy in adult patients 488
Extravasation of chemotherapy in paediatric patients 492
Common Terminology Criteria for Adverse
    Events (CTCAE) 493
Intrathecal administration of chemotherapy 494

Policy for the administration and handling of cytotoxic drugs

Cytotoxic drugs are used in the treatment of cancers and certain other disorders. They act by killing dividing cells, by preventing their division. In addition to malignant cells, they also act on normal cells. Therefore their use poses certain risks to those who handle them. It is important to ensure the safety of staff and patients who come in contact with these drugs.

- Cytotoxic drugs may only be reconstituted in facilities specifically approved for the purpose.
- Staff who prescribe, clinically screen, reconstitute, label, administer, and dispose of cytotoxic drugs must be appropriately trained and assessed as competent and must follow the local approved procedures.
- In areas where cytotoxic drug use is infrequent, a risk assessment must be carried out before a cytotoxic drug is requested. This should assess the availability of appropriate equipment and evidence of training, and demonstrate competence in safe administration of the drugs.
- Oral anticancer medicines must be prescribed, dispensed, administered, and monitored using the same standards as for injectable chemotherapy.

Cytotoxic drug procedures

- Any area in the hospital (including the wards, out-patient or day-case areas, and pharmacy) using cytotoxic drugs should have available current information on the type of agents used. This information should include relevant health and safety information (Control of Substances Hazardous to Health).
- Cytotoxic drugs are occasionally used to treat clinical disorders other than cancer. In such instances, the patient should be referred to a clinical area where cytotoxic drugs are used routinely. Alternatively, a competent practitioner from such an area can administer the drug in the patient's own ward. A trained member of staff must undertake a risk assessment to determine by whom and in what circumstances the drug can be administered.

Prescription, preparation, and reconstitution

- Ideally, all chemotherapy prescriptions are prescribed on an electronic chemotherapy prescribing system. In non-cancer areas, prescriptions may be handwritten on standard prescription charts, and they must be written legibly and signed in indelible black ink. In some cases, prescriptions might be computer-generated, either on an approved chemotherapy chart or on a standard prescription chart.
- Chemotherapy should be prescribed by prescribers experienced in the treatment of neoplastic disorders. Be aware of local policies stipulating who can prescribe chemotherapy.

- The chief pharmacist is responsible for ensuring that cytotoxic drug reconstitution services are provided in appropriate facilities. In exceptional circumstances, they can designate other areas for reconstitution.

Labelling and transportation

- Syringes, infusion devices, and infusion fluids containing cytotoxic drugs must be clearly labelled, to identify the potential cytotoxic hazard, and placed inside a sealed plastic bag,
- Cytotoxic drugs must be packaged and transported in sealed containers identified as containing cytotoxic drugs. The designated cytotoxic drugs reconstitution services must be notified at once if the integrity of a container received is suspect.
- Oral cytotoxic drugs should be transported in the same way as non-cytotoxic medication. In-patient supplies should be labelled as 'cytotoxic' on the normal prescription label.

Administration

- Relevant clinical laboratory results, as defined by chemotherapy protocols, must be reviewed before administration, and appropriate action taken.
- The following checks are advised to be made by two qualified staff members, one of whom must be registered as competent in cytotoxic drug administration, depending on local policy.
  - Visual check of the product (to include signs of leakage, contamination, or breakdown products).
  - The drug has been appropriately stored and is within its expiry date.
  - Patients must be identified positively using three patient identifiers, as defined in the locally approved policy.
  - The following prescription details must be checked:
    — protocol
    — dose
    — diluent (if relevant)
    — route of administration
    — frequency.
  - Staff should use personal protective equipment and clothing if handling and administering cytotoxic drugs. This includes gloves, an apron, and in some cases protection for the face (either goggles or a mask.).

Accidental spillage

- All areas in which cytotoxic agents are stored, prepared, and administered should have a spill kit available for use at all times. These kits are usually obtained from the pharmacy department. The kit includes instructions on how to proceed safely. Staff should be familiar with the instructions before dealing with a spill.
- A trained healthcare professional should deal with the spill immediately. After use, the spillage kit should be replaced.
- Be familiar with your local policy and location of spillage kits in areas using cytotoxic drugs.

Disposal of product waste

- Cytotoxic waste should be disposed of separately to normal clinical waste and marked as being cytotoxic, according to local policy. The incorrect disposal of cytotoxic waste can result in prosecution under the Special Waste Regulations 1996.
- Cytotoxic waste includes vials that have contained cytotoxic drugs, syringes, needles, IV bags, infusion sets used to administer cytotoxic drugs, gowns, and gloves, and urinary catheters and drainage bags from patients undergoing cytotoxic therapy.
- Cytotoxic waste should be disposed of according to local policy and clearly marked with cytotoxic residue tape.
- Hospitals have specific policies on the storage and collection of cytotoxic waste to ensure that it does not enter the normal clinical waste stream.

Disposal of excreta and blood

- Precautions should be taken to prevent occupational skin contact.
- Because cytotoxic drugs have varying half-lives, specific information about them will be found on safety datasheets. If the information is not specified, it is deemed GCP to apply universal precautions for 48h after administration.
- Patients and relatives (particularly pregnant mothers) who handle body fluids at home should be given appropriate advice.
- Gloves must be worn when handling all body fluids (e.g. blood, urine, faeces, colostomy and urostomy bags, nappies) during and after the administration of cytotoxic drugs.
- Linen contaminated with body fluids and cytotoxic drugs must be handled according to the local policy for handling cytotoxic contaminated waste.
- If contamination of the skin, eyes, or mucous membranes is suspected, the area should be rinsed thoroughly with large amounts of water and then washed with soap and water.

Incidents arising from handling and administration of cytotoxic drugs

- Any incident involving prescribing, administration, and disposal of cytotoxic drugs must be reported according to the local incident reporting system.
- The most probable incident for staff is accidental exposure to the drug during the set-up and administration of the drug. This might result from a bag leaking or bursting, or problems with the line *in situ*.
- If there is eye and skin contamination, rinse the affected area with copious amounts of tapwater and seek further treatment, if needed. The occupational health department should be notified of all cases of staff exposure to organize risk assessment and follow-up care plans.
- For patients, the most probable incidents arising are extravasation during treatment (see 🔲 p.486).

Handling cytotoxics during pregnancy

Pregnant staff should refer to their local policy with regard to handling cytotoxic drugs, because this group of drugs is potentially mutagenic, teratogenic, and carcinogenic. A risk assessment must be undertaken for each local area.

See 📖 pp. 190–3 for recommendations on handling potentially teratogenic drugs in pregnancy.

Intrathecal chemotherapy

See 📖 p. 494, 'Intrathecal administration of chemotherapy'.

Further reading

Allwood M et al. (2002). *The Cytotoxics Handbook* (4th edn). Abingdon: Radcliffe Medical Press.
Hyde L, Dougherty L (2008). Safe handling of cytotoxic drugs. In: Doughterty L, Lister S (eds), *The Royal Marsden Hospital Manual of Clinical Procedures* (7th edn). Oxford: Blackwell.
March guidelines: 🔊 http://www.marchguidelines.com

Clinical screening of chemotherapy prescriptions

All chemotherapy prescriptions must be checked and authorized by an oncology pharmacist who has undertaken the appropriate specialist training and local accreditation. Where possible, chemotherapy should be prescribed using an electronic chemotherapy prescribing system.

Validating prescription details

- Check that doses have been correctly calculated and prescribed.
- Ensure that generic drug names have been used and the dosage form is specified.
- Check maximum doses according to the protocol.
- Check patient weight, height, and body surface area (BSA). Ensure that weight has been taken within time frames specified in local protocols—e.g. if it is more than 2 months since a patient has been weighed and no new weight is recorded, ask for the patient to be weighed.
- BSAs are often rounded. Do not query a discrepancy unless it is >0.1m^2 for adults.
- Oncology patients might have their BSA capped at 2m^2 or 2.2m^2, or calculated using ideal body weight. Check the local policy. For example, obese patients—confirm with the prescriber that BSA has not been capped if >2m^2 or >2.2m^2.
- Haematology patients may not have their BSA capped—check the local policy.
- Drug dosages should be expressed in metric notation. The word *units* should never be abbreviated.
- For rounding doses, be aware that the exact dose might have to be rounded to account for tablet or vial size, or dose banded according to local policy.
- Check cumulative doses—e.g. anthracyclines (doxorubicin has a maximum cumulative dose of 450mg/m^2) and bleomycin (maximum cumulative dose of 400,000 IU).
- Check local policy for variation in the dispensed dose compared with the prescribed dose that has been agreed (often 5% variation is agreed).
- Administration rate and route should be specified.
- Administration schedule and duration of treatment should be included.
- For oral anticancer agents, calculate the exact number of tablets or capsules to be supplied and annotate the prescription accordingly.
- Ensure that the appropriate prescriber has signed and dated the prescription.
- Ensure that the infusion fluid and volume are stated and appropriate.
- For routes other than IV, ensure that the route is prescribed in full (e.g. *intrathecal*, not *IT*).

Verification of cycle 1 prescriptions

- Check patient's name, date of birth and hospital/NHS number.
- Check the date the order was generated, and time and date treatments are to be administered.
- Check that the BSA has been calculated correctly:

$$\text{Surface area} = \sqrt{\left(\text{Height}\,[\text{cm}] \times \text{weight}\,[\text{kg}]\,/\,3600\right)}$$

- BSA is often capped at $2m^2$ or $2.2m^2$. Check your local policy.
- Check the patient's ideal body weight (IBW). If the patient is significantly more or less than their IBW, discuss with their doctor. An example of an IBW formula is as follows:
  IBW (kg) men = [(height (cm) − 154) x 0.9] + 50
  IBW (kg) women = [(height (cm) − 154) x 0.9] + 45.5
  IBW calculators are available on the intranet (e.g. www.halls.md/ideal-weight/body.htm).
- Check the patient's treatment against the established protocol.
- Check the frequency of intended cycles and appropriate interval since any previous chemotherapy.
- Ensure that the protocol is the one intended to be prescribed by checking the patient's medical record.
- Check the patient's age, because some doses/protocols are age related.
- Check for verification of dose modification or variance from the protocol and identification of the factors on which treatment modifications are based.
- Confirm the dose per day versus the dose per cycle with the protocol.
- Interpret critical laboratory values to see if a dose modification is required—e.g. impaired renal function, clotting disorders and LFTs (if appropriate for drug).
- Check that the correct drugs have been prescribed and that all calculations have been performed correctly.
- Check if there are any drug interactions between the chemotherapy and the patient's regular medication.
- Check patient's allergies and medication sensitivities.
- Check if there are any drugs contraindicated with the chemotherapy.
- Check for authorized prescriber's name and signature.

Second and subsequent cycles

- Check that the chemotherapy cycle is correct for the protocol.
- Check that the correct cycle was ordered.
- Check that the drugs were prescribed on the correct days and start dates.
- Check that there has been no significant change in the patient's weight that might significantly change the calculated BSA.
- Check response to previous treatment:
  - blood indices—haematology/biochemical
  - tolerability and adverse reactions.
- Check to see if any appropriate modifications have been made in relation to a previous response or critical laboratory values (normally in the protocol).

Clinical check

- What type of malignancy does the patient have? Is the chemotherapy appropriate for the malignancy?
- What is the patient's renal and hepatic function? Do any of the doses need adjusting to take this into account?
- Has the patient had any chemotherapy before? Do any of the drugs have a maximum cumulative lifetime dose (e.g. anthracyclines)?
- Other checks include allergies/reactions to previous chemotherapy and the extent of disease (need for prehydration or allopurinol).
- Check critical laboratory values—if white cell count, neutrophils or Hb are above or below a predefined limit, refer to individual protocols.
- Check to see if any appropriate modifications have been made in relation to previous response or critical tests (normally in protocol).
- Check if any supportive care has been prescribed—e.g. antiemetics.

Endorsing prescriptions

- Amend any abbreviations.
- Annotate generic names.
- Ensure infusion fluid, volume, and rate of administration are stated and appropriate.
- Check that the appropriate route is prescribed.
- For routes other than IV, ensure that the route is prescribed in full—e.g. intrathecal not IT.
- Check that oral doses are rounded up or down to account for tablet size.

Annotations

- Sign and date the prescription to confirm that it is correct, safe, and appropriate.
- The following annotations should be made in the medical record.
  - Date.
  - 'Chemo ordered'—'confirmed' or 'awaiting confirmation (TBC)'.
  - Cycle number and date the cycle is due.
  - Any dose reductions.
  - Other relevant notes.
    — With the first cycle, annotate the drugs, doses, and frequency in the medical record, including reasons for alterations, so that it is clear exactly what the patient has received. Include the BSA, height, and weight that were used to calculate the doses and relevant biochemistry.
    — On the last cycle, record the cumulative dose of anthracyclines or bleomycin received.
  - Clinical pharmacist's signature and contact details.

Further reading

Royal College of Radiologists' Clinical Oncology Information Network (COIN) (2001). Guidelines for cytotoxic chemotherapy in adults. A document for local expert groups in the United Kingdom preparing chemotherapy policy documents. *Clinical Oncology* **13**; s209–48.

Allwood M et al. (2002). *The Cytotoxics Handbook* (4th edn). Abingdon: Radcliffe Medical Press..

British Oncology Pharmacy Association (BOPA) (2010). *Standards for Clinical Pharmacy Verification of Prescriptions for Cancer Medicines:* ℘ http://www.bopawebsite.org

British Oncology Pharmacy Association (BOPA) (2010). *Guidance to Support BOPA Standards for Clinical Pharmacy Verification of Prescriptions for Cancer Medicines:* ℘ http://www.bopawebsite.org

British Oncology Pharmacy Association (BOPA) (2010). *Competencies to Support Verification of Prescriptions for SACT.* ℘ http://www.bopawebsite.org

Chemotherapy dosing

Cancer chemotherapy drugs often have a narrow therapeutic window between the dose that is effective and the dose that can be toxic. Inappropriate dose reduction reduces chemotherapy efficacy. However, if doses are not ↓ in patients with organ dysfunction, this can lead to serious or life-threatening toxicity. It is essential that cytotoxic drugs are dosed correctly and adapted to individual patients to enable the maximum probability of a desired therapeutic outcome, with minimum toxicity.

Before administration of chemotherapy, each patient should be assessed for performance status, renal function, liver biochemistry tests, serum albumin level, and prognosis. Myelosuppression is the most common and dangerous toxicity of cytotoxics, so all patients must have a blood count before each cycle of chemotherapy. Patients should only be administered chemotherapy if their white blood cell count is >3.0 x 10^9/L (or neutrophil count is >1.5 x 10^9/L) and platelet count is >150 x 10^9/L. There can be exceptions to this in some local policies or for patients with haematological malignancies and those undergoing intensive treatment with specialized support.

Doses of cytotoxics are usually calculated on the basis of BSA, which is measured in square metres (m^2). The dose is quoted as units (e.g. milligrams, grams, or international units) per square metre. The patient's BSA is calculated using a nomogram from patient height and weight measurements or using the following calculation:

$$\text{Surface area} = \sqrt{\left(\text{Height}[\text{cm}] \times \text{weight}[\text{kg}]/3600\right)}$$

This practice is derived from the relationship between body size and physiological parameters (e.g. renal function). The performance status of the patient and their renal and liver functions are also taken into account. Prior to each cycle of treatment, toxicities must be recorded using common toxicity criteria. Doses are modified if the patient experiences toxicity to treatment or changes in body weight occur. The size of the reduction depends on the nature and severity of the toxicity, taking into account whether the chemotherapy is palliative or curative in intent.

Obese patients have physiological changes that affect drug disposition, including ↑ blood volume, organ size, and adipose tissue mass. BSA is often 'capped' at 2.0–2.2m^2 in obese patients. The use of ideal body weight can be considered in these settings. However, the possibility of under-dosing needs to be considered in curative patients.

Although it is conventional to prescribe chemotherapy according to BSA, it is acceptable to use pre-prepared standard doses for commonly used drugs to facilitate bulk preparation and rapid dispensing. This is known as 'dose banding'. The rounded dose must be within agreed limits—e.g. within 5% of the calculated dose.

However, there are some exceptions to calculation of doses on the basis of BSA. Drugs whose doses can be calculated using other parameters include the following.
- Asparaginase—the dosage is IU/kg body weight or IU/BSA.
- Bleomycin—IU, either per patient surface area or as a fixed dose.
- Carboplatin—the Calvert equation[1] can be used to calculate the dose of carboplatin in patients with or without renal impairment:

$$\text{dose (mg)} = \text{AUC} \times (\text{GFR} + 25)$$

where AUC is the target area under the plasma concentration curve (AUC is usually in the range 4–7) and GFR is the glomerular filtration rate. For example, the dose of carboplatin for a patient with a GFR of 75mL/min, using an AUC of 5, would be:

$$5 \times (75 + 25) = 500\text{mg carboplatin.}$$

- Cytarabine—dosage in mg/kg for certain indications.
- Floxuridine—dosage in mg/kg.
- Mitomycin—dosage in mg/kg for certain indications.

Some chemotherapy drugs (e.g. anthracyclines) have a maximum recommended cumulative lifetime dose. For example, doxorubicin has a maximum cumulative lifetime dose of 450mg/m^2 and bleomycin has a maximum cumulative lifetime dose of 400,000 IU. If patients receive more than the maximum cumulative lifetime dose, they are at increased risk of potentially life-threatening toxicity.

Frequency of chemotherapy administration

Chemotherapy is administered in various treatment cycles ranging from 1 to 6wks. Cycle frequency is based on cancer type and treatment choice. Frequency and duration of treatment cycles continue to evolve and are not absolute. It is important to always verify treatment selection, frequency, and duration with established protocols. For example, a lot of chemotherapy is administered at 3-week intervals, with up to 8–12 cycles of treatment being administered.

Some examples of exceptions to 3-week administration intervals are as follows:
- Carboplatin—can be administered every 3 or 4 weeks.
- Irinotecan—administered every 2 weeks.
- 5-fluorouracil—can be administered once weekly every 2, 3, or 4 weeks, depending on dosage schedule.
- Mitomycin—administered every 6 weeks.
- Paclitaxel—can be administered once weekly (unlicensed).
- Docetaxel—can be administered once weekly (unlicensed).

1 Calvert AH et al. (1989). Carboplatin dosage: prospective evaluation of a simple formula based on renal function. *Journal of Clinical Oncology* **7**: 1748–56.

Critical tests for chemotherapy to proceed on time

Chemotherapy should only be administered at the full protocol dose if the haematological and biochemical parameters are within the normal range. Biochemical parameters depend on the excreted route of the drug. Creatinine clearance should be monitored for renally cleared drugs and LFTs should be monitored for those drugs metabolized hepatically. Haematological parameters include the white cell count (WCC), absolute neutrophil count (>1.5), and platelet count (>100).

If the biochemical or haematological parameters are not within the normal range, dose reduction or delaying subsequent doses must be considered. Doses are usually reduced by 20–25% initially. Chemotherapy is usually delayed by a week at a time.

Treatment guidelines

Oncology is an evolving field of practice. Treatments are becoming more individualized and targeted on the basis of genetics, tumour markers, and staging of disease. Check your local network protocols for information on cancer treatments locally.

For more detailed information on the management of oncological disorders, refer to the *Oxford Handbook of Oncology*.

Further reading

Allwood M et al. (2002). *The Cytotoxics Handbook* (4th edn). Abingdon: Radcliffe Medical Press.

Murff S (2011). *Safety and Health Handbook for Cytotoxic Drugs*. Government Institutes Inc. U.S.

Hoskin P, Neal A (2009). *Clinical Oncology: Basic Principles and Practice* (4th edn). London: Hodder Arnold.

Brighton D, Wood M (eds)(2005). *The Royal Marsden Hospital Handbook of Cancer Chemotherapy: A Guide for the Multidisciplinary Team*. Edinburgh: Churchill Livingstone.

Summerhayes M, Daniels S (2003). *Practical Chemotherapy: A Multidisciplinary Guide*. Abingdon: Radcliffe Medical Press.

Cassidy J. et al. (eds) (2002). *Oxford Handbook of Oncology*. Oxford: Oxford University Press.

Calvert AH et al. (1989). Carboplatin dosage: prospective evaluation of a simple formula based on renal function. *Journal of Clinical Oncology* **7**: 1748–56.

National Chemotherapy Advisory Group (2009). *Chemotherapy Services in England: Ensuring Quality and Safety*. ℘ http://www.nelm.nhs.uk

National Confidential Enquiry into Patient Outcomes and Death (NCEPOD) Report, November 2008: ℘ http://www.ncepod.org.uk

NPSA-RRR 2008/001 Risks of incorrect dosing of oral anti-cancer medicines, January 2008: ℘ http://www.npsa.nhs.uk

NICE. *Cancer Service Guidance: Clinical Guidelines and Technology Appraisals*: ℘ http://www.nice.org.uk

CPPE Open Learning pack—Cancer: In Relation to Pharmacy Practice, September 2009: ℘ http://www.cppe.manchester.ac.uk

Williamson S, Polwart C (2008). *The Oral Anticancer Medicines Handbook* (3rd edn) (ISBN 978-1-4092-4044-0).

Antiemetics for the prophylaxis of chemotherapy-induced nausea and vomiting

- Nausea and vomiting remain two of the most feared side effects of chemotherapy in cancer patients.
- The goal of antiemetic therapy is to prevent nausea and vomiting completely.
- Antiemetics should be given regularly and prophylactically.
- Combinations of antiemetics are significantly more effective than single agents.
- Clinical practice guidelines ensure appropriate and cost-effective antiemetic use.
- Factors that need to be considered when choosing an antiemetic regimen include the following:
  - The chemotherapy emetic risk (Table 23.1), dose, and schedule.
  - The type of nausea and vomiting being treated—anticipatory, acute, or delayed (Table 23.2).
  - The patient risk of nausea and vomiting (Table 23.3).
  - Other underlying causes of nausea and vomiting (Table 23.4).
  - The mechanism of action and routes of administration of the antiemetic (Tables 23.5–23.10).
  - The adverse effects of the drugs.
  - The cost-effectiveness of the drugs.
  - Whether patients can self-administer the antiemetic.

Chemotherapy drug combinations have an additive emetic effect. If chemotherapy drugs from the same category are combined, the regimen is classified as a higher emetic risk. If drugs are from different categories, the emetic risk is determined according to the most emetic drug in the combination.

Table 23.1 Emetic risk of chemotherapy

High emetic risk	Moderate emetic risk	Low emetic risk	Minimal emetic risk
Altretamine	Actinomycin-D	Bexarotene	Alemtuzumab
Carmustine >250mg/m^2	Amifostine	Capecitabine	Asparaginase
Cisplatin ≥50mg/m^2	Amsacrine	Cyclophosphamide (oral)	Bevacizumab
Cyclophosphamide >1500mg/m^2	Arsenic	Cytarabine	Bleomycin
Dacarbazine	Azacitidine	Docetaxel	Bortezomib
Doxorubicin/epirubicin + cyclophosphamide combination	Busulfan >4mg/day	Doxorubicin 20–59mg/m^2	Busulfan (low dose)
Mustine	Carboplatin	Etoposide	Chlorambucil (oral)
Procarbazine	Carmustine ≤250mg/m^2	Fludarabine	Chlorodeoxyadenosine
Streptozocin	Cisplatin <50mg/m^2	5-Fluorouracil	Cetuximab
	Cyclophosphamide ≤1500mg/m^2	Gemcitabine	Dasatinib
	Cytarabine >1000mg/m^2	Imatinib	Dexrazoxane
	Daunorubicin	Methotrexate 50–250mg/m^2	Erlotinib
	Doxorubicin	Mitomycin	Fludarabine
	Doxorubicin (liposomal)	Mitoxantrone	Gefitinib
	Epirubicin	Paclitaxel	Gemtuzumab
	Idarubicin	Pemetrexed	Hydroxycarbamide
		Teniposide	

(continued)

Table 23.1 (Contd.)

High emetic risk	Moderate emetic risk	Low emetic risk	Minimal emetic risk
	Ifosfamide	Topotecan	Lapatinib
	Irinotecan	Treosulphan	Lenalidomide
	Lomustine	Vorinostat	Melphalan (low dose)
	Melphalan >50mg/m^2		Mercaptopurine
	Methotrexate 250–1000mg/m^2		Methotrexate ≤50mg/m^2
	Oxaliplatin		Rituximab
	Temozolomide		Temsirolimus
	Topotecan		Thalidomide
	Treosulfan		Tioguanine
			Vinblastine
			Vincristine
			Vindesine

Table 23.2 Definitions of chemotherapy-induced nausea and vomiting

Acute nausea and vomiting	Initial 24h after chemotherapy
Delayed nausea and vomiting	>24h after chemotherapy
Anticipatory nausea and anticipatory nausea/vomiting	Days to hours before chemotherapy

Table 23.3 Patient risk factors which predict poor antiemetic control

Patients with more than three or four risk factors should be considered to receive additional antiemetics at the outset.

- Female
- <30 years old
- History of sickness—in pregnancy/travel sickness/with surgery
- Poor control with prior chemotherapy
- Underlying nausea and vomiting
- Anxiety

Note: high alcohol intake can have a protective effect and ↓ risk of emesis.

Table 23.4 Other causes of nausea and vomiting to be considered

- Radiotherapy
- Radiosensitizers
- Infection
- Metabolic disorders
- Electrolyte disturbances
- Constipation
- GI obstruction
- Cachexia syndrome
- Metastases (brain, liver or bone)
- Paraneoplasia
- Emetic medication (e.g. opioids, antibiotics, antifungals, or amifostine)

Table 23.5 Notes on appropriate antiemetic prescribing with chemotherapy

- Antiemetics should be administered regularly, prophylactically, and orally.
- (Serotonin) 5HT-3 receptor antagonists are equally efficacious and should be administered orally, and only for acute nausea and vomiting.
- There is only evidence for the use of 5HT-3 receptor antagonists for an additional day in the delayed phase for cyclophosphamide and carboplatin.
- Neurokinin receptor antagonists (e.g. aprepitant) can be considered as an adjunct to dexamethasone and a 5HT-3 receptor antagonist to prevent acute and delayed nausea and vomiting with cisplatin-based chemotherapy.
- Optimal emetic control in the acute phase is essential to prevent nausea and vomiting in the delayed phase.
- Dexamethasone is not required when steroids are included in chemotherapy regimen and for some haematology regimens.
- Consider administering antiemetics by IV infusion, subcutaneously, rectally, or sublingually (if available in those formulations) if the patient is unable to take oral antiemetics.
- Metoclopramide can be replaced with domperidone if the patient has extra-pyramidal side effects.
- If a patient is already taking antiemetics (e.g. cyclizine or prochlorperazine) for underlying nausea and vomiting before starting on chemotherapy, these drugs could be continued as a substitute for metoclopramide.

Table 23.6 Combinations of oral antiemetics to prevent chemotherapy-induced nausea and vomiting

High emetic risk	
Acutely	Serotonin receptor antagonist oral start 1h before chemotherapy (Table 23.1) on days of chemotherapy
	Dexamethasone 12mg oral once daily, starting on the morning of chemotherapy until 24h after highly emetic chemotherapy
	Continue for the duration of highly emetic chemotherapy administration
	Neurokinin receptor antagonist (e.g. aprepitant 125mg 1h before chemotherapy)
Delayed phase	Dexamethasone 8mg orally daily (single or divided doses) for 3–4 days, which can be reduced to 4mg daily for 1–2 additional days
	Neurokinin receptor antagonist (e.g. aprepitant 80mg daily for 2 days) given in addition to dexamethasone
	Metoclopramide 10–20mg orally four times daily for 3–4 days regularly, then if required
Moderate emetic risk	
Acutely	Serotonin receptor antagonist oral start 1h before chemotherapy (Table 23.1) on days of chemotherapy
	Dexamethasone 12mg oral daily, starting on the morning of chemotherapy until 24h after chemotherapy.
Delayed phase	Dexamethasone 8mg oral daily for 3 days
	Metoclopramide 10–20mg oral four times daily for 3–4 days, if required

Table 23.6 (*Contd.*)

Low emetic risk

Acutely	Dexamethasone 12mg oral daily for days of chemotherapy
	Metoclopramide 10–20mg oral four times daily for 3–4 days

Minimal emetic risk

No routine prophylaxis required

Metoclopramide 10–20mg oral four times daily, if required.

Note: for patients <30 years old, consider domperidone instead of metoclopramide if the patient experiences extrapyramidal side effects.

Table 23.7 Recommended oral daily doses of serotonin 5-HT$_3$ receptor antagonists to be administered 1h before chemotherapy

- Granisetron 2mg daily
- Ondansetron 8mg 1h before chemotherapy and another dose 12h later
- Tropisetron 5mg daily
- Dolasetron 200mg daily

Table 23.8 Recommended IV doses of 5-HT$_3$ receptor antagonists to be administered if patients are unable to tolerate medicines by the oral route

- Granisetron 1mg daily
- Ondansetron 8mg daily
- Tropisetron 5mg daily
- Dolasetron 100mg daily

Table 23.9 Antiemetics for failure of control

- Aprepitant and dexamethasone are the most useful agents for delayed nausea and vomiting
- To ensure absorption of antiemetics administered, consider subcutaneous, IV, or rectal administration if available (e.g. prochlorperazine 25mg rectally 2–4 times daily, or domperidone 30–60mg rectally 4 times daily
- Ensure antiemetics cover full period of nausea and vomiting

Table 23.10 Suggested antiemetics for patients refractory to first-line antiemetics

Acutely

1. Use antiemetics recommended for more emetic chemotherapy (for low or moderate emetic risk regimens)

2. If highly emetic chemotherapy, consider **one** of the following options.

Add **lorazepam 1mg orally/sublingual/IV every 8h** if anxious (sedative and amnesic)

Consider **levomepromazine 6.25–12.5mg orally as a single daily dose** instead of metoclopramide

Replace lorazepam and metoclopramide with **levomepromazine 6.25–12.5mg oral or subcutaneous (in the evening) as a single daily dose (Note: 12.5mg oral = 6.25mg subcutaneous)**

Prescribe regular lorazepam with prochlorperazine 10mg oral four times daily instead of metoclopramide

3. For cisplatin-containing regimens, consider adding a neurokinin receptor antagonist to dexamethasone and a 5HT-3 receptor antagonist on subsequent cycles of chemotherapy (e.g. aprepitant 125mg 1h before chemotherapy, then 80mg daily for 2 days)

Delayed

Dexamethasone 4mg twice daily for up to 1 week after chemotherapy

Consider **levomepromazine 6.25–12.5mg oral as a single daily dose** instead of metoclopramide

Anticipatory

Consider **lorazepam** 1mg oral at night (or dose up to 1mg three times daily) orally if anxious or anticipatory nausea and vomiting.

Further reading

Fauser AA et al. (1999). Guidelines for antiemetic therapy: acute emesis. *European Journal of Cancer* **35**: 361–70.

Gralla RJ et al. (1999). Recommendations for the use of antiemetics: evidence-based, clinical practice guidelines. *Journal of Clinical Oncology* **17**: 2971–94.

Stoner NS (2004). Therapy-induced nausea and vomiting: assessment of severity and indications for treatment. In: Hoy A et al. (eds) *The Effective Prevention and Control of Symptoms in Cancer*, pp.139–44. Cardiff: Clyvedon Press.

Stoner, NS (2004). Evidence for selection and use of antiemetic agents and regimens: therapy-induced nausea and vomiting. In: Hoy A et al. (eds) *The Effective Prevention and Control of Symptoms in Cancer*, pp.145–54. Cardiff: Clyvedon Press.

Herrstedt J (2000). *European Society for Medical Oncology (ESMO) Recommendations for Prophylaxis of Chemotherapy-Induced Nausea and Vomiting*: ℘ http://annonc.oxfordjournals.org/content/20/suppl_4/iv156.full

Antiemetic Subcommittee of MASCC (2006). Prevention of chemotherapy- and radiotherapy-induced emesis: results of the 2004 Perugia International Antiemetic Consensus Conference. *Annals of Oncology* **17**: 20–8.

Kris MG et al. (2006). American Society of Clinical Oncology (ASCO) Guideline for Antiemetics in Oncology: update. *Journal of Clinical Oncology* **24**: 2932–47 (available at: ℘ http://www.asco.org).

National Comprehensive Cancer Network (NCCN) (2008). *NCCN Clinical Practice Guidelines in Oncology Antiemesis v.3*: ℘ http://www.nccn.org

Principles of extravasation

- Extravasation is the inadvertent administration of IV administered vesicants into the tissue instead of into the intended IV compartment. A number of agents used in cancer chemotherapy are extremely damaging if they extravasate or infiltrate into the tissues rather than remaining within the vasculature.
- If left undiagnosed or inappropriately treated, extravasation of chemotherapy can cause necrosis and functional loss of the tissue and limb concerned.
- Extravasation can occur with any IV injection. However, it is only considered to be a problem with compounds that are known to be vesicant or irritant.
- Appropriate treatment of extravasation within 24h should ensure that the patient has no further problems.

Signs and symptoms

- Pain, burning, swelling, erythema, loss of blood return, skin necrosis, inflammation, and discomfort.

Risk factors

Risk factors associated with extravasation include the following.

- Administration technique—↑ risk if staff are inadequately trained.
- Administration device—use of unsuitable cannulae (e.g. cannulae 24h old), large-gauge catheters, unsecured IV devices.
- Location of cannulation site—the forearm is the favoured site.
- Distractions during IV infusion.
- Patient factors:
  - underlying conditions, such as lymphoedema, diabetes, and peripheral circulatory diseases.
  - Patient age—additional precaution required for paediatric and elderly patients.
- Concurrent medication—e.g. steroids and anticoagulants.
- Physical properties of the administered drug–e.g. high vesicant potential of medication infused.

Prevention

- Extravasation is best prevented using one or more of the following techniques.
  - Avoid areas of joint flexion for IV sites.
  - Use smallest gauge catheter possible.
  - Use of central line for slow infusions of high-risk drugs.
  - Administer cytotoxic drugs through a recently sited cannula.
  - Ensure cannula cannot be dislodged during drug administration.
  - Ensure that the cannula is patent before administration by confirming positive blood return through the catheter.
  - Administer vesicants by slow IV push into the side arm of a fast-running IV infusion of a compatible solution.
  - Administer the most vesicant drug first.
  - Assess the site continuously for any signs of redness or swelling.

- • Ensure that the patient is aware of extravasation risks and reports any burning or pain on administration of the drug.
  - • Take time—do not rush.
- • Stop the infusion or injection immediately if an extravasation is thought to have occurred and follow the local extravasation policy.
- • An extravasation policy and kit must be available in all areas where chemotherapy is administered.
- • Check your local extravasation policy, and be aware of the location of extravasation kits.

Further reading

Allwood M et al. (2002). The Cytotoxics Handbook.(4th edn). Abingdon: Radcliffe Medical Press.
National Extravasation Information Service: ℘ http://www.extravasation.org.uk/home.html

Extravasation of chemotherapy in adult patients

A number of agents used in cancer chemotherapy are extremely damaging if they extravasate or infiltrate into the tissues, rather than remaining within the vasculature (Table 23.11). Extravasation might have occurred if there is evidence of the following.

- Any pain or burning on administration, either at the cannulation site or in the surrounding area.
- Swelling, inflammation, redness, or erythema around or above the cannulation site.
- Redness or heat at or around the area.

If the patient makes any complaint, stop the administration and check the site. If extravasation is suspected, the nursing/medical staff should follow the directions:

- The administration of the infusion/injection must be stopped and the cannula left in place.
- The healthcare professional administering the treatment should remain with the patient and ask a colleague to collect the extravasation kit and summon a doctor to examine and prescribe the appropriate treatment, according to the local extravasation policy.
- If a vesicant or exfoliant drug (Table 23.11) has been extravasated, the plastic surgical specialist registrar on-call 24h should be contacted according to the local policy. An emergency intervention/antidote might be required, according to the local policy.
- Disconnect the infusion and aspirate as much of the fluid from the extravasation site, through the cannula if possible, with a 10mL syringe.
- Mark the affected area. If possible take digital images of the site.
- The cannula can then be removed.
- Hydrocortisone 1% cream should be applied topically to the extravasated site twice daily, as long as redness persists, according to local policy.
- The extravasated area should be covered with a sterile gauze dressing. Depending on the drug extravasated and the local policy, heat can be applied to disperse the extravasated drug or the area can be cooled to localize the extravasation. Check the local policy to see whether a heat or cold pack should be used for the extravasated drug. For example:
  - vinca alkaloids—warm pack
  - oxaliplatin—heat pack
  - other vesicant drugs—cold pack
  - non-vesicant drugs—cold pack.
- The site should be elevated while swelling persists.
- Analgesia should be provided, if required.
- For the management of each individual drug, refer to the management plans in the local policy.

Table 23.11 Extravasation classification of anticancer drugs

Vesicants	Exfoliants
Amsacrine	Aclarubicin
Carmustine	Cisplatin
Dacarbazine	Daunorubicin (liposomal)
Dactinomycin	Docetaxel
Daunorubicin	Doxorubicin (liposomal)
Doxorubicin	Floxuridine
Epirubicin	Oxaliplatin
Idarubicin	Topotecan
Mitomycin	**Irritants**
Mitoxantrone	Bortezomib
Chlormethine (mustine)	Carboplatin
Paclitaxel*	Etoposide
Streptozocin	Irinotecan
Treosulfan	Mesna (undiluted)
Vinblastine	Teniposide
Vincristine	**Neutrals**
Vindesine	Asparaginase
Vinorelbine	Bleomycin
Inflammatory agents	Cladribine
Aldesleukin	Cyclophosphamide
Etoposide phosphate	Cytarabine
Fluorouracil	Fludarabine
Methotrexate	Gemcitabine
Pemetrexed	Ifosfamide
Raltitrexed	Interferons
Mesna (diluted)	Interleukin 2
	Melphalan
	Pentostatin
	Rituximab
	Thiotepa
	Trastuzumab

*Classification as vesicant or irritant.

- The following documents should be completed, according to local policy.
  - Standard local documentation for extravasation—file in patient's notes.
  - Record in patient's notes.
  - Local incident form.
- The patient's consultant should be informed within 24h (at the discretion of the specialist registrar on-call).

Follow-up care

- If IV chemotherapy is to be continued on the same day as an extravasation incident, if possible avoid using the limb where the extravasation has occurred.
- Review the extravasation site (suggested at ~24h and at 7 days). If not ulcerated, advise gradual return to normal use. For subsequent cycles of chemotherapy, consider surgical opinion if persistent pain, swelling, or delayed ulceration occurs.
- Inform risk management of the outcome.

Extravasation risk for chemotherapy products

There is no standard test to determine a drug's extravasation risk. The absolute risk is determined by extravasation reports originating from clinical practice and therefore controversy will exist for certain drugs.

Definitions of cytotoxic drug classification

- Vesicants—capable of causing pain, inflammation, and blistering of the local skin, underlying flesh, and structures, leading to tissue death and necrosis. This can result in loss of limb function and mobility.
- Exfoliants—capable of causing inflammation and shedding of skin, but less likely to cause tissue death.
- Irritants—capable of causing pain, inflammation, and irritation, rarely proceeding to breakdown of the tissue. This usually occurs at the administration site and/or along the vein.
- Inflammatory agents—capable of causing mild to moderate inflammation and flare in local tissues.
- Neutral—ostensibly inert or neutral compounds that do not cause inflammation or damage.

Guidelines for the use of hyaluronidase for an extravasated vinca alkaloids

Hyaluronidase may be indicated for a suspected or known extravasation of vinca alkaloids. It should be administered within 1h of the extravasation, before applying hydrocortisone cream. 1500IU of hyaluronidase is diluted in 1mL of water for injection. A 25 or 27 gauge needle is used to administer the dose intradermally or subcutaneously around the peripheral extravasation at approximately five separate sites. Clean the skin and change the needle after each injection. Consider infusing 0.4mL of the dose directly through the affected IV catheter if there is no blood return, prior to removing the catheter.

Guidelines for the use of dexamethasone for an extravasated vesicant drug

Dexamethasone may be indicated for a suspected or known extravasation of a vesicant drug. It should be administered within 1h of the extra-vasation, before applying hydrocortisone cream. 4mg dexamethasone injection is diluted in 1mL of water for injection. After cleaning the skin, a 25 or 27 gauge needle is used to administer the dexamethasone intra-dermally or subcutaneously around the peripheral extravasation. Administer 0.2mL at each site, changing the needle after each injection.

Guidelines for the use of dexrazoxane for an extravasated anthracycline

Dexrazoxane is a DNA topoisomerase II inhibitor licensed for administration after an anthracycline (doxorubicin, epirubicin, daunorubicin, idarubicin) extravasation of ≥3mL. The dose should be administered in the opposite limb over 1–2h within 6h of the extravasation:

- day 1: 1000mg/m^2
- day 2: 1000mg/m^2
- day 3: 500mg/m^2

The dose should be capped at a BSA of 2m^2, with a single dose not exceeding 2000mg.

Suggested contents of an extravasation kit

- Cold/hot packs × 2 (one to be stored in the freezer and one to be microwaved for a hot pack)
- Hydrocortisone 1% cream × 1
- Dexamethasone injection 8mg/2mL
- Hyaluronidase 1500IU injection
- 10mL water for injection × 2
- 2mL syringes
- 10mL syringes
- 25G needles
- Copy of local extravasation policy
- Extravasation incident forms
- Patient extravasation information leaflet
- Consent form for photographs
- Gloves and apron
- Gauze swab and tape
- Alcohol swabs
- Drug chart and pen

Further reading

Allwood M et al. (2002). The Cytotoxics Handbook (4th edn). Abingdon: Radcliffe Medical Press.
European Oncology Nursing Society (2007). Extravasation Guidelines.
  http://www.cancernurse.eu/education/guidelines.html
National Extravasation Information Service: http://www.extravasation.org.uk/home.html

Extravasation of chemotherapy in paediatric patients

Central venous catheters

- The majority of chemotherapy administered to children is given through indwelling central venous catheters.
- It is very unusual for administration of chemotherapy through indwelling central venous catheters to result in any problems with extravasation.
- The very occasional problems that occur with leakage or rupture of indwelling lines must be dealt with on their individual merits, taking account of such factors as site of the leak, type of drug being administered, and volume of drug thought to have been extravasated.

Peripheral catheters

- The same principles regarding extravasation apply to paediatric patients as for adult patients. However, treatment will differ and should be according to a local policy.
- The cannula should be sited on the dorsum of the hand or foot, and NEVER sited at the antecubital fossa or any other deep vein that cannot be carefully monitored.
- During the administration of bolus chemotherapy, very careful attention must be paid to ensure that there is no evidence of extravasation at the time of the injection, with intermittent careful aspiration throughout to demonstrate patency and correct positioning.
- Administration must be stopped immediately if there is swelling around the site of the cannula. Some patients can experience discomfort during IV injection and therefore pain is a less reliable sign of extravasation. Some drugs can induce marked amounts of flare, even when being delivered safely into the vein, and therefore the presence of flare is not an indication that extravasation is occurring.
- Infusion chemotherapy should be administered using a pressure-monitoring pump, with the pressure limit set as low as possible.
- Antidotes are usually avoided in paediatric extravasations because some antidotes can cause more damage than the extravasation itself.
- Suggested contents for a paediatric extravasation kit:
  - hot pack
  - cold pack
  - copy of local extravasation policy
  - extravasation documentation forms.
- Problems of extravasation are most likely to occur with the administration of vincristine or vinblastine. Extravasations with vincristine or vinblastine should be regarded as an emergency. If there is an extra-vasation of either of these two drugs, it is appropriate to call the plastic surgeons so that the site of the extravasation can be extensively irrigated. Arrangements should be made quickly for the patient to be taken to theatre and anaesthetized and the area irrigated.
- Lead consultant for the patient or the haematology/oncology consultant in charge at the time should be notified of the event immediately.

Further reading
Allwood M et al. (2002). *The Cytotoxics Handbook* (4th edn). Abingdon: Radcliffe Medical Press.

Common Terminology Criteria for Adverse Events (CTCAE)

The CTCAE are a standardized classification developed by the National Cancer Institute (NCI) used for the side effects of chemotherapy drugs. The adverse events are graded from 0 (none) to 5 (death) for all possible side effects. The CTCAE are used in cancer clinical trials, adverse drug reporting, and publications to ensure uniform capture of toxicity data. The full CTCAE table is available from the website ℘ http://ctep.cancer.gov/forms; select link 'CTCAE v.3'.

Intrathecal administration of chemotherapy

Background

- Intrathecal chemotherapy is mainly used to treat CNS complications of haematological malignancy.
- Only three chemotherapy drugs are licensed to be given intrathecally: cytarabine, methotrexate, and hydrocortisone.
- However, other non-cytotoxic drugs can be administered by this route and include bupivicaine, opioids, baclofen, clonidine, gentamicin, hydrocortisone, and vancomycin.

Safe practice

- In the UK, there is a national policy that encompasses a range of standards that hospitals must comply with to enable staff to administer intrathecal chemotherapy.[1]
- To prevent inadvertent mix-up with other drugs, intrathecal chemotherapy is segregated from IV chemotherapy. The separate delivery and locations for these drugs help to ensure that IV drugs are never present in the same location as intrathecal medications.
- To facilitate this, intrathecal medications should only be administered in a designated location, such as an anaesthetic room, at a standard time by competent registered staff. In this way, the pharmacy can release intrathecal medications to the doctor immediately before they are needed.
- Also, at least two health professionals should independently verify the accuracy of all intrathecal doses before administration.

Frequently asked questions

Which drugs are contraindicated for use through the intrathecal route?
Vinca alkaloids (e.g. vincristine, vinblastine, vinorelbine, and vindesine) must never be given by this route. Vincristine is the most commonly used drug of this group.

Neurotoxicity of vincristine
Vincristine and the other vinca alkaloids do not pass through the blood–brain barrier. They are always used intravenously. Peripheral neurotoxicity is one of the main side effects, which ↑ in a cumulative fashion with the total dose of treatment. Hence, when vinca alkaloids are inadvertently injected into the cerebrospinal fluid (CSF) the outcome is normally fatal. Since 1975, 14 people have died in the UK because vincristine was mistakenly given intrathecally—i.e. as a spinal injection.

How should vincristine to be labelled?
The label will state 'For IV use only—fatal if given by other routes'. The dose is be diluted to a fixed volume of 50mL for all adults and to a fixed concentration of 0.1mL/mL for paediatric patients.

1 🖰 http://www.dh.gov.uk

Explain the intrathecal route of administration?

Chemotherapy is injected into the area of the lower spine into the CSF. This injection is also termed 'spinal' or subarachnoid. It is mainly indicated when patients show clinical signs that their disease has spread into the CNS. Drugs can also be administered through an Ommaya reservoir, discussed later in this section.

Why have people been given the wrong drug intrathecally?

The main problem occurs as a result of inexperienced health professionals becoming involved in the process with the result that the drug vincristine (intended solely for the IV route) is administered in error using the intrathecal route. This results in immediate neural damage that normally results in death.

How are intrathecal products labelled?

The label on the product states that the drug is intended for intrathecal use only. The product is packaged and transported in a separate container from other IV chemotherapy products and collected by the person who is going to give the drug.

What range of volumes is administered intrathecally?

Generally, the volume administered varies with the dose, but the typical volume tends to be 5mL.

Who is allowed to administer intrathecal products?

Until 2008, only doctors who were registered were allowed to administer chemotherapy products intrathecally. However, staff must be appropriately trained, deemed competent by a designated lead trainer, and registered for the administration task . Obviously, anaethetists also administer intrathecal products, but are not allowed to administer cytotoxic chemotherapy intrathecally unless they are deemed competent and are authorized on the trust's register. Senior hospital officers can only be involved in administration if a risk assessment has been undertaken and a waiver that endorses their involvement has been signed by the chief executive.

What is an Ommaya reservoir?

It is a small plastic dome-like device with a small tube. The reservoir is placed under the scalp and the tube is placed into the ventricles so that it connects with the CSF. The Ommaya reservoir is permanent, unless there are complications. This device allows certain drugs to be administered into the CSF and allows CSF sampling without repeated need for lumbar puncture.

How are intrathecal products administered?

A spinal needle is inserted past the epidural space until the dura is pierced and enters the CSF, which should flow from the needle. When CSF appears, care is needed not to alter the position of the spinal needle while the syringe for chemotherapy is being attached. The syringe is attached firmly to the hub of the needle and then injected slowly. When the injection is complete, the needle is removed.

Collecting

The staff member who is to administer the intrathecal chemotherapy should collect the drug in person by presenting the intrathecal prescription and any other chemotherapy prescriptions for that patient. The person must check the drug against the prescription before accepting the drug. It must be released only by a pharmacist authorized to do so. The drug should be carried to the patient from pharmacy in a dedicated container.

Administering

Frequently asked questions about administering include the following.

Where can intrathecal chemotherapy be administered?
This must be done only in designated areas.

When can intrathecal chemotherapy be administered?
This can only be done at designated times that have been approved locally, and must be undertaken within normal working hours.

Who checks the intrathecal chemotherapy at the bedside?
This should be done by a staff nurse authorized to perform this task. A final check must always be done by the administering doctor just before injection.

How should intrathecal chemotherapy be administered?
Access to the CSF should be obtained by a standard lumbar puncture procedure to obtain free flow of CSF. Injection of the chemotherapy must only be performed when the physician is confident that the spinal needle is in the intrathecal space. If assistance from an anaesthetist is required to perform the lumbar puncture, the chemotherapy must only be injected intrathecally by an authorized doctor, as outlined.

Pertinent points for nursing staff

For nurses to be able to check intrathecal drugs, they have to have received specific training related to these drugs and must be registered locally after competency assessment.

Pertinent points for pharmacists

Clinically screening prescriptions

Pharmacists must have been assessed as competent and registered to screen intrathecal chemotherapy. Follow the chemotherapy screening protocol.

Releasing the product to medical staff

Only pharmacists who have been authorized and registered are involved in this process. The staff member who is due to administer the intrathecal product presents the correct prescriptions to an authorized pharmacist who releases the product provided that there is documented evidence that any IV chemotherapy intended on the same day has already been administered.

Therapy-related issues: nutrition and blood

Administration sets 498
Intravenous (IV) administration pumps and other devices 500
Management of magnesium imbalance 504
Management of phosphate imbalance 506
Management of hypokalaemia 508
Guidelines for the treatment of hypocalcaemia 512
Prescribing IV fluids 514
Nutritional support in adults 519
Normal nutritional requirements 520
Practical issues concerning parenteral nutrition 522
Children's parenteral nutrition regimens 526
Enteral feeding 532
Drug administration in patients with feeding tubes 536
IV therapy at home 540

Administration sets

A standard administration set, which does not have a filter chamber, is suitable for most IV infusions except the following.

- Blood and blood products—a blood administration set has an integral filter chamber.
- Platelets—a special administration set is usually supplied with platelets.
- Neonates and paediatrics—a burette should be used.

Rates

These sets deliver different number of drops/mL:

- Standard administration set—20 drops/mL.
- Blood administration set—15 drops/mL.
- Burette—60 drops/mL.

Note: an amiodarone infusion alters the surface tension of the infusion, resulting in a different number of drops/mL.

Changing administration sets

Administration sets should normally be changed every 24h as a precaution on microbiological grounds, although a number of studies have shown that, during administration of crystalloid infusions, there is not an ↑ in infection rates if administration sets are left unchanged for up to 72h. Contamination of infusion fluid during manufacture is extremely rare. However, if drugs are added to infusion fluids at ward level, the risk of microbial contamination is high and sets must be changed every 24h.

Administration sets should be changed every 24h for the following:

- parenteral nutrition
- blood and blood products
- infusions to which drugs have been added.

Calculating flow rates

If an infusion depends on gravity for its flow, there will be a limitation to its rate and accuracy of delivery. The rate of administration also needs to be calculated, using the following formula:

$$\text{no of drops/min} = \frac{\text{quantity to be infused(mL)} \times \text{no of drops/mL}}{\text{no of hours over which infusion is to be delivered} \times 60\,\text{min}}$$

The number of drops/mL depends on the administration set and the viscosity of the fluid. If greater safety is required, a burette administration set can be used, particularly if large bolus volumes could be harmful (e.g. in children or in patients with cardiac failure).

The burette set has a discreet 150–200mL chamber that can be filled from the infusion bag, as necessary, depending on the flow rate. This enables the nurse to ensure that the patient receives no more than the prescribed hourly rate.

Peripheral venous access devices

- Provides a relatively easy method for obtaining immediate IV access.
- Used for short-term drug and/or fluid administration and blood transfusion. Principal problems associated with peripheral cannulae are infection, occlusion, phlebitis, and extravasation.

For central venous access see 📖 p.540.

Size of cannula

The size of cannula is relevant to the potential trauma it may cause to the vein in which it rests. Cannula size relates to the diameter and is stated in gauge size, where the increase in gauge number is inversely proportional to the diameter of the cannula (Table 24.1).

The cannula should be considered as a wound with direct entry to the vascular system and must be treated as any other wound using an aseptic technique.

Dressings should be changed only if they are bloodstained or have become wet or stained, or when fluid has collected at the insertion point. If they are dry and intact it is preferable to leave them alone to minimize exogenous infection or dislodgement of the cannula at the site.

If there are any signs of inflammation or pain, the cannula should be removed. If it is not in regular use, removal should also be considered. Most institutions recommend that peripheral cannulae should not remain in place for longer than a specified period (e.g. 48h).

Table 24.1 Cannula sizes

Size (gauge)/actual diameter (mm)	Colour	Use	Flow rate (mL/min)
22G/0.8mm	Blue	For small fragile veins	35
20G/1mm	Pink	For IV drug and fluid administration in patients who have fragile veins	60
18G/1.2mm	Green	Standard size for IV drug and fluid administration	100
16G/1.7mm	Grey	For patients requiring rapid IV fluid replacement	200
14G/2mm	Brown	Used in theatre for rapid transfusion	350

Intravenous (IV) administration pumps and other devices

Classification

The Medical Devices Agency (MDA) has developed a classification for pumps according to the perceived risk and suitability of a device for a specific clinical purpose.

- Neonatal—the highest risk category.
- High-risk infusions—infusion of fluids in children, where fluid balance is critical, or the infusion of drugs (e.g. cardiac inotropes) or cytotoxic drugs where consistency of flow and accuracy are important.
- Lower-risk infusions—delivery of simple electrolytes, parenteral nutrition, and infusional antibiotics.

Neonatal

The required characteristics of neonatal devices are as follows.

- High accuracy.
- Consistency of flow delivery, with very low flow rates.
- Flow rate increments in mL/h.
- Very short occlusion and low-pressure alarm times.
- Very low bolus volume on release of occlusion.

High-risk infusion pumps

The required characteristics of high-risk infusion pumps are as follows.

- High accuracy.
- Consistency of flow delivery.
- Short occlusion and low-pressure alarm times.
- Low bolus volume on release of occlusion.

Lower-risk infusion pumps

The characteristics of lower-risk infusion pumps are as follows.

- Lower accuracy over the long and short terms.
- Less consistent flow.
- Rudimentary alarm and safety features.
- Higher occlusion alarm pressure.
- Poorer overall occlusion alarm response.

IV pumps and syringe drivers are increasingly being used to control infusions in general wards, in addition to specialist clinical areas. Operators have a responsibility to ensure that they are fully conversant with any device being used. Training is provided initially by company representatives, although long-term local on-the-job competency training is the usual method employed.

There is a continuing expanding range of infusion devices, which vary slightly in design. However, there are normally a number of common features that operators need to be familiar with to understand the appropriate clinical use of each device.

Most devices require a specific administration set, cassette, or syringe. The use of the incorrect type can have a detrimental effect on patient care. If a pump is designed to use a variety of sets or syringes, it normally must be programmed with information regarding the type and size being used.

Devices can be grouped into four main types.

- Infusion devices using a syringe:
  - syringe infusion pumps
  - syringe drivers
  - anaesthetic pumps
  - patient-controlled analgesia pumps.
- Infusion devices using gravity controllers:
  - drip-rate controllers
  - volumetric controllers.
- Infusion pumps:
  - drip-rate pumps
  - volumetric pumps
  - patient-controlled analgesia pumps.
- Ambulatory pumps:
  - continuous infusion
  - multimodality pumps
  - patient-controlled analgesia pumps.

Syringe infusion pumps

These are devices in which a syringe containing fluid or a drug in solution is fitted into the pump and the plunger of the syringe is driven forwards at a predetermined rate. These pumps are usually set to run at mL/h.

Application

Designed for the accurate delivery of fluids at low flow rates. Therefore syringe pumps are ideally selected for the safe infusion of fluids and drugs to neonates or children and drugs to adults. Often used in anaesthesia and critical care areas. Commonly used for the administration of patient-controlled analgesia.

Gravity controllers

Electronic devices that achieve the desired infusion rate on the principle of restricting flow through the administration set by an infusion force that depends on gravity (drip-rate control) or via a dedicated rate-controlling administration set.

Application

Suitable for most low-risk infusions such as IV fluids (e.g. sodium chloride or glucose 5% solutions). Not recommended for total parenteral nutrition (TPN).

Volumetric pumps

Application

Preferred for larger flow rates. They usually weigh between 3 and 5kg, and are designed to be 'stationary'. Volumetric pumps have the facility to work off mains power or a battery. The infusion rate is set using mL/h and most devices can be programmed to between 1 and 1000mL/h, although if used at rates <5mL/h, accuracy might ↓. Most pumps use a linear peristaltic pumping action.

The pump can often be programmed to stop infusing after a set volume, which useful if it is necessary to give a proportion of an infusion bottle or bag.

Ambulatory pumps

Small portable devices

They can use a small syringe but most use a reservoir bag of volume 100–250mL. Pumps are preprogrammable.

Implanted pumps

Implanted pumps have been developed for those ambulatory patients who need long-term low-volume therapy. These pumps are small and are implanted subcutaneously. The drug is then infused through an internal catheter into a vein, an artery, or an area of dedicated tissue.

Disposable pumps

These are non-electronic devices, which are generally very lightweight and small. Usually very 'user-friendly', requiring the minimum of input from the patient. They do not require a battery.

Disposable pumps work on a variety of principles.
- An elastomeric balloon, which is situated inside a plastic cylinder. When the balloon is filled with the infusion fluid, the resulting hydrostatic pressure inside the balloon is enough to power the infusion. The drug is infused through a small-bore administration set, which usually has a rate restrictor at the patient end.
- SideKick® exerts mechanical pressure from a spring-loaded device.
- SmartDose® works by generation of CO_2 in the space between a rigid plastic outer cylinder and the infusion bag.

Management of flow control devices

Any technical equipment will only function optimally if maintained appropriately and standardized, because devices are often moved with patients through various wards and departments. Care should be taken to comply with the manufacturer's instructions regarding storage of their product.

Management of magnesium imbalance

- The normal range of magnesium is 0.7–1.0mmol/L.

Hypomagnesaemia

Causes of hypomagnesaemia

- Malnutrition
- Burns
- Trauma
- Alcoholism
- Medications—e.g. amphotericin B, cisplatin, cyclosporin, loop diuretics

Complications of hypomagnesaemia

- Hypokalaemia
- Hypocalcaemia
- Tetany
- Seizure
- Arrhythmias
- Cardiac arrest

Preparations for replacement

- Magnesium glycerophosphate tablets (4mmol)
- Magnesium hydroxide mixture (14mmol/10mL)
- Magnesium sulphate 50% solution 5g in 10mL (20mmol/10mL)

Mild hypomagnesaemia (0.5–0.7mmol/L) or asymptomatic patients

- Magnesium glycerophosphate tablets (4mmol): one or two tablets three to four times daily. Unlicensed, but shows greatest absorption and least side effects (diarrhoea).
- Magnesium hydroxide mixture (14mmol/10mL): 5–10mL three to four times daily. Dosing can be increased up to 50mmol orally, but can be limited by side effects.

Moderate to severe hypomagnesaemia (<0.5mmol/L) or symptomatic patients

- Magnesium sulphate injection of 10–20mmol (2.5–5g) in 1L infusion fluid over 12h daily until serum magnesium is within the normal range.
- The volume of fluid is not critical but consider the following.
  - The maximum peripheral concentration is 20% (20mmol in 25mL) because the injection has a very high osmolality.
  - The maximum rate is 150mg/min (20mmol over a period of 40min).
- Magnesium sulphate is compatible with sodium chloride 0.9% solution, glucose 5% solution, and sodium chloride/glucose solution.

Monitoring

Magnesium levels for symptomatic patients should be checked daily until corrected. Note that plasma levels might be artificially high while magnesium equilibrates with the intracellular compartment. However, if toxicity is suspected, treatment should be discontinued.

Hypermagnesaemia

Causes of hypermagnesaemia
- Renal insufficiency
- Hypothyroidism
- Medications (lithium)

Complicaitons of hypermagnesaemia
- Hypotension
- Bradycardia
- Confusion
- Respiratory depression
- Coma

Non-pharmacological treatment
- Treat underlying disorder
- External cardiac pacing (symptomatic)
- Mechanical ventilation (symptomatic)
- Dialysis (use only in emergency situations unless patient is already on dialysis)

Pharmacological treatment
- 1000mg calcium gluconate: slow IV push over 10min
- Hydration with sodium chloride 0.9% solution (200mL/h)
- Add calcium gluconate 1000mg to each litre of fluid
- Loop diuretics (e.g. furosemide 40mg IV push) to maintain urine output

Monitoring
- Serum magnesium every 2h until normalized and patient is asymptomatic

Management of phosphate imbalance

- The normal range of phosphate is 0.8–1.45mmol/L.

Hypophosphataemia

Causes of hypophosphataemia
- Malnutrition
- Increased urine excretion of phosphorus
- Hyperparathyroidism
- Refeeding syndrome
- Medications

Complications of hypophosphataemia
- Myalgias
- Peripheral neuropathy
- Paralysis
- Rhabdomyolysis
- Seizures
- Acute respiratory failure

Tratment of hypophosphataemia (Table 24.2)
- Mild hypophosphataemia: 0.61–0.79mmol/L
- Moderate hypophosphataemia: 0.41–0.60mmol/L
- Severe hypophosphataemia: <0.40mmol/L

Table 24.2 Treatment of hypophosphataemia

	Moderate (0.4–0.6mmol/L) Asymptomatic	Moderate (0.4–0.6mmol/L) Symptomatic	Severe (<0.4mmol/L)
Patient able to tolerate oral or enteral therapy	Phosphate-Sandoz® effervescent tablets: 2 tabs twice daily (16mmol phosphate/tab)	Oral therapy not appropriate	
Patient on IV therapy only	20mmol phosphate as sodium glycerophosphate in 0.9% sodium chloride or 5% glucose over 12h. Dilution volume ≤50mL must be administered via central access	20mmol phosphate as sodium glycerophosphate in 0.9% sodium chloride or 5% glucose over 6h. Dilution volume ≤50mL must be administered via central access.	

- Oral supplementation should be considered as first line in all patients who can tolerate oral therapy and who do not have a sodium restriction.
- Check plasma calcium. If high, seek specialist advice prior to supplementation.
- Half the dose in renal impairment and in patients <40kg.

Monitoring
Serum levels need to be checked 6h after the end of the infusion to enable time for distribution.

Hyperphosphataemia

Causes of hyperphosphataemia
- Renal insufficiency
- Acidosis
- Hypoparathryoidism
- Tumour lysis syndrome
- Medications—e.g. phosphate supplements, bisphosphonates

Complications of hyperphosphataemia
- Calcium–phosphate complex formation and deposit in muscle
- Tetany
- Mortality

Non-pharmacological treatment
- Treat underlying condition
- Dialysis—use only in emergency situations, unless patient is already on dialysis

Pharmacological treatment
- Phosphate binders.
    - Calcium carbonate 1250mg oral three times daily with each meal.
    - Calcium acetate 1000mg oral three times daily with each meal (adjusted to requirements).
    - Sevelamer 800–1600 mg oral three times daily with each meal.
    - Aluminium-based products are not usually recommended because of aluminium toxicity.

Seek specialist information for dosing schedule.

Monitoring
- Serum phosphorus levels until normal.
- Serum calcium levels.

Management of hypokalaemia

Causes of hypokalaemia
- Excessive loss through GI tract or kidney
- Hypomagnesaemia
- Intracellular shift
- Medications—e.g. diuretics

Complications of hypokalaemia
- Nausea/vomiting
- Weakness/fatigue
- Constipation
- Paralysis
- Respiratory failure
- Arrhythmias
- Sudden death

Treatment of hypokalaemia
Treatment is summarized in Table 24.3.

Risks associated with IV potassium
- Rapid administration of IV potassium or administration of concentrated IV potassium can result in hyperkalaemia paralysis, respiratory failure, arrhythmias, and asystole
- Potassium should NOT be administered undiluted or by IV push
- Peripheral administration of potassium may lead to burning, phlebitis, and necrosis, less concentrated solutions should be used peripherally.

Safety measures for IV potassium
- In July 2002, the National Patient Safety Agency (NPSA) in the UK issued a patient safety alert to prevent further fatalities following accidental overdose with IV potassium chloride concentrate that had been misidentified for sodium chloride 0.9% solution and water for injections.
- The risks associated with IV potassium chloride are well known. Potassium chloride, if injected too rapidly or in too high a dose, can cause cardiac arrest within minutes. The effect of hyperkalaemia on the heart is complex—virtually any arrhythmia could be observed.
- The true incidence of potassium-related fatalities and incidents is unknown.
- The alert identified safe medication practice recommendations concerning the prescribing, distribution, storage, and preparation of potassium chloride solutions in hospitals.
- The NPSA recommended withdrawal of concentrated potassium solutions from ward stock to be replaced by ready-to-use infusion products.
- The NPSA recommended that new control arrangements be introduced in critical care areas continuing to use potassium chloride concentrate ampoules and development of the use of pre-filled potassium syringes.

- Although recommendations have ↓ the risk to patients, staff still need to be vigilant to minimize and prevent harm to patients from incompetent/dangerous practice.

Minimizing risk: points pharmacists should encourage

- Labelling: the labelling format used differs between different manufacturers. The font size of K⁺ details should be ↑ to improve identification. Historically, there has been a reliance on specifying the K⁺ concentration as a percentage rather than mmol/volume on products as the primary focus. The latter should become main emphasis in future.
- Storage: decanting from boxes should be discouraged. Although most ward areas have limited storage space, it is GCP to segregate K⁺-containing bags from other infusion fluids.
- Develop and publish a local range of infusions (e.g. Table 24.4)
- Staff competency needs to be established for IV fluid administration.

Concentrated K⁺-containing products

Critical areas, high-dependency areas, and cardiac theatres that are allowed to store ampoules of potassium chloride locally should have a risk assessment performed periodically to overview the prescribing, ordering, storage, and administration processes. Other areas, such as general theatres, should not have access to concentrated ampoules of K⁺.

Training development

The process from prescribing through to administration needs to be mapped and used as a backbone to develop multidisciplinary training.

Table 24.3 Treatment and monitoring of hypokalaemia

Serum potassium level (mmol/L)	Degree of hypokalaemia	Treatment
3.0–3.4	Mild or asymptomatic hypokalaemia	Oral potassium replacement is preferred for patients who are asymptomatic
		IV replacement: 40mmol in 1L of sodium chloride 0.9% solution or glucose 5% solution administered peripherally (or centrally) over at least 6h
<3.0	Severe or symptomatic hypokalaemia	IV replacement with 40mmol in 500mL sodium chloride 0.9% solution or glucose 5% solution administered peripherally (or centrally) over at least 4h or over at least 2h through a central line with continuous ECG monitoring of heart rate and rhythm; repeat according to serum potassium levels
Monitoring	Serum potassium level every 1–6h if severe or symptomatic or if IV treatment ongoing	Testing serum magnesium may be indicated if hypokalaemia is resistant to treatment, and magnesium correction warranted if low

Table 24.4 Suggested example of formulary for K^+-containing IV fluids

Approved name	Manufacturer	Bag price*	Notes
Potassium chloride 20mmol in 50mL sodium chloride 0.9% in pre-filled syringe	NHS manufacturer	£6	20mmol in 50mL (critical care only)
Potassium chloride 0.15%, glucose 10% (500mL)	Baxter	£6	10mmol in 500mL
Potassium chloride 0.15%, glucose 10% sodium chloride 0.18% (500mL)	IVEX	£5	10mmol in 500mL
Potassium chloride 0.15%, glucose 2.5%, sodium chloride 0.45% (1000mL)	Fresenius Kabi	£5	20mmol in 1L
Potassium chloride 0.15%, glucose 4% sodium chloride 0.18% (1000mL)	Fresenius Kabi	£1	20mmol in 1L
Potassium chloride 0.15%, glucose 5% (1000mL)	Fresenius Kabi	£1	20mmol in 1L
Potassium chloride 0.15%, sodium chloride 0.9% (1000mL)	TPS	£1	20mmol in 1L
Potassium chloride 0.15%, sodium chloride 0.9% (500mL)	TPS	£1	10mmol in 500mL
Potassium chloride 0.3%, glucose 4%, sodium chloride 0.18% (1000mL)	Fresenius Kabi	£1	40mmol in 1L
Potassium chloride 0.3%, glucose 5%, sodium chloride 0.18% (500mL)	Fresenius Kabi	£1	20mmol in 500mL
Potassium chloride 0.3%, glucose 5% (1000mL)	Fresenius Kabi	£1	40mmol in 1L

Table 24.4 (Contd.)

Approved name	Manufacturer	Bag price*	Notes
Potassium chloride 0.3%, sodium chloride 0.9% (1000mL)	Fresenius Kabi	£1	40mmol in 1L
Potassium chloride 0.3%, sodium chloride 0.9% (500mL)	Fresenius Kabi	£1	20mmol in 500mL
Potassium chloride 0.6%, sodium chloride 0.9% (500mL)	Baxter	£5	40mmol in 500mL
Potassium chloride 0.6%, sodium chloride 0.9% (1000mL)	Baxter	£5	80mmol in 1L
Potassium chloride 3%, sodium chloride 0.9% (100mL)	Baxter	£4	40mmol in 100mL

*Prices listed as guide only. Cost will vary locally.

Guidelines for the treatment of hypocalcaemia

- The normal range of total calcium is 2.15–2.60mmol/L.
- The normal range of ionized calcium is 1.1–1.4mmol/L.

Causes of hypocalcaemia

- Malabsorption, inadequate intake, vitamin D deficiency
- Hypoalbuminaemia
- Hyperphosphataemia
- Hypomagnesaemia
- Pancreatitis
- Hypoparathryroidism

Complications of hypocalcaemia

- Dysrhythmias
- Muscle cramping
- Paresthesiae
- Seizures
- Stridor
- Tetany

Non-pharmacological treatment

Treat the underlying disorder. The most common cause of low total serum calcium is hypo-albuminaemia. Therefore it is important to measure ionized calcium or correct the total serum calcium using the formula

$$Ca_{corrected} = [(40 - Alb_{measured}) \times (0.02)] + Ca_{measured.}$$

Preparations for replacement

- Calcium gluconate 10% (0.1g/mL)—injection contains 0.22mmol/mL of calcium.
- Calcium chloride 14.7% (0.147g/mL)—injection contains 1mmol/mL of calcium.
- Calcium solutions (especially calcium chloride) are irritants and care should be taken to prevent extravasation.

Dilution

- A calcium gluconate 10% injection can be given undiluted, or diluted in glucose 5% solution or sodium chloride 0.9% solution.
- A calcium chloride 14.7% solution should ideally be diluted in at least twice its volume of glucose 5% solution or sodium chloride 0.9% solution for peripheral administration. Calcium chloride can be given un-diluted by central line administration only.

Emergency elevation of serum calcium in symptomatic patients

- Give 2.25mmol IV stat over 10min.
- This is equal to either of the following:
  - 10mL of calcium gluconate 10% solution
  - 2.25mL of calcium chloride 14.7% solution.

Hyperkalaemia and disturbance of ECG function

- 2.25–4.5mmol of calcium over 10–20min, depending on dose (up to a maximum rate of 0.2mmol/min).
- This is equal to either of the following:
  - 2–4mL of calcium chloride 14.7% injection
  - 10–20mL of calcium gluconate 10% injection.
- Titrate dose according to ECG.

Monitoring

For symptomatic patients calcium and albumin levels should be checked every 4h until corrected. Serum phosphate and magnesium levels should be monitored periodically.

Suggested dosing in asymptomatic hypocalcaemic patients

IV infusion to give 9mmol daily, which might need to be repeated at intervals of 1–3 days, as follows.

- 40mL of calcium gluconate 10% injection over 4h can be given neat or diluted in glucose 5% solution or sodium chloride 0.9% solution.
- 9mL of calcium chloride 14.7% injection over 4h diluted in 100mL of glucose 5% solution or sodium chloride 0.9% solution.

If the patient is absorbing oral medication, consider the use of soluble calcium tablets in divided doses.

Prescribing IV fluids

The aim of fluid therapy is to facilitate the patient's recovery by maintaining the following:
- blood volume
- fluid and electrolyte balance
- renal function.

Three phases need to be considered when planning a suitable fluid regimen:
- maintenance
- correction of pre-existing dehydration
- abnormal losses—e.g. fluid management of the surgical patient.

Fluids for maintenance
- A patient who is unable to take fluid by mouth needs a basic IV regimen. In temperate climates, this is $1.5L/m^2$ surface area of fluid or 30–40mL/kg body in 24h.
- Basic electrolyte requirements are sodium (1mmol/kg body weight daily) and potassium (1mmol/kg body weight daily).
- The patient can manage with lower sodium intakes because of efficient conservation processes. However, if there are obligatory losses of K^+ and insufficient replacement, patients become K^+ depleted.
- Remember that febrile patients will have ↑ insensible losses.

Correction of existing dehydration
- Identify the compartment(s) from which the fluid has been lost and the extent of the losses.
- Check fluid charts, and note any loss from drains or catheters.
- Most body fluids contain salt (Table 24.5), but at lower levels than plasma. Thus replacement requires a mixture of sodium chloride and glucose.
- Clinical history and examination are vital but can be assisted by the measurement of changes in electrolytes, packed cell volume (PCV), and plasma proteins.
- Patients with heart failure are at greater risk of pulmonary oedema if over-hydrated. They also are unable to tolerate ↑ salt load because sodium retention accompanies heart failure.
- Patients with liver failure, despite being oedematous and often hypo-natraemic, have ↑ total body sodium. Therefore sodium chloride is best avoided in fluid regimens.

Abnormal losses: fluid management of the surgical patient
Planning an IV fluid therapy regimen
- Ensure adequate preoperative hydration.
- Minimize insensible losses during surgery:
  - humidify inspired gases, minimize sweating by ensuring adequate anaesthesia, and, where possible, cover the patient to ensure adequate ambient temperature.
- Replace losses, such as blood loss.

Preoperative considerations

For routine elective surgery, the patient is kept NBM for 6–12h and takes little oral fluid for 6h postoperatively. A fluid deficit of 1000–1500mL arises, but this will be quickly corrected when the patient is drinking normally. IV fluid therapy is not required for many routine operations in adults, provided that the patient is not dehydrated. IV therapy is indicated preoperatively if the patient is likely to be NBM for >8h. Anaesthetists might set up an IV infusion of Hartmann's solution just before induction. On return to the surgical ward, this should be switched to sodium chloride or glucose as required, because there is no evidence that further treatment with Hartmann's solution has a clinical benefit compared with other crystalloids.

Perioperative considerations and blood loss

Operative blood loss of up to 500mL can be replaced with crystalloid solution (remembering that four times as much crystalloid solution will be needed). Use the following replacement fluids for blood loss:
- <500mL—use crystalloid solution
- 500–1000mL—use colloid solution
- >1000mL or Hb <10gdL—use whole blood.

Other replacement fluid is more appropriate if there is excess fluid loss from a specific compartment.

Hartmann's solution causes the least disturbance to plasma electrolyte concentrations and avoids postoperative fluid depletion. An allowance of 1mL/kg body weight/h should be begun at the start of anaesthesia to replace essential losses intraoperatively.

Table 24.5 Composition of gastrointestinal body fluid

	Volume (L/24h)	Na$^+$ (mmol/L)	K$^+$ (mmol/L)	Cl$^-$ (mmol/L)	HCO$_3^-$ (mmol/L)	pH
Saliva	0.5–1.5	20–80	10–20	20–40	20–60	7–8
Gastric juice	1.0–2.0	20–100	5–10	120–160	0	1–7
Bile	0.5–1.0	150–250	5–10	40–120	20–40	7–8
Pancreatic juice	1.0–2.0	120–250	5–10	10–60	80–120	7–8

Postoperative considerations

- Normal fluid requirement is 2–3L/24h.
- Electrolyte requirements: Na$^+$, 2mmol/kg body weight; K$^+$, 1mmol/kg body weight.
- Low urine output (night after surgery) almost always results from inadequate fluid replacement, but might be a consequence of the anaesthetic technique. (K$^+$ is not normally administered during the first24h in such patients.) Check JVP/CVP for signs of cardiac failure and consider fluid challenge, if appropriate.
- Check operation notes for extent of bleeding in theatre.
- Losses from gut—replace NGT; aspirate volume with sodium chloride 0.9% solution.

- Losses from surgical drains—replace significant losses. However, calculate total fluid loss (24h) as follows:
  - estimate skin and lung loss = (10 × body weight)mL.
  - estimation of stool losses = 50mL.
  - estimation of urine losses, normally measured directly.
  - drain loss/NGT loss.

Design a fluid regimen
- Calculate fluid losses and replace them (as outlined).
- Calculate Na^+ and K^+ requirements.
- Measure plasma U&Es if patient is ill.
- Start oral fluids as soon as possible.

For example, a fluid regimen for a 60kg patient would be calculated as follows.
- Fluid losses:
  - patient urine output 1500mL
  - fluid losses = (10 × 60) + 1500 + 50mL = 2150mL
  - NGT loss = 1000mL.
- Na^+ requirement = 2 × 60 = 120mmol.
- K^+ requirement = 1 × 60 = 60mmol.
- Volume of sodium chloride 0.9% solution that will provide sodium requirement = 1000mL (154mmol Na^+).
- Amount of K^+ required = 60mmol
- Remember that glucose 5% solution can be considered as isotonic water and will be used to make up the difference for the patient's fluid requirement.
- NGT replacement = 1000mL sodium chloride 0.9% solution.

Hence, a suitable 24h regimen for a 60kg patient with 1.5L urinary output and 1L NGT losses would be as follows:
- 2 × 1000mL sodium chloride 0.9% solution + 20mmol potassium chloride.
- 1000mL glucose 5% solution + 20mmol potassium chloride.
- Each bag runs for a period of 8h.
- Start oral fluids as soon as reasonable, depending on the patient's condition/indication for surgery.

Special conditions that need more specialist fluid knowledge
- Haemorrhagic/hypovolaemic shock
- Septic shock
- Heart or liver impairment
- Excessive vomiting

Fluid balance

During a lifetime, the water content and fluid compartments within the body alter. In infants, fluid content is 70–80% of body weight. This progressively ↓, reaching 60% of body weight at age 2 years. In adults, the fluid content accounts for 60% of body weight in ♂ and 55% in ♀, and the ratio of extra-cellular fluid (ECF) to intracellular fluid (ICF) is 1:3.

For example, the fluid content of a 70kg ♂ is as follows:
- total fluid = 42L
- ICF – 67% of body water = 28L
- ECF – 33% of body water = 14. (25% of intravascular space = 3.5L; 75% of interstitium = 10.5L).

Compartment barriers

- The fluid compartments are separated from one another by semi-permeable membranes through which water and solutes can pass. The composition of each fluid compartment is maintained by the selectivity of its membrane.
- The barrier between plasma and the interstitium is the capillary endo-thelium, which allows free passage of water and electrolytes but not large molecules such as proteins.
- The barrier between the ECF and the ICF is the cell membrane.

Transport mechanisms

- Simple diffusion: movement of solutes down concentration gradients.
- Facilitated diffusion: again depends on concentration gradient differences, but also relies on the availability of carrier substances.
- Osmosis: movement of solvent through semipermeable membranes.
- Active transport: e.g. Na^+/K^+ exchange pump.

Osmolality

- Osmotic pressure is generated by colloids impermeable to the membrane.
- Water distributes across in either direction if there is a difference in osmolality across the membrane.
- Osmolarity is the number of osmoles per litre of solution.
- Osmolality is the number of osmoles per kilogram of solvent or solution.
- The osmolality of blood is 285–295mOsm/L.

Tonicity

Molecules that affect the movement of water (e.g. sodium and glucose) are called 'effective osmoles' and contribute to compartment osmolality (sometimes termed 'tonicity'). The normal range of serum osmolality is 285–295mOsm/L. The measured osmolality should not exceed the predicted value by >10mOsm/L. A difference of >10mOsm/L is consid-ered an osmolal gap. Causes of a serum osmolal gap include the presence of mannitol, ethanol, methanol, ethylene glycol, or other toxins (usually small molecules) in very high concentrations. (The propylene glycol in lorazepam can cause hyperosmolarity and hyperosmolar coma in some patients, particularly when lorazepam is used as a continuous infusion.)

Serum osmolality is calculated as follows:

serum osmolality = $[2 \times (Na^+ + K^+)] + (glucose/18) + (BUN/2.8)$

where BUN is blood urea nitrogen. Na^+ and K^+ are in mmol/L, and glucose and BUN are in mg/dL. To convert glucose from mmol, divide by a factor of 0.05551. To convert BUN from mmol, divide by a factor of 0.3569.

Knowledge of fluid distribution

- Glucose 5% solution distributes through the ECF with a resultant fall in ECF osmolality, water distributes into the cells, and thus glucose 5% solution distributes throughout the body water.
- Conversely, a person marooned on a life raft with no water loses water from all compartments.
- Sodium chloride 0.9% solution contains 154mmol/L of sodium with an osmolality of 300mOmol/L. When infused, most of the solution stays in the ECF, which is of a similar osmolality.
- Conversely, if water and electrolytes are lost together (e.g. severe diarrhoea), fluid is mainly lost from the ECF.
- With ECF losses, sodium and water are lost together, so the sodium concentration in the remaining ECF does not change.
- However, protein and red cells are not lost so their concentration rises.
- If plasma alone is lost, only the PCV rises.
- Extra fluid for continuing losses should resemble as closely as possible the fluid that has been lost.

The body is normally in positive water balance (Table 24.6), with the kidney adjusting for varying intakes and losses by altering water clearance. The kidney requires 500mL of water to excrete the average daily load of osmotically active waste products at maximal urinary concentration.

Table 24.6 Fluid balance—average daily water balance

Input (mL of water)	Output (mL of water)
Drink: 1500	Urine: 1500
In food: 800	Insensible losses (lungs and skin): 800
Metabolism of food: 200	Stool: 200
Total: 2500	Total: 2500

Nutritional support in adults

Parenteral support

Poor nutritional status is a major determinant of a patient's morbidity (as a consequence of depressed cell-mediated immunity and wound healing) and mortality.

The decision to provide nutritional support must be as a result of a thorough clinical assessment of the patient's condition. Parenteral nutritional support should be for patients who are malnourished or likely to become so, and in whom the GI tract is not sufficiently functional to meet nutritional needs or is inaccessible.

Appropriate indications for parenteral nutrition

- Short bowel syndrome.
- GI fistulae.
- Prolonged paralytic ileus.
- Acute pancreatitis if jejunal feeding is contraindicated.
- Conditions severely affecting the GI tract, such as severe mucositis following systemic chemotherapy.

Guide to calculating parenteral nutritional requirements in adults

Nutritional assessment

Assessment is essential for the correct provision of nutritional support. A variety of techniques are available to assess nutritional status. Some of the common criteria used to define malnutrition are recent weight loss and changes in body mass index (BMI).

Identifying high-risk patients

- Unintentional weight loss—5–10% is clinically significant.
- ↓ oral intake—can result from vomiting, anorexia, or NBM.
- Weight loss—take oedema, ascites or dehydration into consideration.

Body mass index

$$BMI = \frac{Weight\,(kg)}{Height^2\,(m)}$$

Normal
♀ 20–25
♂ 22–27

BMI is useful for identifying malnourished underweight patients, but a normal BMI does not rule out malnutrition, especially in an increasingly obese population.

Normal nutritional requirements

The Schofield equation is used typically in the UK; the Harris–Benedict and Ireton–Jones equations are commonly referred to in US texts.

It is always best to be cautious and start low and titrate up, depending on tolerance and clinical response. Use actual bodyweight if BMI >30kg/m²: A useful starting point in obese patients is to use 75% of body weight or alternatively feed to basal metabolic rate (BMR), without stress or activity factors added.

Macronutrients

- Calories
- Schofield equation
- Calculate BMR (W = weight in kilograms) (Table 24.7).

Add activity factor and stress factor as follows.
- Activity:
  - bedbound/immobile: +10%
  - bedbound mobile/sitting: +15–20%
  - mobile: +25% upwards.
- Stress: percentage added for stress varies widely depending on the clinical condition, but it is typically in the range 0–30%.

Harris–Benedict equation

♂: BMR = 66.473 + (13.751 × BW) + (5.0033 × HT) − (6.755 × age)
♀: BMR = 655.0955 + (9.463 × BW) + (1.8496 × HT) − (4.6756 × age)

where BW is body weight in kilograms, HT is height in centimetres, and age is in years.

Total caloric requirement is obtained by multiplying the BMR by the sum of the stress and activity factors. Stress conditions and activity factors need to be factored to calculate specific requirements).

Composition of parenteral nutrition regimens

- If possible, a balance of glucose and lipids should be used to provide total amount calories calculated.
- Glucose provision should be within the glucose oxidation rate (GOR) if possible.
- Normal GOR is 4–7mg/kg body weight/min.

Nitrogen

- Normal nitrogen requirements are 0.14–0.2g/kg body weight.
- Requirements in catabolic patients can be in the range 0.2–0.3g/kg body weight.
- Non-renal nitrogen losses should be taken into consideration— e.g. wound, fistula, and burn losses.

Electrolytes

- Sodium (normal range 0.5–1.5mmol/kg body weight).
  - Sensitive to haemodilutional effects. Actual low sodium level is usually only as a result of excessive losses, and a moderately low level is unlikely to be clinically significant.
  - Renal excretion can be a useful indicator. Aim to keep urine sodium >20mmol/L.

- Potassium (normal range 0.3–1.0mmol/kg body weight).
  - Affected by renal function, drugs, or excessive losses.
- Calcium (normal range 0.1–0.15mmol/kg body weight).
  - Sensitive to haemoconcentration and haemodilution. Minimal supplementation generally adequate in short-term parenteral nutrition.
- Magnesium (normal range 0.1–0.2mmol/kg body weight).
  - Renally conserved. Minimal amounts generally suffice unless patient has excessive losses.
- Phosphate (normal range 0.5–1.0mmol/kg body weight).
  - Influenced by renal function, re-feeding syndrome, and onset of sepsis.

Trace elements and vitamins

Commercial multivitamin and mineral preparations (e.g. Solivito N®, Decan®, Additrace®, and Cernevit®) are suitable for most patients in the short to medium term. Requirements for long-term patients are dictated by monitoring.

Table 24.7 Calculation of BMR

♀ (kcal/day)		♂ (kcal/day)	
18–29yrs	(14.8W) + 692	18–29yrs	(15.1W) + 692
30–59yrs	(8.3W) + 846	30–59yrs	(11.5W) + 873
60–74yrs	(9.2W) + 687	60–74yrs	(11.9W) + 700
>75yrs	(9.8W) + 624	>75yrs	(8.3W) + 820

How specific clinical conditions can affect parenteral nutrition requirements and provision

Re-feeding syndrome

- Start with low calories/day (max 20kcal/kg body weight/day).
- Monitor and supplement potassium, magnesium, and phosphate as required.
- Ensure adequate vitamin supply, especially thiamine.

Acute renal failure

- Consider fluid, potassium, and phosphate restriction.
- Sodium restriction can also help to ↓ fluid retention.

Chronic renal failure

- Influenced by dialysis status.
- Consider need for nitrogen, potassium, and phosphate restriction.

Acute liver failure

- Use dry body weight to calculate requirements (especially if ascites is present).
- Patients might require sodium and fluid restriction. Protein restriction is not necessary.
- Provision of nutrition usually outweighs risks of abnormal LFTs.

Congestive cardiac failure

- Consider need for sodium and fluid restriction.

Practical issues concerning parenteral nutrition

The identification and selection of patients who require parenteral nutrition, and the subsequent provision and monitoring of this treatment, consist of a number of overlapping phases.

If there is concern with regard to a patient's nutrition they should be referred to the ward dietician for a full assessment.

Initiation of parenteral nutrition

Once referred to the nutrition support team, the patient will be formally assessed and, if it is felt appropriate, line access will be planned. For short-term parenteral nutrition (7–10 days), this will usually be a peripherally inserted venous catheter (PICC). A tunnelled central line will be used if the anticipated duration of parenteral nutrition is longer or peripheral access is limited.

Before initiating parenteral nutrition, baseline biochemistry should be checked (Table 24.8) and fluid and electrolyte abnormalities corrected. In those at risk of developing re-feeding syndrome. Additional IV vitamins might be required.

Early monitoring phase

During the first week of parenteral nutrition (and subsequently if the patient is 'unstable' with respect to fluid and electrolyte or metabolic issues) the patient is monitored intensively. This consists of a minimum set of mandatory ward observations, and appropriate blood and other laboratory tests. The aim is to optimize nutritional support, while remaining aware of the other therapeutic strategies in the patient's overall care plan.

It might be necessary to modify either nutritional support or the overall patient care plan to obtain the best patient outcomes.

Stable patient phase

After the patient is stabilized on parenteral nutrition a less intensive monitoring process is required.

Re-introduction of diet

At a certain point, diet or enteral feed is usually introduced in a transitional manner. Liaison with the ward dietician is essential and, if appropriate, reduction or cessation of parenteral nutrition is recommended.

Cessation of parenteral nutrition

Parenteral nutrition is usually stopped when oral nutritional intake is deemed adequate for the individual patient. As a general rule, cessation of parenteral nutrition is determined by a variety of factors and is a multi-disciplinary decision.

Table 24.8 Suggested monitoring guide (please refer to local guidelines)

	Baseline	New patient or unstable	Stable patient
Blood biochemistry			
Urea and creatinine	Yes	Daily	Three times weekly
Sodium	Yes	Daily	Three times weekly
Potassium	Yes	Daily	Three times weekly
Bicarbonate	Yes	Daily	Three times weekly
Chloride	Yes	Daily	Three times weekly
LFTs: bilirubin	Yes	Daily	Three times weekly
ALP	Yes	Daily	Three times weekly
AST or ALT	Yes	Daily	Three times weekly
Albumin	Yes	Daily	Three times weekly
Calcium	Yes	Daily	Three times weekly
Magnesium	Yes	Daily	Three times weekly
Phosphate	Yes	Daily	Three times weekly
Zinc	Yes	Weekly	Every 2 weeks
Copper	Yes	Monthly	Every 3 months
CRP	Yes	Three times weekly	Three times weekly
Full blood count	Yes	Three times weekly	Weekly
Coagulation			
APTT	Yes	Weekly	Weekly
INR	Yes	Weekly	Weekly
Lipids			
Cholesterol	Yes	Weekly	Weekly
Triglycerides	Yes	Weekly	Weekly

LFT, liver function test; ALP, alkaline phosphatase; AST, aspartate amino-transferase; ALT, alanine aminotransferase; CRP, C-reactive protein; APTT, activated partial thromboplastin time.

IV access

Peripheral cannulae (Venflons®) should not be used routinely for the administration of parenteral nutrition. They should only be used in the short term for the administration of 'peripheral formulated' parenteral nutrition.

PICC lines are usually used for medium- to long-term venous access (2–6 months).

Tunnelled cuffed central venous catheters (CVs) are inserted via the subclavian (or jugular) vein for long-term feeding.

A dedicated single-lumen line is the safest route for parenteral nutrition administration. There is a greater risk of infection the more times a line is manipulated. Aseptic technique should be used. Nothing else should be given through this lumen, nor should blood be sampled from the line under normal circumstances (it might be appropriate for blood sampling in patients receiving parenteral nutrition at home).

If a multilumen line must be used for clinical reasons, one lumen should be dedicated for parenteral nutrition use only. Again, ideally, nothing else should be given through this lumen, nor should blood be sampled from it.

Prescribing parenteral nutrition

Patients' nutritional requirements are based on standard dietetic equations. A regimen close to a patient's requirements should be provided in a formulation prepared to minimize risk.

Nitrogen

Protein in parenteral nutrition is provided in the form of amino acids. Individual nitrogen requirements are calculated.

Carbohydrate and lipid

The energy in parenteral nutrition is generally described as non-protein calories (i.e. the figure excludes the energy provided from amino acids).

Total energy intake is best given as a mixture of glucose and lipid, usually in a ratio of 60:40. This might be varied if clinically important glucose intolerance develops or if there is a requirement for a lipid-free parenteral nutrition bag.

Volume

The overall aim is to provide all fluid volume requirements, including losses from wounds, drains, stomas, fistulae, etc., through parenteral nutrition. However, if these losses are large or highly variable, they should be managed separately.

Electrolytes

These are modified according to clinical requirements, with particular regard to extra-renal losses. Electrolytes should be reviewed daily initially and modified as necessary. Monitoring of urinary electrolyte losses is useful.

Vitamins, minerals, and trace elements

These are added routinely on a daily basis. Extra zinc or selenium might be required in patients with large GI losses. Patients on long-term parenteral nutrition will have routine micronutrient screening (Table 24.8).

Other medications

No drug additions should be made to parenteral nutrition on grounds of stability, unless stability work is undertaken. Additions of certain drugs (e.g. heparin) are known to lead to incompatibility.

Recommended monitoring/care (early monitoring phase)

- Daily weight (before starting parenteral nutrition and daily thereafter).
- Take temperature and BP reading every 4–6h. (Also observe for clinical evidence of infection and general well-being.)
- Accurate fluid-balance chart and summary (to maintain accurate fluid balance and homeostasis). Bag change should be undertaken at the same time of day.
- Capillary glucose monitoring (BMS) every 6h during the first 24h, and then twice or once daily until stable (generally, the glucose target should be 4–10mmol/L). Return to BMS every 6h when parenteral nutrition is being weaned off.
- Daily assessment for CVC/PICC site infection or leakage. Change dressing for CVCs at least every 72h and more frequently if loose, soiled, or wet. Change PICC dressings weekly.
- 24h urine collections for nitrogen balance and electrolytes should be undertaken according to local practice.

Storage of parenteral nutrition on ward

Bags not yet connected to the patient must be stored in a refrigerator (at 2–8°C). Bags stored in a drug refrigerator must be kept away from any freezer compartment to prevent ice crystal formation in the parenteral nutrition.

Bags that have been refrigerated should be removed at least 1–2h before being hung and infused, to enable the solution to reach room temperature. Bags connected to the patient should be protected from light using protective covers.

Children's parenteral nutrition regimens

Parenteral nutrition in children

Infants and children are particularly susceptible to the effects of starvation. The small preterm infant (1kg) contains only 1% fat and 8% protein, and has a non-protein caloric reserve of only 110kcal/kg body weight With growth, the fat and protein content rises, so a 1-year-old child weighing 10kg will have a non-protein calorie reserve of 221kcal/kg body weight All non-protein content and one-third of the protein content of the body is available for calorific needs at a rate of 50kcal/kg body weight/day in infants and children.

A small preterm baby (<1.5kg) has sufficient reserve to survive only 4 days of starvation, and a large preterm baby (>3kg) has enough for ~10–12 days. With ↑ calorific requirements associated with disease this might be reduced dramatically to <2 days for small preterm infants and perhaps 1 week for a large preterm baby.

Indications for parenteral nutrition

Some children require short-term parenteral nutrition in the following clinical situations:
- major intestinal surgery
- chemotherapy
- severe acute pancreatitis
- multiorgan failure in extensive trauma, burns, or prematurity.

Others will need long-term parenteral nutrition if there are prolonged episodes of intestinal failure—e.g. in the following clinical situations:
- protracted diarrhoea of infancy
- short bowel syndrome
- gastroschisis
- chronic intestinal pseudo-obstruction.

Nutritional requirements (Table 24.9)

Fluid requirements also depend on the child's size, abnormal losses (e.g. diarrhoea, fever), surgical procedures, and disease state. The requirements for fluid to body weight are much greater in very small children than in older children and adults. Infants have a much larger body surface area relative to weight than older patients. Infants lose more fluid through evaporation and dissipate much more heat per kilogram. The use of radiant heaters and phototherapy further ↑ a neonate's fluid loss, resulting in ↑ fluid requirement. Children with high urinary outputs, ↑ ileostomy or gastrostomy tube outputs, diarrhoea, or vomiting should have replacement fluids for these excessive losses in addition to their maintenance fluid requirements.

The child's weight and assessment of intake and output can be used to estimate hydration status. It is important that children receiving parenteral nutrition are weighed regularly (initially daily, then twice or three times weekly with growth plotted when their condition stabilizes) and their fluid balance is monitored when parenteral nutrition is prescribed.

Energy sources

The body of a child requires energy for physical growth and neurological development.

Carbohydrate

Glucose is the carbohydrate source of choice in parenteral nutrition. To prevent hyperosmolality and hyperinsulinaemia, glucose infusions are introduced in a stepwise manner. In infants, glucose is introduced at 5–7.5% glucose and ↑ by 2.5% each day to an upper limit on glucose infusion rate of 4–7mg/kg body weight/min. In older children parenteral nutrition is started at 10–15% and ↑ daily to 20%, as tolerated.

The amount of glucose depends on the type of feeding line inserted. The glucose concentration in parenteral nutrition infused peripherally is limited to 12.5%. If central access is available, up to 20% glucose can be infused. Infusion of parenteral nutrition with glucose concentrations >20% has been associated with cardiac arrhythmias.

The infant with very low birthweight has low glycogen reserves in the liver and a diminished capacity for gluconeogenesis. Hepatic glycogen is depleted within hours of birth, depriving the brain of metabolic fuel. Thus providing exogenous glucose through parenteral nutrition is a priority. Preterm infants, especially those with birthweights <1000g, are relatively glucose intolerant because of insulin resistance. Infusion of glucose >6mg/kg body weight/min may lead to hyperglycaemia and serum hyper-osmolality, resulting in osmotic diuresis. Tolerance to glucose improves on subsequent days. It is generally recommended that the glucose infusion rate does not exceed 9mg/kg body weight/min for premature infants after the first day of life and that ↑ is implemented gradually as the infant develops.

Table 24.9 Estimated average requirements for fluid, energy, protein, and nitrogen

Age (yrs)	Fluid (mL/kg/day)	Energy (kcal/kg /day)	Protein (g/kg/day)	Nitrogen (g/kg/day)
Preterm	150–200	130–150	3.0–4.0	0.5–0.65
0–1	110–150	110–130	2.0–3.0	0.34–0.46
1–6	80–100	70–100	1.5–2.5	0.22–0.38
6–12	75–80	50–70	1.5–2.0	0.2–0.33
12–18	50–75	40–50	1.0–1.3	0.16–0.2

Lipids

- Regimens require fat as a source of essential fatty acids. Fat is an important parenteral substrate because it is a concentrated source of calories in an isotonic medium, which makes it useful for peripheral administration.
- Fat is a useful substitute for carbohydrate if glucose calories are limited because of glucose intolerance. It is available as emulsions of soybean, soybean–safflower oil mixtures, or olive oil. The major differences are their fatty acid contents.
- Essential fatty acid deficiency can develop in the premature newborn during the first week of life on lipid-free regimens. There is a maximum lipid utilization rate of 3.3–3.6g/kg body weight/day. Above these values, there is ↑ risk of fat deposition 2° to the incomplete metabolic utilization of the infused lipid.
- IV fat should be commenced at a dose not exceeding 1g/kg body weight/day and ↑ gradually to a maximum of 3g/kg body weight/day, depending on age. Tolerance should be assessed by measuring serum triglyceride and free fatty acid concentrations.

Nitrogen

Nitrogen is needed for growth, the formation of new tissues (e.g. wound healing), and the synthesis of plasma proteins, enzymes, and blood cells.

Requirements vary according to age, nutritional status, and disease state. Infants and children experiencing periods of growth have higher nitrogen requirements than adults. Low-birthweight infants have relatively high total amino acid requirements to support maintenance, growth, and developmental needs.

Amino acid intakes of 2.0–2.5g/kg body weight/day result in nitrogen retention comparable to the healthy enteral-fed infant. Rates of up to 4g/kg body weight/day might be required. Because the amino acid profile varies between commercial brands, their nitrogen contents are not equivalent and protein requirements are calculated as grams of amino acids rather than grams of nitrogen in children.

Choice of amino acid solution

The proteins of the human body are manufactured from 20 different amino acids. There are eight essential amino acids. Premature infants and children are unable to synthesize/metabolize some of the amino acids that are 'non-essential' for adults. The use of amino acid solutions designed for adults have resulted in abnormal plasma amino acid profiles in infants. Infants fed with adult amino acid solutions have been shown to develop high concentrations of phenylalanine and tyrosine and low levels of taurine.

Paediatric amino acid solutions

Amino acid solutions specifically designed for neonates have been developed, as follows.

- Higher concentration of branch-chain amino acids (leucine, isoleucine and valine) and lower content of glycine, methionine and phenylalanine.
- Higher percentage of amino acids essential for preterm infants, with wider distribution of nonessential amino acids.
- Contain taurine.

The amino acid preparations available are based on either the amino acid profile of human milk (Vaminolact®) or placental cord blood (Primene®).

Electrolytes
Normal baseline electrolyte requirements are shown in Table 24.10.

Trace elements
Requirements for trace elements are shown in Table 24.11

Table 24.10 Normal baseline electrolyte requirements

Electrolytes	Requirements according to age (mmol/kg body weight/day)	
	Infants	Children
Sodium	2.0–3.5	1.0–2.0
Potassium	2.0–3.0	1.0–2.0
Calcium	1.0–1.5	0.5–1.0
Magnesium	0.15–0.3	0.1–0.15
Phosphate	0.5–1.5	0.12–0.4
Chloride	1.8–1.5	1.2–2

Table 24.11 Requirements for trace elements

Element	Requirements according to age (micrograms/kg body weight/day)		
	Preterm	Infants	Children
Zinc	100–500	50–100	50–80
Copper	30–60	20–50	20
Selenium	n/a	2–5	2
Manganese	n/a	1	1
Iron	100–200	20–100	100

Vitamins

Requirements for vitamins are shown in Tables 24.12 and 24.13.

Administration of nutrition

- The aqueous phase runs over a period of 24h and the solution is filtered using a 0.2µm filter.
- Lipid normally runs over a period of 20–24h and is filtered using a 1.2µm filter, although some centres prefer not to use filters.
- The weight used for calculation is usually the actual weight of the child.

Complications

Catheter-related

Complications could be due to catheter insertion (e.g. malposition, haemorrhage, pneumothorax, air embolism, or nerve injury) or might occur subsequently (e.g. infection, occlusion, or thromboembolism).

Metabolic-related

In stable patients with no abnormal fluid losses or major organ failure, severe biochemical disturbances are unusual.

Parenteral-nutrition-associated cholestasis

The aetiology seems to be multifactorial, including the absence of enteral feeding, overfeeding, prematurity, surgery, and sepsis. It might progress to cirrhosis. Excessive calories, particularly glucose overload, can lower serum glucagon concentrations, which ↓ bile flow. Early initiation of oral calorie intake is the single most important factor in preventing or reversing cholestasis. Small intestinal bacterial overgrowth, which often occurs in the presence of intestinal stasis, can impair bile flow, leading to cholestasis.

Monitoring children receiving parenteral nutrition in hospital

Requires clinical and laboratory monitoring, observations, and assessment of growth. Growth is conveniently assessed by accurate measurement of weight and height, and development assessment is plotted over time. Fluid balance, temperature, and basal metabolism need to be assessed daily.

Laboratory monitoring

- Initial assessment—daily for first 3–4 days, then twice weekly.
- Full blood count.
- Blood test: sodium, potassium, urea, glucose.
- Calcium, magnesium, phosphate, bilirubin, ALP, AST, ALT, blood glucose albumin, triglycerides, cholesterol.
- Copper, zinc, selenium, vitamins A and E: baseline measurement.
- Urine: sodium and potassium (baseline).
- Continued monitoring depends on the child's clinical condition.

Table 24.12 Requirements for water-soluble vitamins

Vitamin	Requirements according to age		
	Preterm	Infants	Children
B_1 (mg)	0.1–05	0.4–1.5	1.0–3.0
B_2 (mg)	0.1–0.3	0.4–1.5	1.0–3.0
B_6 (mg)	008–0.4	0.1–1.0	1.0–2.0
B_{12} (micrograms)	0.3–0.6	0.3–30	20–40
C (mg)	20–40	20–40	20–40
Biotin (micrograms)	5–30	35–50	150–300
Folate (micrograms)	50–200	100–200	100–200
Niacin (mg)	2–5	5–10	5–20

Table 24.13 Requirements for fat-soluble vitamins

Vitamin	Preterm	Infant	Children
A (micrograms)	75–300	300–600	500–800
D (micrograms)	5–10	10–20	10–20
E mg	3–8	3–10	10–15
K (micrograms)	5–80	100–200	N/a

Enteral feeding

Enteral feeding should be considered in patients with a functioning GI tract who are unable to meet requirements with ordinary diet, food fortification, and/or oral nutritional supplements.

Enteral nutrition is contraindicated in patients with intestinal obstruction, paralytic ileus, GI ischaemia, intractable diarrhoea, and diffuse peritonitis. Enteral access device selection is based on several patient-specific factors, including GI anatomy, gastric emptying, tube placement duration, and aspiration potential.

Post-pyloric feeding is indicated if there is gastric outflow obstruction or severe pancreatitis, or if the patient is at risk from aspiration with intragastric feeding.

Types of tube feeding

Intragastric feeding
- Nasogastric
- Percutaneous endoscopic gastroscopy (PEG)

Post-pyloric feeding
- Nasojejunal
- Nasoduodenal
- PEG
- Percutaneous endoscopic jejunostomy
- Surgically placed jejunostomy

Feeding tube specific issues

Site of delivery
- Gastric tubes end in the stomach, whereas jejunal tubes end in the jejunum.
- Sterile water must be used for jejunal tubes because of gastric acid barrier bypass.

Number of differences between tubes apart from site of feed delivery
- Bore size—fine-bore tube is designed for administration of feeds, and wide-bore tube is designed for aspiration
- Number of lumens
- Rate of flow
- Length

Complications of tubes
- Removal by patient
- Oesophageal ulceration or strictures
- Incorrect positioning of tube.
- Blockage

Categories of feed
Polymeric feeds
Contain whole protein, carbohydrate, and fat, and can be used as the sole source of nutrition for those patients without any special nutrient requirements. Standard concentration is 1kcal/mL with 40–50g/L protein, but they can vary in energy density (0.8–2kcal/mL) and can be supplemented with fibre, which can help improve bowel function if this is problematic.

Elemental feeds
Contain amino acid and glucose or maltodextrins; fat content is very low. Used in situations of malabsorption or pancreatic insufficiency. Because of their high osmolality, they should not be used in patients with short bowel syndrome.

Disease-specific feeds and modular supplements
Certain clinical conditions require adjustment in diets—e.g. high-energy low-electrolyte feeds for patients requiring dialysis, and low-carbohydrate and high-fat diets for patients with CO_2 retention (for certain patients on ventilators) as carbohydrate leads to more CO_2 production compared with calorific equivalent amounts of protein or fat.

Modular supplements are used for a variety of conditions—e.g. malabsorption and hypoprotein states. They are not nutritionally complete and hence are not suitable as the sole source of food. These feeds contain extra substrates that are claimed to alter the immune and inflammatory responses. These substrates include glutamine, arginine, RNA, omega-3 fatty acids, and antioxidants.

Administration of tube feeds
For intragastric feeds, diet can be delivered at a continuous rate over a period of 16–18h daily. Alternatively, intermittent boluses of 50–250mL can be administered by syringe over a period of 10–30min 4–8 times a day, although complications such as aspiration and delayed gastric transit times have been reported more frequently with this approach.

Post-pyloric feeding is generally performed by continuous infusion because it is deemed more physiological.

Complications from feeds
Diarrhoea
Diarrhoea is the most common complication associated with enteral nutrition, occurring in 21–72% of patients. Severe diarrhoea can cause life-threatening electrolyte changes and hypovolaemia. Management is by excluding other explanations (e.g. colitis, laxative use, antibiotics, and malabsorption).

Concomitant medications need to be rationalized. Antidiarrhoeal medications (codeine phosphate and/or loperamide) are often useful and fibre can help in some cases.

If diarrhoea persists after treatment, consider switching to the post-pyloric route.

Constipation

Usually a result of a combination of inadequate fluid, dehydration, immobility, and drugs. If functional pathology is excluded, management is by laxatives, suppositories, and fibre-containing feeds.

Vomiting, aspiration, or reflux

Both nasogastric and post-pyloric feeding can ↑ the risk of aspiration. Both can interfere with oesophageal sphincter function, and wide-bore tubes cause more problems than fine-bore tubes. Standard antiemetics and prokinetics are usually effective.

Metabolic complications

Re-feeding syndrome

Excess carbohydrate stimulates insulin release, which leads to intracellular shifts of phosphate, magnesium, and potassium that can lead to cardiac arrhythmias or neurological events. Emaciated patients must have their feed introduced gradually at a rate of 20kcal/kg body weight and electrolytes replaced in accordance with daily blood levels.

Vitamin/trace element deficiencies

Incidence is rare as commercially available feeds are nutritionally complete. Patients being fed over extended periods should be monitored appropriately.

Hyperglycaemia

Important in the critically ill. It is imperative that blood glucose is monitored and controlled because good glycaemic control reduces mortality rates in the critically ill.

Drug administration in patients with feeding tubes

The administration of medication to patients with feeding tubes can be challenging, and a number of issues need to be considered in parallel with the patient's medical problems. These issues include the following:

- The continued need for the patient's regular medicines and the consequences of medication withdrawal or administration delay, both medically and legally.
- The intention to tube feed and subsequent compliance of the patient to retain the tube.
- Institutional ability to site percutaneous tubes.
- Availability and appropriateness of different formulations of medication.

Formulation difficulties

Pharmacists will be involved in influencing the choice of medication formulation on the basis of their training and experience.

Is there a formulation available for use by a licensed route? Use alternative routes of administration, if appropriate (i.e. buccal, intramuscular, intravenous, intraosseous, transdermal, topical, nebulized, rectal, subcutaneous, sublingual, etc.)

Pharmacists should also be able to calculate the cost implications of the different formulations and, importantly, should facilitate long-term choice, particularly if the parenteral route cannot be used in the long term.

- Is there a commercial oral solution, suspension, or soluble solid dose form?
- Oral liquid—dilute with 10–30mL sterile water or enteral formula if hyperosmolar.
- Oral immediate-release tablet—crush to fine powder and mix with 10–30mL water
- Oral immediate-release capsule—open capsule and crush contents to fine powder. Mix with 10–30mL sterile water.
- Oral soft gelatin capsule (e.g. acetazolamide, nifedipine)—remove liquid contents with a needle and syringe. Then mix with 10–30 mL of sterile water
- IV liquid preparation—draw dose into an amber oral syringe prior to administration
- Soluble tablets dissolved in 10mL of water are often the best option for tube-fed patients.
- Refer to specific manufacturer's advice for feed-tube administration.
- Remember to shake liquid preparations before administration.
- Viscous liquids might have to be diluted with water to ↓ tube blockage.
- Liquids with high osmolality or sorbitol content can lead to diarrhoea.
- Does the crushed tablet or capsule contents disperse fully or form a workable suspension that will not clog or block the feeding tube?
- Is the parenteral formulation of the product suitable for enteral use?
- Osmolality concerns for parenteral product.
- Additives in injections might make administration through a tube unsuitable.
- Is there a therapeutic substitute that can be administered via a tube?

Administration of medication through a tube

- Do not add medication directly to the feed.
- Only administer one medication at a time.
- Use an oral syringe if possible.
- Flush the tube with 50mL water immediately after stopping the feed.
- Add the volume of water used to fluid balance charts.
- Draw identified formulation into appropriate 50mL syringe.
- Attach the tube and apply gentle pressure.
- Flush with a minimum 15mL of water between different medicines.
- Flush with 50mL of water after the last medication.
- If drug is to be taken on an empty stomach, for gastric tubes, stop feed for 30min before the dose and resume feeding 30min afterwards. These measures are not relevant for jejunal tubes.
- Add the total volume of flushes and medicine to fluid balance chart.

Specific drug/tube feeding problems

Drug-specific issues

- Absorption could be unpredictable because the tube might be beyond the main site of absorption for the specific drug.
- Formulation issues of medication being administered through feeding tubes.
- Crushing destroys the formulation properties of tablets, altering peak and trough levels.
- Detrimental clinical effect for certain slow-release products (e.g. nifedipine LA), causing severe hypotension if inadvertently given crushed.

Adsorption onto feeding tubes

Examples are phenytoin, diazepam, and carbamazepine. Dilute with at least 50mL of water and flush the tube well.

Interactions causing blockage

Antacids and acidic formulations could cause precipitation because of an acid–base reaction.

Feed ↓ drug absorption

- Phenytoin—50–75% reduction in serum levels when given with enteral nutrition. Hold tube feeding for 2h before and after each dose as well as flushing the tube before and after each phenytoin dose.
- Fluoroquinolones (ciprofloxacin, levofloxacin, moxifloxacin)—give enterally via large-bore feeding tube. Crush tablets and mix with 20–30mL of water prior to administration. Hold tube feeding for 2h before and 4h after administration. Ciprofloxacin suspension should not be administered via the feeding tube. It has a thick consistency that may clog the tube, and since it is an oil-based suspension it does not mix well with water.
- Warfarin—reductions in absorption may occur because enteral feeding solutions may bind warfarin.

Drug–feed interactions

If vitamin K is in present in the feed it means that doses of warfarin might need to be amended (monitor INR).

Bioequivalence

Different formulations might necessitate adjustment of dose (e.g. phenytoin tablets and liquid).

Further reading

Beckwith MC et al. (2004) A guide to drug therapy in patients with enteral feeding tubes: dosage form selection and administration methods. *Hospital Pharmacy* **39**: 225–37.

℘ http://www.bapen.org.uk

IV therapy at home

Patients who are medically stable but require prolonged courses of IV drugs (usually antimicrobials) can benefit from IV therapy at home. Suitable indications or therapies are as follows:
- bone infections
- endocarditis
- cystic fibrosis
- cytomegalovirus infection
- total parenteral nutrition
- immunoglobulins.

The advantages of treating these patients at home are as follows:
- releases hospital beds for other patients
- avoids patient exposure to hospital-acquired infection
- ↑ patient autonomy
- improved patient comfort and convenience
- some patients can to return to work or study while therapy continues.

Despite the potential benefits, IV therapy at home should not be undertaken lightly. All IV therapy is potentially hazardous and complications, such as line sepsis or blockage, are potentially more probable and risky in the community.

It is recommended that a multidisciplinary home IV team is set up to oversee the process and that guidelines are drawn up to ensure that home IV therapy is done safely and effectively.[1]

Home IV therapy team

The following people should be included in the team. They may not have hands on involvement in every patient but should be available for advice and support.
- Clinician with an interest in home IV therapy (e.g. microbiologist, infectious diseases physician)
- Home IV therapy specialist nurse(s)/community liaison nurse(s).
- Pharmacist.
- Community representative (GP or community nurse).

24-hour access to key member(s) of the team (usually the specialist nurse and/or a clinician) is essential.

For individual patients, the medical and nursing team responsible for the patient's care should liaise with the home IV team and be involved in assessment, discharge planning, and follow-up.

IV access

Venous access through short peripheral lines (Venflons®) is unsuitable for home delivery because it is designed for short-term use and should be replaced every 48–72h. Peripheral access is also unsuitable for irritant or hyperosmolar infusions (e.g. TPN). Central venous access is preferred for the following reasons.

1 Nathwani D, Conlon C (1998). Outpatient and home parenteral antibiotic theraphy (OHPAT) in the UK: a consensus statement by a working party. *Clinical Microbiology and infection* **4**: 537–51.

- It can remain in place for prolonged periods.
- It can be used for irritant or hyperosmolar infusions.
- It is easier for patients to self-administer through a central line.

Three types of central IV access are used for home IV therapy.
- *Central line* (e.g. *Hickman*® or *Groshong*®)—the line is inserted, usually through the subclavian vein, and is threaded through a sub-cutaneous tunnel to exit on the chest wall. The tip lies in the superior vena cava or just inside the right atrium. Central lines are inserted under general or local anaesthetic. In some hospitals specialist nurses insert central lines. Central lines might have one or more lumens, but for IV therapy at home a single lumen line is recommended to ↓ complications. These lines can remain in place for many months.
- *Port-A-Cath*®—a central venous access device, consisting of a small reservoir (the port) attached to a catheter. The port is implanted into the chest wall, with the catheter inserted into the subclavian or internal jugular vein. The reservoir is covered with a thick rubber septum, which is accessed through the skin using a special needle known as a Huber® needle. Port-A-Caths® are inserted under general anaesthetic. They can remain in place for years. Because of the cost and complexity of insertion, Port-A-Caths® are only suitable for patients who require prolonged or repeated IV therapy (e.g. cystic fibrosis patients).
- *Peripherally inserted central catheters (PICCs)*—these are fine flexible catheters inserted into the basilic or cephalic vein at the ante-cubital fossa, in a similar manner to peripheral venous access. Using a guidewire, the catheter is threaded up the axillary vein and into a central vein. PICC lines are inserted under local anaesthetic and are the least complex of the three types to insert. They can remain in place for several weeks or months. PICC lines are the least costly and complex and therefore are usually the preferred type of access.

To preserve the patency of central lines and avoid septic complications, guidelines should give advice on handling the line, including the following.
- Aseptic technique for drug administration.
- Flushing the line between doses.
- Use of heparinized saline to avoid clot formation within the line.
- Dressing and cleaning the insertion site.
- Care of the line when not in use.
- Procedure if the line is blocked or damaged.
- Procedure if there are signs of infection/cellulitis around the insertion site or signs/symptoms of sepsis.

Assessment and discharge planning

The home IV team should take responsibility for assessing whether the patient is suitable for IV therapy at home and for planning the discharge jointly with other nursing/medical staff caring for the patient. It is important that sufficient time is allowed to ensure that assessment, training, and general organization of the discharge are carried out adequately. Guidelines should advise a minimum of 48h notice, and ideally longer.

Patients should have the following characteristics:
- medically stable
- not likely to misuse the line
- psychologically able to cope with IV therapy at home
- willing to have IV therapy at home
- able to recognize problems and act accordingly.

The patient's home circumstances must also be taken into account.
- Is there another responsible adult who can support the patient and, if necessary, contact medical services themselves?
- Does the patient have a telephone?
- Are there reliable water and electricity supplies?
- Is there somewhere cool, dry, and safe to store drugs (out of reach of children)?
- Does the patient have a fridge, if needed, for drug storage (and do children have unsupervised access to this fridge)?
- Are there children or other people in the house who might be distressed by seeing drugs being administered IV?
- Does the patient have some means of transport to out-patient appointments?

Procedures for children receiving IV therapy at home are much the same as those for adults, but special attention must be paid to ensuring that home circumstances are suitable and that parents do not feel too pressured, especially if they are responsible for administering the drugs.

The discharge plan should be written in the patient's medical records (Table 24.14). A copy should be supplied to the GP, and patients should be provided with written information on the drugs, their administration, and their side effects, and given monitoring and emergency contact details.

Drug selection and administration

Drug selection primarily depends on the condition being treated. Ideally, drugs that are administered once daily should be used. In most UK schemes, IV infusions are avoided and wherever possible drugs are administered by slow IV push because this is a less complex and time-consuming method of drug administration. Where IV infusion cannot be avoided (e.g. vancomycin), the drug should be administered through a volumetric pump rather than a gravity drip. In some situations, it can be more appropriate to use an ambulatory infusion device such as an elastomeric pump (e.g. Homepump®) or other system (e.g. Sidekick®), rather than a volumetric pump. Discussion of these devices is beyond the scope of this chapter.

Guidelines should give advice on drug administration. Issues that must be considered are as follows.
- Who will administer the drug—e.g. patient, carer, community nurse?

- What training will they require?
- Who will do the training?

Many patients or their carers are capable of administering IV therapy provided that they receive suitable training and support. However, if therapy is only to continue for a week or less it is probably not worth the time taken to train a patient or carer. In some areas community nurses can administer the drugs, but they might also need additional training. Training is usually provided by a specialist nurse.

Training should include recognition of adverse effects and what action to take. This includes possible allergic or anaphylactic reactions. Protocols for administration of drugs by patients/carers or for community nurses to treat anaphylaxis should be in place and an 'anaphylaxis kit' kept in the patient's home. These protocols should follow UK Resuscitation Council guidelines.[1]

It is recommended that the first one or two doses of the drug should be administered in hospital so that the patient can be monitored for acute side effects.

Guidelines should include procedures for disposal of clinical waste (e.g. used dressings), sharps, and empty vials. These should follow local practice—e.g. some areas might accept sharps boxes for disposal in the community, whereas others might require them to be returned to the hospital.

Table 24.14 Checklist of information to be included in the discharge plan

Patient	Vascular access device	Treatment
Relevant past medical history	Type of device	Pathology and infecting organism
Problems/side effects experienced	When inserted or placed, and by whom	Details of antimicrobial regimen, drug, dose, etc
Frequency and timing of clinic visits during treatment	If centrally placed, where is the tip?	Administration details
Blood monitoring and frequency	Possible complications—signs, symptoms, prevention, and management	Side effects
Length of time on treatment	Day-to-day care of the line	Monitoring requirements and action required if results are abnormal
Finish/review date for treatment	Who to contact if there are any difficulties with the device	
How to access help	Who will remove the device and how	

[1] *UK Resuscitation Council Guidelines:* ℘ http://www.resus.org.uk/pages/mediMain.htm

Community support

The patient's GP should be willing for the patient to go home with IV therapy. Even if they are not administering the drug, community nurses might be involved in other aspects of patient care and so should be kept informed. Good communication between the home IV therapy team and community healthcare workers is essential. Contact details for the hospital clinician and specialist home IV therapy nurse should be provided, including out-of-hours contact details.

Follow-up

Before discharge, follow-up arrangements should be planned. This should include the following.

- What to do if the patient has a significant ADR—who is responsible for managing this?
- Blood tests for monitoring ADR and TDM.
  - Who will take blood?
  - What tests are required?
  - Frequency.
  - How will the results be communicated and to whom?
  - Who will act on the results?
- The specialist home IV therapy nurse will usually be the main point of contact.
- The referring team should follow up the patient with respect to presenting indication, in addition to follow-up from the home IV therapy team.
- Duration of IV therapy is usually decided before discharge. It should be agreed which team is responsible for review of this and for provision of oral follow-on therapy.
- The home IV therapy team is usually responsible for line removal (as appropriate) at the end of the IV course.

The role of the pharmacist

The pharmacist is an important member of the home IV team. Their role includes the following responsibilities.

- Advice on drug stability and compatibility.
- Advice on drug administration, including infusion rates, and ambulatory infusion devices.
- Ensuring the supply of IV and ancillary drugs on discharge.
- Ensuring that follow-on oral therapy is prescribed.
- Provision of anaphylaxis kits.
- Liaison with homecare companies
- Supporting the training of patients, and community nurses.

The American Society of Health System Pharmacists has published guidelines on the pharmacist's role in home care which includes home IV therapy.[1] It should be borne in mind that these guidelines reflect the US system of healthcare and so some aspects might not be relevant to non-US pharmacists.

---

1 American Society of Health System Pharmacists (2000). ASHP guidelines on the pharmacist's role in home care. *Amercan Journal of Health Systems Pharmacy* **57**: 1252–7.

Drugs for home IV therapy at home fall into the 'hospital at home' category and, as such, all supplies should come from the hospital. Thus community pharmacists are rarely involved in IV therapy at home. However, it is important that hospital pharmacists liaise with their community colleagues as appropriate—e.g. where oral follow-on therapy might be prescribed by the GP.

Homecare companies

A number of companies provide support services for home IV therapy. The service may range from supply of drugs and ancillaries direct to the patient's home to provision of the IV drug in an ambulatory infusion device to full nursing support. Pharmacists should ensure that they are familiar with the services being provided by the homecare companies used and that local procedures are complied with.

Therapy-related issues: musculoskeletal diseases

Rheumatoid arthritis 548
Gout 556

Rheumatoid arthritis

Rheumatoid arthritis (RA) is an autoimmune disease which causes joints lined with synovium to become inflamed, swollen, stiff, and painful, and leads to joint erosion. It is a multisystem disorder which can affect many organs including the eyes, lungs, heart, and blood vessels. The aim of treatment is to decrease pain and inflammation, prevent joint damage, and ultimately induce remission of disease.

Disease-modifying anti-rheumatic drugs (DMARDs) (Table 25.1)

- DMARDs should be started early, ideally within 3 months of the onset of persistent symptoms.
- Use a combination of at least two, usually including methotrexate.
- If a single DMARD is used, increase the dose rapidly to a therapeutic level.
- Unless contraindicated, use analgesics and NSAIDs as needed to relieve pain.
- When the disease is controlled, DMARDs can be cautiously reduced.

Common characteristics of DMARDs

- May take up to 3 months for full therapeutic effect. Therefore short-term glucocorticoids may be required in this period (IA, IM, or oral).
- Can cause adverse effects. Safety monitoring is required (see Table 25.1).
- Live vaccines should be avoided, but annual influenza and pneumococcal vaccines are recommended.
- Caution with exposure to chickenpox/shingles.

Biological therapies (Table 25.2)

Biological therapies offer major new options in the treatment of rheumatoid arthritis and their role is rapidly evolving. In England and Wales the use of these therapies is determined by NICE guidance.

- Biological therapies are associated with increased risk of serious infection and their use is contraindicated in patients with current infections.
- Screen patients for mycobacterial infections before biological therapies are initiated—if necessary give anti-TB prophylaxis.
- Can exacerbate heart failure—assess patients prior to initiation.
- Caution is required in patients with demyelinating diseases as anti-TNF therapies have been associated with demyelinating syndromes in a few cases.

Ankylosing spondylitis

Ankylosing spondylitis is an inflammatory disease affecting the spine and causing back pain, stiffness, and joint fixation. The large peripheral joints can also be affected.

- Conventional treatment is with physiotherapy and NSAIDs only.
- Methotrexate, and occasionally sulfasalazine, are used for peripheral disease.
- Anti-TNF therapies may be used for patients who have persistent active disease that has not responded to conventional therapy (Table 25.2).

Psoriatic arthritis

Psoriatic arthritis is a chronic inflammatory arthropathy of variable and unpredictable course associated with psoriasis of the skin or nails.

- Traditional standard therapy is with NSAIDs and corticosteroid injections.
- Methotrexate, leflunomide, and sulfasalazine are the DMARDs of choice (only leflunomide is specifically licensed). The risks of hepatotoxicity are slightly greater than for the same drugs used in RA and monitoring is essential.
- Patients with poor response may be changed to alternative DMARDs (e.g. ciclosporin).
- Etanercept, adalimumab, or infliximab may be used (in accordance with NICE guidelines) in patients with active and progressive psoriatic arthritis not responsive to adequate trials of at least two DMARDS either individually or in combination.

Vasculitis

The vasculitides comprise a group of diseases featuring inflammation and necrosis of blood vessels. They include temporal arteritis, Wegener's granulomatosis, Churg–Strauss syndrome, and vasculitis secondary to RA, systemic lupus erythematosus, or Sjögren's syndrome. Treatment depends on the extent and severity of disease.

Treatment of acute phase of the disease

- Cyclophosphamide may be given at a dose of 10–15mg/kg IV in pulses every 2–3wks for 3–6 months, or 2mg/kg daily taken orally, with monitoring of white blood cells and neutrophils and reductions in dose or frequency for renal impairment and age.
- Mesna is given in conjunction with cylophosphamide to prevent bladder toxicity. Patients are advised to maintain a fluid intake of ~3L/day on the day of treatment.
- Antiemetics will be needed with cyclophosphamide.
- Corticosteroids may be given prior to the cyclophosphamide as either IV methylprednisolone 10–15mg/kg or high-dose oral prednisolone.
- Co-trimoxazole 480–960mg three times weekly should be given as prophylaxis against *Pneumocystis jirovecii*.
- Patients on high-dose corticosteroids will require bone protection with a bisphosphonate and calcium and vitamin D supplements and may also require a PPI. Fluconazole or nystatin may be required as prophylaxis against oral candidiasis.

Maintainence therapy

After the cyclophosphamide course is complete, azathioprine or methotrexate may be given as maintenance therapy.

Further reading

♫ http://www.nice.org.uk; musculoskeletal section.
♫ http://www.rheumatology.org.uk; guidelines.
♫ http://www.arthritisresearchuk.org

Table 25.1 Disease-modifying anti-rheumatic drugs

DMARD	Dose	Other clinical information	Suggested Monitoring regimen
Methotrexate	7.5–10mg weekly ↑ to 25mg weekly	Folic acid 5mg may be given 3–4 days after the methotrexate, ↑ as necessary, but avoiding the day of methotrexate. Patient information and shared care card should be given as per NPSA alert. NSAIDs may be continued with regular monitoring; however, over-the-counter NSAIDs should be avoided. May be changed to subcutaneous route for maximum bioavailability and improved tolerability. The strength and form of methotrexate must be clearly stated.	FBC, LFTs, U&Es, ESR, and CRP every 2wks for 3 months, then monthly.
Sulfasalazine	500mg daily ↑ by 500mg weekly to 1g twice daily. Maximum 3g daily.	May colour urine orange and stain soft contact lenses yellow. May be used in pregnancy (up to 2g/day) and breastfeeding.	FBC, U&Es, LFTs, ESR, and CRP monthly for 3 months, then every 3 months.
Hydroxychloroquine	200–400mg daily	Visual acuity should be monitored annually by an optometrist and patients advised to report any visual disturbances. May be continued in pregancy	Regular blood monitoring is not required.
Leflunomide	10–20mg daily Occasionally 30mg daily	Long elimination half-life. Teratogenic—women planning to have children should discontinue leflunomide for 2 years or have cholestyramine washout procedure. Men should stop leflunomide 3 months before trying to father a child.	FBC, LFTs, U&Es, ESR, CRP, BP, and weight monthly for 6 months, then 2 monthly.

Drug	Dose	Notes	Monitoring
Azathioprine	1mg/kg/day for 4–6wks ↑ to 2–3mg/kg/day	If patient started on allopurinol reduce azathioprine dose to 25% of original dose.	FBC, LFTs, U&Es, CRP, and ESR weekly for 6wks, fortnightly until stable, then monthly.
Ciclosporin	2.5mg/kg/day in 2 divided doses for 6wks. ↑ at 2–4wk intervals to maximum 4mg/kg/day	Bioavailability varies with formulation—prescribe by brand name. Reduce diclofenac dose by 50%. Avoid colchicines, St John's wort, and doses of simvastatin >10mg.	U&Es, FBC, ESR, CRP, BP, and urinalysis fortnightly for 3 months, then monthly. LFTs monthly. Lipids every 6 months.
Mycofenolate	500mg daily ↑ by 500mg weekly to 1–2g daily. Maximum 3g daily	Used to treat vasculitis.	FBC weekly for 6wks, then monthly LFTs, U&Es, ESR, and CRP monthly.
Gold	10mg test dose. 50mg IM weekly until total of 1g, then review.	Given by deep IM injection. Patients should be observed for 30min after injection because of risk of anaphylaxis. Benefit not usually seen until cumulative dose of 500mg given. Stop if no response after 1g	FBC and urinalysis before each injection. CRP, ESR, and U&E at least 3 monthly.
Penicillamine	125mg daily ↑ by 125mg every 4wks to 500mg daily in divided doses. Maximum 1g daily	Stop if no response after 3 months on maximum dose	Urinalysis with blood tests every 2 weeks FBC, U&Es, ESR, CRP, and LFT every 2wks until stable, then monthly.

Table 25.2 Biological therapies

Biological	Dose	Action	Licence in rheumatology	NICE approval
Infliximab	RA—3mg/kg by IV infusion over 2h at 0, 2, and 6wks, then every 8wks with methotrexate. Can ↑ in steps of 1.5mg/kg to 7.5mg/kg AS and PA—5mg/kg at 0, 2 and 6wks, then every 6–8wks. In PA use with methotrexate	TNF-α inhibitor	RA—severe active progressive RA. when response to DMARDs including methotrexate has been inadequate (see NICE Critera) AS—where conventional therapy has been inadequate PA—where response to DMARDs has been inadequate	RA—for patients with inadequate response to 2 DMARDs including methotrexate AS—not recommended PA—when response to 2 DMARDs has been inadequate
Etanercept	RA—25mg twice weekly or 50mg weekly SC in combination with methotrexate unless not tolerated or contraindicated AS and PA—25mg twice weekly or 50mg weekly SC	TNF receptor fusion protein	RA—when response to DMARDs including methotrexate has been inadequate. Severe active progressive RA AS—where conventional therapy has been inadequate PA—where response to DMARDs has been inadequate	RA—for patients with inadequate response to 2 DMARDs including methotrexate AS—Severe active AS when 2 NSAIDs have not been effective PA—when response to 2 DMARDs has been inadequate

Drug	Action / Dosing	Indications
Adalimumab	RA—40mg every 2wks SC with methotrexate unless not tolerated or contraindicated AS, PA, PJIA—40mg every 2wks	TNF-α inhibitor	RA—when response to DMARDs including methotrexate has been inadequate. Severe active progressive RA AS—where conventional therapy has been inadequate PA, PJIA—where response to DMARDs has been inadequate	RA—for patients with inadequate response to 2 DMARDs including methotrexate AS—severe active AS when 2 NSAIDs have not been effective PA—when response to 2 DMARDs has been inadequate
Rituximab	RA—1g by IV infusion 30min after 100mg IV methylprednisolone. Followed by a further dose after 2wks. May be repeated after 6 months. In combination with methotrexate	Depletes B lymphocytes	RA (adults) with severe active RA and inadequate response or contraindication to other DMARDs including one or more tumour necrosis inhibitors	RA (adults) with severe active RA and inadequate response or contraindication to other DMARDs including one or more tumour necrosis inhibitors
Certolizumab	RA—400mg SC at 0, 2, and 4wks, then 200mg every 2wks in combination with methotrexate	TNF-α inhibitor	RA—when response to DMARDs including methotrexate was inadequate	RA—for patients with inadequate response to 2 DMARDs including methotrexate. The manufacturers provide the first 12 weeks treatment free of charge

(continued)

Table 25.2 (Contd.)

Biological	Dose	Action	Licence in rheumatology	NICE approval
Tocilizumab	RA—8mg/kg (minimum 480mg) by IV infusion over 1h every 4wks. In combination with methotrexate	Inhibits interleukin-6	RA—in patients who have responded inadequately to or are intolerant of DMARDs or TNF antagonists	RA—for patients with moderate or severe active RA that has responded inadequately to one or more anti-TNFs and whose RA has responded inadequately to rituximab or in whom rituximab is contraindicated or not tolerated
Abatacept	RA—<60kg 500mg, 60–100kg 750mg, >100kg 1000mg IV as a 30min infusion at 0, 2, and 4wks, then every 4wks. In combination with methotrexate PJIA—<75kg 10mg/kg, >75kg as adult dosing	Attenuates T-lymphocyte activation	RA—in patients who have responded inadequately to or are intolerant of DMARDs, including at least one TNF inhibitor PJIA—severe PJIA age ≥6 years with insufficient response to DMARDs including at least one TNF inhibitor	RA—for patients with severe active RA with inadequate response to or intolerance of other DMARDs including at least one anti-TNF and who have a contraindication to or intolerance of rituximab or methotrexate
Anakinra	RA—100mg daily SC	Inhibits interleukin1	RA—in combination with methotrexate in patients with inadequate response to methotrexate alone	Not recommended

RA, rheumatoid arthritis; AS, ankylosing spondylitis; PA, psoriatic arthritis; PJIA, polyarticular juvenile idiopathic arthritis.

Gout

Treatment of an acute attack of gout

- NSAIDs at maximum dose for 1–2 weeks, unless contraindicated. For patients at increased risk of peptic ulceration gastroprotection can be added or a COX-2 inhibitor used (e.g. etoricoxib 120mg daily). Aspirin or salicylates at analgesic doses should not be used because of reduced uric acid excretion, but low-dose aspirin may be continued.
- Colchicine may be used as an alternative or in addition to an NSAID. Give 500micrograms every 4–6h until pain relief is achieved, a total dose of 6mg is reached, or side effects become limiting (commonly sickness and diarrhoea) Note interactions with ciclosporin and erythromycin.
- If NSAIDs are contraindicated or ineffective or if gout is refractory, corticosteroids may be needed. Intra-articular corticosteroid injections may be useful if only one joint is affected. Systemic corticosteroids may be needed for polyarticular disease.
- Allopurinol and uricosurics should not be started during an acute attack or for 2–3 weeks after the attack has resolved. However, they should be continued in patients who are already taking them.
- Simple analgesics may be used in addition if necessary.
- Diuretics should be stopped if prescribed for hypertension. If an alternative antihypertensive is required, losartan should be considered as it has modest uricosuric effects. Diuretics for heart failure should be continued.

Lifestyle changes

- During an acute attack the joint should be rested. Ice packs and splinting may be of benefit.
- If obese, a weight reduction programme should be adopted, but high-protein low-carbohydrate diets should be avoided. Once the acute attack has subsided, moderate exercise should be encouraged.
- Alcohol should be restricted to <21 units per week for males and <14 units per week for females, particularly avoiding beer.
- Foods with a high purine content, such as red meat, offal, game, shellfish, and yeast extracts, should be avoided.

Management of chronic or recurrent gout

- Allopurinol should be started at 50–100mg daily and increased by 100mg every 2–4wks until symptom control is achieved, serum urate <0.3 or 0.36mmol/L, or the maximum dose of 900mg daily in divided doses is reached. Allopurinol lowers urate levels by inhibiting xanthine oxidase. It is metabolized principally to oxipurinol which has a $t_{1/2}$ of 13–30h and can accumulate in renal impairment. Therefore reduced dosing is required. Withdraw immediately if a rash develops. Note interactions with azathioprine, mercaptopurine, and coumarins.
- A uricosuric may be used in patients with normal renal function and no history of renal stones if allopurinol is not tolerated. Sulfinpyrazone 100–200mg daily may be used, increasing over 2–3 weeks to 600mg daily. Probenecid 1–2g daily is available (in the UK) on a named patient basis.

- Febuxostat is a selective inhibitor of xanthine oxidase which may be used in patients who are intolerant of allopurinol or for whom allopurinol is contraindicated. It is started at 80mg daily and may be increased to 120mg daily after 2–4 weeks if serum urate >0.36mmol/L.
- Colchicine 0.5mg twice daily or low-dose NSAIDs should be given at the same time as allopurinol to prevent an acute attack and continued for 1 month after normal serum urate is achieved.
- Fenofibrate should be considered for patients with hyperlipidaemia, as this has a uricosuric effect.

Further reading

British Society for Rheumatology and British Health Professionals in Rheumatology (2007). *Guidelines for the Management of Gout:* ℜ http://www.rheumatology.org.uk

Zhang W et al. (2006). Eular evidence-based recommendations for gout. Part II: Management, report of a taskforce of the Eular Standing Committee for International Clinical Studies Including Therapeutics (ESCISIT). *Annals of the Rheumatic Diseases* **65** :1312–24.

Therapy-related issues: skin

Wound care 560
Eczema 566
Psoriasis 572

Wound care

The skin is the largest organ of the body and has the primary function of protecting underlying tissues and organs. Breaching this barrier exposes the underlying tissues and organs to:

- mechanical damage
- dehydration
- microbial invasion
- temperature variations.

The ideal wound dressing replicates the skin's protective qualities, in addition to promoting wound healing.

Factors affecting the healing process

For a wound to heal the following factors are required.

- Moist environment, but not excessively wet.
- Warmth.
- Oxygen.
- Nutrition.
- (Relatively) free from contamination with microbes or foreign bodies, including slough and necrotic tissue.

A wound dressing should provide all these factors.

Some patients experience delayed wound healing and can develop chronic wounds (e.g. leg ulcers) despite good wound care. This might be caused by patient-related factors which inhibit wound healing, and these must be addressed as far as possible (Table 26.1).

Classification of wounds

Various wound classifications exist. For the purposes of wound care, the following descriptions are the most useful because they correspond to dressing choice. Note that some wounds may show more than one of the following features.

- Epithelializing or granulating—a clean red or pink wound, usually shallow with minimal exudates.
- Sloughy—yellow slough covers part or all of the wound. This might be a dry or wet wound. Note that visible bone or tendon appears yellow.
- Necrotic—dead tissue creates a black, dry, leathery eschar.
- Infected—yellow or greenish in colour, with possible surrounding cellulitis of unbroken skin. The wound might have an offensive smell.
- Exuding—all the features listed so far (except necrotic) might produce exudates to varying degrees. High levels of exudates can lead to maceration of surrounding skin.
- Cavity—the wound might form a deep or shallow cavity. Sinuses are narrow cavities which can extend to some depth, including tracking to bone or between two wounds.
- Malodorous—fungating tumours and infected and necrotic wounds can all have an offensive smell.

These classifications broadly represent the stages of wound healing. Thus, as the wound heals, the type of dressing appropriate to the wound can change. Slough and necrotic tissue are effectively foreign bodies that inhibit wound healing. After these have been removed, the underlying tissue should be granulating. Patients should be warned that as debridement occurs the wound might appear to become bigger before it starts to heal. Occasionally pain associated with the wound can ↑ as the wound heals because damaged nerve endings also heal.

It is important to review wound care on a regular basis. Frequency of reviews (and dressing changes) depends on the severity and nature of the wound. An infected or highly exuding wound might require daily dressing changes, but a granulating wound might only require re-dressing every few days. It is important to avoid renewing a dressing unnecessarily becuase this can expose the wound to cooling, dehydration, or mechanical damage. It is good clinical practice to prepare a wound care chart (Table 26.2). This ensures that all staff are informed about the nature of the wound, which dressings are being used, and the frequency of dressing changes/review. Including photographs of the wound enables progress (or deterioration) to be monitored.

Table 26.1 Patient factors that inhibit wound healing

- Poor perfusion, e.g. peripheral vascular disease
- Older age (usually linked to poor nutrition or other disease)
- Concurrent disease, e.g. diabetes, cancer or anaemia
- Drugs, e.g. steroids, cytotoxics or NSAIDs
- Smoking
- Immobility

Table 26.2 Wound care plan

Patient's name: _____	Date: _____
Photograph/diagram (number each wound and use numbering scheme when describing wounds):	**Description of wound(s)**
Dressings (number, as above):	**Frequency of dressing changes:**
Other information (e.g. analgesia required with dressing changes):	
Review date: _____	
Signature: _____	

Selection of wound dressing

There is no universal wound dressing and different types of dressing suit different wounds. The ideal dressing satisfies all the requirements described in Table 26.3 according to the environment in which it is being used. Dressings are divided into the following two categories.

- Primary dressings—applied directly to the wound surface.
- Secondary dressings—placed over the primary dressings to hold them in place and/or provide additional padding or protection.

It is less important for secondary dressings to satisfy the ideal requirements.

Each time a dressing is changed, it exposes the wound to contamination, dehydration, and cooling. Thus, ideally, the frequency of primary dressing changes should be kept to a minimum. Secondary dressings can be changed more frequently, without disturbing the primary dressing.

Wound care has advanced greatly since the introduction of 'interactive' dressings. These dressings provide active wound management, usually by interacting with the wound surface (e.g. alginates form a gel on contact with exudates) rather than simply acting as a barrier. Selection of the correct dressing is important both to ensure that the wound is healed as efficiently as possible and to ensure cost-effective use because interactive dressings are usually more expensive than non-interactive dressings (Table 26.4).

Table 26.3 Characteristics of the ideal wound dressing

- Maintain moist environment
- Manage excessive exudates
- Allow oxygenation
- Provide a barrier to micro-organisms
- Maintain a warm environment (~37°C)
- Not shed particles or fibres
- ↓ or eliminate odour
- Cost-effective
- Acceptable to the patient

Table 26.4 Matching the dressing to the wound

Dressing type	Examples	Suitable for:	Comment
Alginate	ActivHeal® alginate Sorbsan® Sorbsan® Plus Kaltostat®	Exuding, sloughy Ribbon or rope—cavity or sinus	'Plus' versions have a highly absorbent backing, suitable for highly exuding wounds
Foams	ActivHeal® Foam Lyofoam® Allevyn®	Exuding or highly exuding wounds	Avoid adhesive versions on fragile skin
Films and membranes	Opsite® Tegapore®	Shallow, granulating	
Hydrocolloid	ActivHeal® hydrocolloid Granuflex® Comfeel® Tegasorb®	Sloughy, light to medium exudates	Not suitable for infected wounds or if frequent dressing changes required Avoid on fragile skin
Hydrofibres	Aquacel®	Sloughy, medium to high exudates Ribbon—cavity or sinus	
Hydrogels	ActivHeal® hydrogel Intrasite® Granugel®	Dry, sloughy	Always requires secondary dressing
Low-adherent	Melolin® NA® NA Ultra®	Dry, lightly exuding, granulating	Even 'non-adherent' versions can stick to wound, causing trauma on removal
Odour-absorbing	Clinisorb® Carbopad® VC	Malodorous	Apply over primary dressings
Padding	Gamgee®	Highly exuding	Secondary dressing only
Paraffin gauze	Jelonet®	Granulating	

Use of topical antimicrobials

These agents are not usually recommended because of the risk of development of resistance and high incidence of local sensitivity reactions (which could ultimately lead to systemic allergic reactions). There is little evidence that topical antimicrobials work, and infection should be treated systemically.

The following preparations are recommended for particular situations.
- Povidone iodine preparations, as either impregnated dressings (Inadine®) or solutions (Betadine® aqueous) can be used on wounds infected with bacteria, fungi, or protozoa. These should be stopped as soon as the infection is under control as povidone iodine has been shown to inhibit wound healing.
- Silver, either as silver sulfadiazine cream (Flamazine®) or as silver-impregnated dressings (AquacelAg®), is active against Gram-negative infection (e.g. *Pseudomonas infection* in burns) and MRSA. These preparations are often used inappropriately for any 'infected' wound. Use should be restricted because they are expensive and excessive use of the cream can cause irreversible black skin staining (argyria) because of deposition of silver into the skin.
- Metronidazole gel is used to inhibit anaerobic bacteria which cause the malodour associated with fungating tumours or necrotic wounds. Liberal application of metronidazole suppresses bacterial growth and thus ↓ odour. The surrounding skin should be protected from the gel to avoid maceration. Excessive use could (theoretically) lead to the emergence of metronidazole resistance. Where metronidazole gel is unavailable (e.g. in developing countries), the tablets can be crushed to a fine powder and sprinkled over the wound or mixed with an aqueous gel (e.g. KY® jelly) before application.

Other special wound care agents

Chlorinated desloughing agents

These agents, such as Eusol® and Chlorasol®, are no longer recommended. Although effective for debriding sloughy wounds, they are potential irritants and can delay healing because of cell toxicity and ↓ capillary blood flow. With more modern desloughing dressings available, the disadvantages of these agents outweigh the benefits.

Sugar paste and honey dressings

These can be used on sloughy, infected, and/or malodorous wounds. The antibacterial effect of the sugar or honey ↓ odour. Bacterial growth is inhibited because of the ↑ osmotic pressure in the wound, and honey (especially manuka honey) has some inherent antimicrobial effect. These dressings debride sloughy wounds and can promote angiogenesis. Pharmaceutical quality honey should be used as it is prepared according to set standards and gamma irradiated to reduce the risk of bacterial contamination. Sugar pastes are made from preservative-free icing or caster sugar. Thin pastes can be used in wounds with small openings, using a syringe to dribble the paste into the wound, and thick pastes are used for larger cavity wounds. The disadvantage of these dressings is that they might require frequent changes—twice daily or more.

Vacuum-assisted closure (VAC)

VAC therapy is a form of wound care where negative pressure is applied to a special porous dressing which is placed in the wound cavity or over a flap or graft. VAC helps to remove excess exudates and mechanically draws the edges of the wound inwards, promoting healing. It is suitable for any chronic open wound or acute and traumatic surgical wounds, and is used in plastic surgery to promote healing of grafts and flaps. VAC therapy should not be used on infected wounds (including those involving osteomyelitis) unless these are being treated with systemic anti-microbials. VAC is unsuitable for fistulae, which connect with body cavities or organs, and malignant or necrotic wounds, and should be used with caution on bleeding wounds.

Larval (maggot) therapy

Larvae of the common greenbottle are used in the management of necrotic or sloughy wounds. To feed, the larvae produce proteolytic substances that degrade dead tissue but have no adverse effect on living tissue.

Larvae are supplied either in a gauze bag—various sizes contain different numbers of larvae—or loose. The former presentation is often more acceptable to patients (and nurses) and can be used on cavity wounds, where it might be difficult to locate and retrieve free larvae.

Larvae should usually be used within 48h of receipt, otherwise they will die because of lack of nutrients, and will generally survive for 3–5 days feeding on the wound. During this time, they ↑ in size, and as long as they are still active and increasing in size, they are still effective.

The gauze bag or individual larvae are applied directly to the wound and covered with a non-adherent dressing, which is soaked in saline to ensure that the larvae are kept moist (but not drowning!). A non-occlusive secondary dressing should be used to cover them to prevent them from drying out and to ensure that they have sufficient O_2 to survive. Most interactive dressings are unsuitable (and unnecessary) for use on a wound being treated with larvae because they might kill them by ↑ osmotic pressure or ↓ O_2 supply. During treatment, the amount of exudate can ↑ and appear greenish in colour, but this is normal. It might be necessary to protect surrounding healthy skin from maceration caused by ↑ exudates by applying a barrier film such as Cavilon®.

Further reading

🔗 http://www.worldwidewounds.com: A peer-reviewed online wound care journal, sponsored by industry but with a code of practice to limit bias.

Eczema

Eczema is an inflammatory skin condition. It nearly always causes itching but its appearance can vary, depending on the site, cause, and severity, and whether it is acute or chronic. Signs can include dryness, scaling, erythema, oedema, weeping, crusting, papules, and vesicles. The terms eczema and dermatitis are interchangeable.

- There are a number of different types of eczema (Table 26.5), but the most common is atopic eczema which affects 15–20% of school children and 2–10% of adults.[1]
- Atopic eczema often affects the face and hands in infants, and the face, neck, wrist, and elbow and knee flexures in children.
- Discoid/nummular eczema affects the limbs with round coin-shaped lesions.
- Gravitational eczema affects the lower legs.
- Pompholyx eczema produces itchy vesicles which can form on the fingers, palms, and soles.
- Seborrhoeic eczema often affects the scalp, face, back, presternal area, groin, and armpits.
- Allergic contact dermatitis is usually caused by a delayed hyper-sensitivity reaction to an allergen, although it can be an immediate reaction. Nickel and latex are common causes, but it should be noted that some medicines and excipients can act as allergens (e.g. neomycin, benzocaine, chlorocresol).
- Irritant contact dermatitis is caused by substances that damage the skin—e.g. acids, alkalis, solvents, and detergents. Once the causative irritant or allergen has been identified, steps should be taken to try and avoid it, or if that is not possible to minimize the risk of exposure.
- Photodermatitis is caused by the interaction between light and chemicals absorbed by the skin.

Emollients

- Emollients should be used to rehydrate the dry skin usually associated with eczema.
- Soap should be avoided as it dries the skin—use an emollient soap substitute instead. Emollient bath oils can be added to bath water to enhance rehydration and ensure that the whole skin is treated.
- Aqueous cream is suitable as a soap substitute, but not as an emollient.[2]
- They can be used on wet skin as a soap substitute or after drying.
- They should be applied liberally and as frequently as possible.
- They should be applied in the direction of hair growth by smoothing rather than rubbing in.
- Ointments are better for dry scaly skin, but are also more greasy and difficult to wash off.

1 Primary Care Dermatology Society and British Association of Dermatologists (2009). *Guidelines for the Management of Atopic Eczema*: ℘ http://www.bad.org.uk
2 Tsang M, Guy RH (2010). Effect of aqueous cream on human stratum corneum *in vivo*. *British Journal of Dermatology* **163**: 954–8.

- Creams are better for wet weeping eczema and can help with pruritus because of the cooling effect as the water evaporates.
- Ensure sufficient supplies of emollients—600g/wk for an adult and 250g/wk for a child.
- Numerous generic and proprietary brands are available. It is important to find one that the patient is happy with and confident using.
- Some emollients may contain sensitizers, such as lanolin, or preservatives which can cause allergies and further exacerbate the eczema.
- Use of emollients should be continued even after the eczema has cleared.

Table 26.5 Classification of eczema

Exogenous	Endogenous
Allergic contact dermatitis	Atopic
Irritant contact dermatitis	Discoid/Nummular
Photodermatitis	Gravitational/Stasis/Venous
	Pompholyx
	Seborrhoeic

The fingertip unit

Some patients or their carers may be inclined to undertreat eczema because of fear of medication side effects. Others may overtreat to keep it away. In order to standardize the amount used, the fingertip unit has been devised. It is defined as the amount of cream or ointment that can be applied to the terminal phalanx of an adult index finger and is ~500mg. The fingertip unit should not be used for emollients, which should always be used liberally. Table 26.6 shows the number of fingertip units which should be used to cover various parts of an adult's body. Table 26.7 shows the number of fingertip units which should be used to cover various parts of a child's body at different age ranges.

Corticosteroids

Topical corticosteroids are an effective treatment for eczema and are the first-line treatment for atopic eczema exacerbations.[1] If not used correctly, there is a significant risk that their use will be ineffective or will cause adverse effects. Poor adherence is a major cause of treatment failure in atopic eczema.[2] The risks can be minimized and adherence improved by the following.

- Tailoring potency to the severity of the eczema, using the least potent corticosteroid that effectively controls the disease.
- Explaining how and when to step treatment up or down, including the maximum period of time to treat a flare before potency should be stepped down or healthcare advice should be sought to review the eczema.
- Using weaker corticosteroids on the face, genitals, and flexures.
- Labelling topical corticosteroids with the potency class on the tubes when they are dispensed.[3]
- Treating secondary infections promptly. Oral treatment is often necessary. There is only limited evidence to support corticosteroid/anti-infective combination creams and ointments.
- Applying emollient first and then waiting for at least 30min until the emollient has been absorbed before applying the corticosteroid.
- Applying gently in the direction of hair growth.
- Counselling on using thinly, the fingertip unit, and how much to apply.
- Counselling on how long to apply, how often to apply (no more than twice daily), and where to apply.
- Counselling on adverse effects and what to do if they notice them, but also reassuring the patient or carer that adverse effects are rare when the treatment is used correctly.

1 NICE (2004). Technology Appraisal 81: Frequency of Application of Topical Corticosteroids for Atopic Eczema. ℳ http://www.nice.org.uk
2 Beattie PE, Lewis-Jones MS (2003). Parental knowledge of topical therapies in the treatment of childhood atopic dermatitis. *Clinical and Experimental Dermatology* **28**: 559–53.
3 NICE (2007). *Clinical Guideline 57: Atopic Eczema in Children*: ℳ http://www.nice.org.uk

Table 26.6 The fingertip unit and how to assess the quantity of topical agents needed to cover a given body surface area in adults[*]

Area to be treated	No. of fingertip units	Approximate BSA (%)
Scalp	3	6
Face and neck	2.5	5
One hand (front and back) including fingers	1	2
One entire arm including entire hand	4	8
Elbows (large plaque)	1	2
Both soles	1.5	3
One foot (dorsum and sole), including toes	1.5	3
One entire leg including entire foot	8	16
Buttocks	4	8
Knees (large plaque)	1	2
Trunk (anterior)	8	16
Trunk (posterior)	8	16
Genitalia	0.5	1

[*]Menter A et al. (2009). Guidelines of care for the management of psoriasis and psoriatitic arthritis. Section 3: Guidelines of care for the management and treatment of psoriasis with topical therapies. *Journal of the American Academy of Dermatologists* **60**: 643–59.

Table 26.7 The fingertip unit in children[*]

Age	Face and neck	Arm and hand	Leg and foot	Trunk (front)	Trunk (back) including buttocks
3–6mo	1	1	1.5	1	1.5
1–2 yrs	1.5	1.5	2	2	3
3–5 yrs	1.5	2	3	3	3.5
6–10 yrs	2	2.5	4.5	3.5	5.5

[*]MeReC (1999). Using topical corticosteroids in general practice. *MeReC Bulletin* **10**: 21–4.

Topical calcineurin inhibitors

Topical tacrolimus and pimecrolimus are licensed for treating atopic eczema only. Their use in the UK is restricted to second-line treatment after corticosteroids have failed or the risks of further adverse effects (e.g. irreversible skin atrophy) are unacceptable. They are not recommended for treating mild atopic eczema.[1] Patients or carers should be given the following advice.

- To use thinly, and how much to apply with reference to the fingertip, unit.
- That it is common to get initial skin irritation at the site being treated (e.g. burning, itching, feeling of warmth), but this usually subsides.
- Emollients should not be used within 2h of applying tacrolimus.
- Excessive exposure to UV light should be avoided.
- The medication may cause intolerance to alcohol (flushing and skin irritation).

Other topical treatments

- Wet wraps are wet bandages applied to the areas affected by eczema. A dry bandage layer is put over the top. The eczema may have been pretreated with emollients and/or topical corticosteroids. Wet wraps cool the eczema, enhance the absorption of the corticosteroid, and act as a barrier to scratching.
- Bandages containing ichthammol (to reduce itching), zinc oxide, or coal tar are used to treat lichenification.
- Potassium permanganate 0.1% solution can be used to treat eczema when it is weeping and wet. Care must be taken because it stains skin, clothes, and baths.
- Ketoconazole shampoo and coal tar shampoos are effective treatments for seborrhoeic eczema.

---

1 NICE (2007). *Technology Appraisal 82: Tacrolimus and Pimecrolimus for Atopic Eczema:* ℘ http://www.nice.org.uk

Psoriasis

Psoriasis is a chronic inflammatory skin disease characterized by raised erythematous scaly plaques. The vast majority of cases are managed in primary care or the dermatology out-patient setting. It is relatively common, with a prevalence of 1.5% in the UK population.[1]

It is not known why psoriasis develops but there is a strong genetic component. A number of factors are known to trigger or exacerbate it, including drugs, so it is essential to establish a full and accurate drug history. Drugs recognized to worsen psoriasis or precipitate a relapse include:

- lithium
- chloroquine/hydroxychloroquine
- β-blockers
- ACE inhibitors
- terbinafine
- mepacrine
- bupropion
- ethanol
- NSAIDs

There is no known cure for psoriasis; treatments are aimed at suppressing symptoms and inducing remission. Some treatments may be relatively safe but unpleasant or inconvenient to use. Other treatments, although well tolerated, have risks of severe toxicity to the liver, bone marrow, kidney or unborn fetus, and may even increase the risk of malignancy. Thus it is essential to tailor treatment to each individual patient based on their age, sex, occupation, personality, general health, and resources, and their perception and understanding of the disease.[2] The success of treatment depends on patient concordance, and all patients need to be carefully counselled on their treatment to ensure adherence. A list of the treatment options available is shown in Table 26.8.

Emollients

- Emollients have a beneficial effect in psoriasis.[3]
- They are particularly useful in inflammatory psoriasis and palmoplantar plaque psoriasis.
- Apply liberally and frequently to soften and reduce scaling.

See 📖 pp.566–7, 'Emollients' in 'Eczema', for counselling points.

---

1 Gelfand JM et al. (2005). Prevalence and treatment of psoriasis in the United Kingdom. *Archives of Dermatology* **141**: 1537–41.

2 British Association of Dermatologists & Primary Care Dermatology Society (2009). *Recommendations for the Initial Management of Psoriasis:* 🔊 http://www.bad.org.uk/Portals/_Bad/Guidelines/Clinical%20Guidelines/BAD-PCDS%20Psoriasis%20reviewed%202010.pdf

3 Menter A et al. (2009). Guidelines of care for the management of psoriasis and psoriatitic arthritis. Section 3. Guidelines of care for the management and treatment of psoriasis with topical therapies. *Journal of the American Academy of Dermatology* **60**: 643–59.

Coal tar

- This has been an effective treatment for psoriasis for many years.
- Smelly, messy, and stains skin and clothing.
- Difficult to apply, resulting in reduced concordance.
- Tar-based shampoos are the first-line treatment for scalp psoriasis.

Salicylic acid

- A topical keratolytic agent.
- Used for hyperkeratotic psoriasis of the palms, soles, and scalp where penetration of other topical agents will be prevented by significant scaling leading to treatment failure.

Dithranol

- A very effective treatment for chronic plaque psoriasis.
- Like coal tar, its use has declined in recent years because of the widespread availability of more cosmetically acceptable treatments.
- Burns normal skin and is oxidized to a dye which stains skin and anything else it comes into contact with (e.g. hair, clothes, bed linen, and bathroom fittings).

Table 26.8 Treatment options for psoriasis

Topical therapies	Systemic therapies
Emollients	Psoralen + ultraviolet A radiation
Coal tar	Acitretin
Salicylic acid	Methotrexate
Dithranol	Ciclosporin
Corticosteroids	Biological agents
Vitamin D analogues	
Tazarotene	
Ultraviolet B radiation	

Topical corticosteroids
- Effective treatment for some forms of psoriasis.
- Non-irritant compared with coal tar and dithranol.
- Clean and easy to use.
- Limited by adverse effects which include causing rebound exacerbation of psoriasis on discontinuation and precipitating unstable forms of psoriasis.
- Long-term use can also cause tachyphylaxis.
- Rarely used for widespread chronic plaque psoriasis, but reserved for delicate areas, such as the face, genitals, and flexures, or more resistant areas such as the scalp, palms, and soles.
- Use on the face, genitals, and flexures should be limited to mild potency topical corticosteroids—e.g. hydrocortisone 1%.
- Potent topical corticosteroids can be used initially on the scalp, palms, and soles, with the strength adjusted according to clinical improvement.

The British Association of Dermatologists has made the following recommendations concerning the use of topical corticosteroids in psoriasis.[1]
- No more than 100g moderate or higher potency preparations should be applied per month.
- Attempts should be made to rotate topical corticosteroids with alternative non-corticosteroid preparations.
- Use of potent or very potent preparations should be under dermatological supervision.
- Patients should be counselled on the use of the fingertip unit to ensure that they know how much ointment or cream to apply.
- No topical corticosteroid should be used regularly for more than 4wks without critical review.
- Potent corticosteroids should not be used regularly for more than 7 days.

Vitamin D and its analogues
- Calcipotriol, a vitamin D analogue, is first-line treatment for plaque psoriasis.
- Easy to apply.
- Does not smell or stain.
- Lacks many of the adverse effects of topical corticosteroids.
- Calcipotriol can irritate the skin, particularly in sensitive areas such as the scalp, face, and flexures, but this rarely leads to withdrawal of treatment.
- Calcitriol and the topical vitamin D analogue tacalcitol are both less irritant than calcipotriol.
- Avoid vitamin D and its analogues in patients with calcium metabolism disorders.
- Do not exceed maximum doses cited in the *BNF* or hypercalcaemia can develop.

---

1 British Association of Dermatologists (2008). *Topical corticosteroids*: ℜ http://www.bad.org.uk/site/1117/Default.aspx

Tazarotene

- A topical retinoid.
- Effective treatment for mild to moderate plaque psoriasis involving up to 10% BSA.
- Local irritation is common, necessitating careful application, avoidance of normal skin, and titration of gel strength.
- Often used in alternation with a topical corticosteroid.
- Patients need counselling on washing hands after use, avoiding contact with sensitive areas, avoiding excessive exposure to UV radiation, and not applying cosmetics or emollients within 1h of application.

Ultraviolet B (UVB) radiation

- An effective treatment of guttate psoriasis or plaque psoriasis that is unresponsive to topical treatment.
- Broadband UVB is less effective than narrowband (311 ± 2nm) therapy.
- Treatment is usually three times weekly, and 10–30 doses are required to achieve clearance.
- Dosage can be based on the minimal erythema dose or skin type.
- Used alone or combined with other treatments (e.g. tar, dithranol, calcipotriol, and oral retinoids) to enhance their effect.
- Increased risk of cutaneous malignancies.

Ultraviolet A radiation and psoralen

- Topical or systemic administration of a psoralen followed by exposure to ultraviolet A radiation (PUVA) is an effective treatment for most forms of psoriasis and is used in some centres.
- There is no licensed psoralen available in the UK.
- Increased risk of cutaneous malignancies.
- It can be combined with acitretin or calcipotriol.

Patients receiving UVB or PUVA treatment should not be prescribed photosensitizing agents such as:
- amiodarone
- nalidixic acid
- ofloxacin
- chlorpromazine
- tacrolimus
- tetracyclines
- voriconazole.

Acitretin

- An oral retinoid.
- Least effective of the systemic therapies when used alone, but it also lacks many of their toxicities.
- Often used in combination with topical therapies or PUVA.
- Commonly causes drying of the skin and lips, which can be countered with regular use of emollient and lip salve.
- Less frequently, it also dries the mucous membranes and conjunctiva.
- Stringent controls are in place when acitretin is used in female patients of child-bearing age because of its teratogenicity which can continue for up to 2 years after cessation of treatment.

Methotrexate

- An effective treatment for severe psoriasis which cannot be controlled with topical therapies alone.
- Most patients are managed adequately with 7.5–15mg methotrexate weekly.
- Can cause haematological, renal and liver, toxicity, which necessitates careful counselling of the patient on adverse effects and frequent monitoring of blood tests.
- Contraindicated in pregnancy.
- Men should be advised to avoid fathering children during therapy and for 3 months afterwards.
- Pharmacists screening prescriptions for methotrexate should ensure that they comply with local or national guidelines.

Ciclosporin

- Licensed in the UK for severe psoriasis when conventional therapy is ineffective or inappropriate.
- Efficacy has been fully demonstrated.
- Dose used is 2.5–5mg/kg/day.
- Blood pressure and renal function should be monitored during treatment.

Cytokine modulators

- Adalimumab, etanercept, infliximab, and ustekinumab are all licensed and approved in the UK by NICE for the treatment of severe plaque psoriasis which has failed to respond to standard systemic treatments.
- Pharmacists have an important role to play in all patients on systemic immunosuppressants by:
  - counselling
  - monitoring
  - identifying important drug interactions
  - preventing prescribing errors.

Therapy-related issues: palliative care

Anorexia and cachexia 578
Constipation 578
Fatigue 579
Hypercalcaemia of malignancy 580
Mouth care 581
Noisy breathing 581
Insomnia 582
Spinal cord compression 582
Malignant bowel obstruction 583
Syringe drivers and compatibility of medicines 584
End-of-life pathways 585
Anaemia 586

Anorexia and cachexia

The dictionary definition of anorexia is a lack of appetite (for food). Cachexia is involuntary weight loss which can progress to an emaciated state. The majority of palliative care patients experience cachexia at some stage, and this difficult condition requires determination of the cause, if possible, and development of careful management. A number of Cochrane reviews have been published which summarize a fairly large volume of literature. The following interventions may be considered.

• Megestrol—evidence for effectiveness in stimulating appetite at doses ranging from 160 to 1600mg daily.
• Medroxyprogesterone acetate—evidence of greater weight gain and appetite than placebo at doses of 300—800mg daily.
• Corticosteroids—some evidence for improvement in appetite but not weight gain.
• Eicosapentanoic acid—somewhat heterogeneous literature with an unclear picture for benefit. Possibly worth trying if other treatments fail.

Constipation

Constipation is a common symptom in palliative care patients. It is related to opioid analgesic use, reduced food intake, and reduced activity. A patient diary can be helpful in determining the severity of the condition.

There is a lack of good-quality evidence for the effectiveness of laxatives, so a pragmatic approach is required. In general, it is necessary to combine an increase in fibre with a stool softener and probably a stimulant in order to maintain good bowel function. Choices can be based on local formularies. Rectal laxatives may be necessary for hard impacted faeces. This is not a pleasant option for either patient or care staff, but may be the only option for some cases.

A more recent and more expensive option is the use of peripheral opioid receptor antagonists. At the time of writing, only methylnaltrexone was licensed for use in the UK, administered by injection. The license is for opioid constipation in palliative care patients where other laxatives have failed. Methylnaltrexone is added to other laxative treatment. Doses should be reduced in renal failure.

Other drugs such as Alvimopan are under development and may prove useful. A Cochrane review of these agents suggested that there is currently insufficient evidence for the use of naloxone or nalbuphine.

Fatigue

- Fatigue is among the most common symptoms in palliative care patients. It is not easily defined, but is commonly described by words such as lethargy, muscle weakness, tiredness, and mood disturbance.
- A number of assessment tools exist and these are useful to monitor both decline and improvement.
- A number of Cochrane reviews and other systematic reviews show benefit from a range of interventions. These include cognitive behavioural therapy (CBT), erythropoietin and similar agents, and exercise.
- A systematic review has shown that Chinese herbal medicine is not effective.
- Patients who are able to undertake therapeutic exercise regimes may find these to be helpful.

Hypercalcaemia of malignancy

- This is a common complication, especially in breast and lung cancer and in myeloma, and often occurs with bone metastases.
- Mild hypercalcaemia—corrected serum calcium 2.7–3.0mmol/L.
- Moderate to severe hypercalcaemia—corrected calcium ≥3.0mmol/L.

Signs and symptoms

- Nausea
- Vomiting
- Thirst
- Polyuria
- Constipation
- Headache
- Impaired consciousness.

The patient may be severely dehydrated and in renal failure.

Management[1]

- Mild, asymptomatic—rehydrate and observation. Recheck calcium after 24h.
- Symptomatic—ensure hydration. Treat with bisphosphonates.
- Moderate to severe—urgent rehydration up to 3–6L in 24h and bisphosphonates.
- Stop any drugs that increase calcium levels—e.g. thiazide diuretics, lithium, calcium, and vitamin D supplements.

Bisphosphonates inhibit osteoclastic bone resorption. A significant decrease in serum calcium is generally observed 24–48h after IV administration and normalization is usually achieved within 3–7 days. If the patient is not normocalcaemic within this time a further dose can be given. Pamidronate should be infused at a concentration ≤60mg/250mL and a rate ≤60mg/h. Renal failure is a relative contraindication to the use of bisphosphonates and the dose should be administered at ≤20mg/h. The patient may be maintained on 4-weekly infusions or, for example, sodium clodronate orally 1.6–3.2g daily in divided doses.

Resissitant hypercalcaemia not responding to pamidronate or recurring frequently can be treated with zolendronic acid 4mg IV depending on renal function. With repeated use of bisphosphonates, be aware of the rare possibility of osteonecrosis of the jaw.

In severe hypercalcamia or with severe symptoms, calcitonin rapidly lowers serum calcium within hours, but the effect only lasts for hours and wears off altogether after a few days. Calcitonin 4–8IU/kg SC or IM every 6–12h for 2 days can be given along with bisphosphonate.

---

1 Twycross R (2007). *Palliative Care Formulary* (3rd edn): ☞ http://palliativedrugs.com

Mouth care

Patients find mouth problems very distressing, and careful attention should be paid to dental hygiene and risk factors for dry mouth.

Dry mouth

- Check for candidiasis.
- Ice-chips, fresh pineapple, sugar-free gum. Rinse with 0.9% saline.
- Artificial saliva and topical saliva stimulants, preferably with neutral pH.
- Review medicines as some (e.g. hyoscine and tricyclic antidepressants) exacerbate dry mouth.

Sore mouth

- Candidiasis—fluconazole 50mg orally once daily or nystatin 100 000IU four times daily for 7 days.
- Soak dentures overnight and ensure that they are thoroughly cleaned.
- A coated tongue can be cleaned by allowing a quarter of a 1g effervescent ascorbic acid tablet to dissolve on the tongue up to four times daily for a week.
- Mucositis—chlorhexidine or benzydamine mouthwashes.
- Stomatitis—choline salicylate gel or hydrocortisone 2.5mg pellets.
- Systemic analgesia may be needed if severe.

Noisy breathing

Noisy breathing (sometimes called death rattle) occurs in significant numbers of people who are dying. The cause of noisy breathing remains unproven, but it is presumed to be due to an accumulation of secretions in the airways. It is managed either physically (repositioning and clearing the upper airways of fluid with a mechanical sucker) or pharmacologically. There are a number of treatment options (mainly anticholinergic drugs with some trials of atropine, hyoscine butylbromide, hyoscine hydrobromide, and glycopyrronium) but studies have found no difference in efficacy between these. A Cochrane review was unable to demonstrate any real effectiveness, and these treatments remain time-honoured rather than evidence-based.

Insomnia

Insomnia is a common problem in palliative care. Daytime sleepiness can lead to nighttime wakefulness therefore so called 'sleep hygiene' is an important consideration. A sleep log may be useful to assess how much sleep is actually achieved. There are many contributing factors to insomnia including anxiety, pain, medications, or limb movements. Pharmacists can help by reviewing those medicines that can induce sleep during the daytime e.g tricyclic antidepressants for neuropathic pain and shifting the dose to later in the day. Ensure adequate pain relief is provided at night. Discourage the use of stimulants including caffeine in the evening. Consider sleep medication only after other issues have been considered and dealt with. There is no evidence that palliative care patients benefit from any different hypnotics that other patients so a general approach to use what is familiar is suggested.

Spinal cord compression

This is a complication of advanced cancer with tumour mass or bone compressing the dural sac and contents. This is a poor prognostic sign, with average survival of 4–6 months. 90% of patients present with back pain and 50% also have some neurological deficit—usually leg weakness with possible bowel or bladder involvement. Investigate with MRI of the whole spine or CT. Speed is of the essence to preserve mobility if the patient is ambulant at diagnosis.

Management

- Dexamethasone 16mg stat, then 8mg twice daily to reduce pain and spinal oedema. First 48h are crucial for the majority of clinical benefit. Taper steroids as appropriate thereafter.
- Radiotherapy within 24h if possible.
- Surgery if single site and patient has good performance status.

Malignant bowel obstruction

This is a complex problem which occurs mainly in patients with advanced gynaecological and gastrointestinal cancers. The condition can range from a partial to a complete obstruction. Symptoms can include nausea and vomiting as well as abdominal distension and pain. In complete obstruction no faeces or flatus are passed. Surgery is usually the first option, but many patients may not be fit for such an intervention and other interventions such as stents may be tried.

Drug therapy includes antiemetics, usually parenteral metoclopramide, anticholinergics such as hyoscine, or other drugs to reduce the persistent nausea that can accompany this condition.

Other interventions include the use of octreotide which may prevent damage to the intestine such as oedema or necrosis and may improve intestinal transit. The beneficial effects seem to be seen in the early stages of obstruction.

Syringe drivers and compatibility of medicines

The syringe driver is a simple and cost-effective method of delivering a continuous subcutaneous infusion (CSCI), which can be used to maintain symptom control in patients who are no longer able to take oral medication because of persistent nausea and vomiting, dysphagia, or bowel obstruction, or are in end-of-life care. Commonly used medicines in syringe drivers are opioid analgesics, antiemetics, antisecretories, and anxiolytics. In addition to the CSCI, each of the medicines should be prescribed prn for breakthrough symptoms and used to calculate the doses for the next driver. The prescription should be reviewed every 24h. Literature sources for compatible combinations of medicines are limited and the following is a guide for combinations known to be compatible when made up to 21mL with water for injection over 24h.

Two medicine combinations

Up to **50mg morphine sulphate** may be combined with **one** of the following medicines.
- Cyclizine up to a maximum dose of 150mg.
- Haloperidol up to a maximum dose of 10mg.
- Metoclopramide up to a maximum dose of 75mg.
- Midazolam up to a maximum dose of 30mg.
- Hyoscine butylbromide up to a maximum dose of 120mg.

Three medicine combinations

Up to **30mg of morphine sulphate** may be combined with the following medicines.
- Cyclizine (up to150mg) and haloperidol (up to 2.5mg).
- Cyclizine (up to 150mg) and midazolam (up to 20mg).
- Midazolam (up to 30mg)and metoclopramide (up to 40mg).
- Midazolam (up to 30mg) and haloperidol (up to 5mg).
- Midazolam (up to 30mg) and hyoscine butylbromide (up to 80mg).
- Haloperidol (up to 5mg) and hyoscine butylbromide (up to 80mg).

Any other combinations or diluents should be confirmed against the references in the 'Further reading' listing in this section or referred for specialist advice.

Further reading

Dickman A et al. (2005). *The Syringe Driver* (2nd edn). Oxford: Oxford University Press.
Trissel LA (2009). *Handbook on Injectable Drugs* (15th edn). Bethesda, MD: American Society of Health System Pharmacists.

End-of-life pathways

- Pharmacists need to be aware of the existence of these pathways which have been pioneered by clinicians in Liverpool.
- The Liverpool Care Pathway is an integrated care pathway that is used at the bedside to improve quality of the dying in the last hours and days of life in any setting.
- It is a means of transferring the lessons learnt in the care of the dying from hospices to other clinical areas.
- It is recommended as a best practice model by the UK Department of Health.

Anaemia

Anaemia is a decrease in red blood cells (RBC), haematocrit, or haemo-globin (Hb) because of:
- blood loss—e.g. GI bleed.
- deficient RBC production (erythropoesis)—e.g. iron deficiency, vitamin B_{12} deficiency.
- excessive RBC destruction (haemolysis)—e.g. G6PD deficiency (see 📖 p.200, 'G6PD deficiency', Chapter 10.

Anaemia is not a diagnosis in its own right but a manifestation of an under-lying disorder (e.g. NSAID-induced GI bleed), and so should be investi-gated to determine the cause. A low Hb is defined as <13.5g/dL in ♂ and <11.5g/dL in ♀ but symptoms are uncommon until Hb <7g/dL, although they may occur at higher Hb if there is an acute ↓ or limited cardiopulmo-nary reserve.

Signs and symptoms
- Fatigue
- Dyspnoea
- Faintness
- Headache
- Pallor (including conjunctival pallor)

Haematological investigations
- Mean cell volume (MCV) – a measure of RBC size.
- Mean corpuscular haemoglobin (MCH)—a measure of the amount of Hb in RBCs
- Mean corpuscular haemoglobin concentration (MCHC)—a measure of the concentration of Hb in RBCs
- Haematocrit—a measure of the percentage of blood that is RBCs.

These investigations can help to indicate the mechanism of anaemia and thus help determine the cause (Table 27.1).
- Microcytic anaemia (i.e. MCV is low) indicates altered haem or globin synthesis.
- Macrocytic anaemia (i.e. MCV is high) indicates impaired DNA synthesis.
- Normocytic anaemia results from insufficient or inadequate response to erythropoietin.
- Hypochromic anaemia (i.e. MCH and MCHC are low).

Table 27.1 Some causes of anaemia based on the MCV

Microcytic/ hypochromic	↓MCV, ↓ MCHC (e.g. Fe deficiency) Thalassaemia Anaemia of chronic disease
Macrocytic	↑ MCV Reticulocytis (polychromasia on blood film) B_{12} or folate deficiency Chronic liver disease Hypothyroidism Alcohol Myelodysplasia
Normocytic/ normochromic	↔ MCV, MCHC Anaemia of chronic disease (e.g. chronic infection, inflammation) Inflammatory disease or malignancy Acute blood loss Renal failure Myeloma

Iron-deficiency anaemia

Iron is present in the body at ~ 50mg/kg of which ~60% is in RBCs, 30% in body stores (as ferritin and haemosiderin), 5% in muscle cell myoglobin and 5% in various enzymes or bound to transferring. Dietary intake is needed to replace normal losses:

- 0.5–1mg/day in faeces, urine, sweat
- 0.5–0.7mg/day (averaged over the month) in menstruating women.

Pregnant women need an additional 1–2mg/day.

Dietary intake comes from haem iron (in meat and fish) and non-haem iron (in grains, fruit, and vegetables). Haem iron is better absorbed than non-haem iron but the absorption of the latter may be ↑ by ascorbic acid or citric acid. Iron is mostly absorbed in the duodenum and jejunum, and the excess is excreted in the faeces.

A low Hb does not necessarily mean low iron and a full blood count as well as iron studies should be conducted to determine whether it is iron-deficiency anaemia and so iron supplements are required (Table 27.2).

Treatment

Treatment includes finding and treating the underlying cause (e.g. GI bleed, menorrhagia) as well as correcting the deficiency. Hb should be ↑ by 1–2g/L every day and continued for 3 months after normalization of Hb to replenish iron stores. Different iron salts contain different amounts of elemental iron (Table 27.3), but the aim is to give 100–200mg elemental iron per day (e.g. as ferrous sulphate 200mg three times daily). Other salts are sometimes better tolerated but may be more expensive. Modified release or enteric-coated preparations supposedly improve tolerability, but may not be released until after the duodenum where absorption is poor.

Parenteral iron (as iron dextran or iron sucrose complex) has no advantage over oral iron as it replenishes Hb, at the same rate although

iron stores are replenished more quickly, and it has been associated with hypersensitivity reactions. It is used in specific situations:
- haemodialysis patients
- intolerance to oral iron
- poor compliance
- continuing blood loss
- documented malabsorption (e.g. IBD).

Prophylaxis with oral or parenteral (if fits listed criteria) iron may be given if there are risk factors for iron deficiency—e.g. pregnancy, malabsorption conditions (e.g. gastrectomy), haemodialysis.

Blood transfusion is not usually necessary in most patients unless Hb <7g/dl. It is potentially hazardous with a risk of transfusion reactions (hypersensitivity type symptoms), fluid overload potentially leading to heart failure, and haemolytic reactions due to blood group or Rhesus factor incompatibility. Fevers and mild allergic reactions are also fairly common, although rarely serious. Therefore transfusion should only be carried out in the following situations:
- acute situation (e.g. haemorrhage)
- comorbidity (e.g. IHD, heart failure, COPD)
- patient symptomatic.

Vitamin B$_{12}$ deficiency/pernicious anaemia

Vitamin B$_{12}$ is found in meat and dairy products but not in plants. Signs and symptoms include:
- general symptoms of anaemia
- glossitis
- angular cheilosis
- peripheral neuropathy.

Causes include dietary (e.g. vegans), malabsorption (e.g. gastrectomy, Crohn's disease), lack of intrinsic factor (necessary for absorption). ↑Hb, ↑MCV, and ↓B$_{12}$. Treatment is with parenteral vitamin B$_{12}$ (hydroxo-cobalamin)—initially alternate day injections for 2wks to replenish stores and then every 3 months. Pharmacists need to be aware of the need for continuing maintenance injections in long-stay patients. Oral maintenance with cyanocobalamin is an option only if the deficiency is due to diet alone.

Folate deficiency

Folate is found in most foods, especially green vegetables, but it can be destroyed by cooking. Causes of folate deficiency include:
- dietary deficiency
- malabsorption
- increased requirements (e.g. pregnancy)
- increased losses (e.g. malignancy)
- other causes (e.g. prematurity, folate antagonist drugs)

Folate deficiency is relatively common in patients with grossly deficient diets as stores are only sufficient for 3–4 months. Clinical presentation is similar to vitamin B$_{12}$ deficiency but:
- there is a more rapid onset of symptoms
- neuropsychiatric disorders are rare.

Table 27.2 Interpreting plasma iron studies

	Iron	TIBC	Ferritin
Iron deficiency	↓	↑	↓
Anaemia of chronic disease	↓	↓	↑
Chronic haemolysis	↑	↓	↑
Haemochromatosis	↑	↓ (or ↔)	↑
Pregnancy	↑	↑	↔
Sideroblastic anaemia	↑	↔	↑

TIBC, total iron-binding capacity.

Table 27.3 Ferrous iron content of different iron tablets

Iron salt	Tablet strength	Ferrous iron content
Ferrous fumarate	200mg	65mg
Ferrous gluconate	300mg	35mg
Ferrous sulphate	300mg	60mg
Ferrous sulphate, dried	200mg	65mg

Treatment

Treatment is with folic acid 5mg daily and patients should be encouraged to increase dietary intake. Coexisting vitamin B_{12} deficiency should be corrected.

Folate deficiency in pregnancy can lead to neural tube defects. Women who are pregnant or planning a pregnancy should be advised to take folate supplements:

• 400micrograms daily before conception and for the first 12 weeks gestation.
• 5mg daily in women with diabetes or sickle cell disease, or on anti-convulsants.

Therapy-related issues: miscellaneous

Introduction to critical care 592
Delirium/acute confusional state 596
Stress ulcer prophylaxis 598
Motility stimulants 600
Mechanical ventilation 602
Vasoactive agents 604
Renal replacement therapy 606
Treatment of alcohol withdrawal 610
Dealing with poisoning enquiries 614
Drug desensitization 618
Drug interference with laboratory tests 620
Therapeutic drug monitoring (TDM) in adults 622

Introduction to critical care

For the purposes of critical care in the UK, patients are grouped into one of four levels of care, an allocation that changes according to severity of illness and degree of actual or potential organ support required by the patient.

- Level 0 patients have needs that can be met by normal ward care.
- Level 1 patients have needs that can be met on an acute ward with additional advice and support from the critical care team. They are at risk of their condition deteriorating, or have recently been relocated from higher levels of care.
- Level 2 patients require more detailed observation or intervention, including support for a single failing organ system or postoperative care, and include patients stepping down from higher levels of care (formerly known as high dependency unit (HDU) patients).
- Level 3 patients require advanced respiratory support alone or basic respiratory support together with support of at least two organ systems. This level includes all complex patients requiring support for multi-organ failure (formerly known as intensive care unit (ICU) patients).

This classification has meant that critical care has come to define a type of therapy, rather than a specific place where such therapy is administered. Critical care teams work in ICUs, HDUs, specialist surgical units, recovery areas, and perioperative care, and on general wards with outreach teams. Therefore critical care encompasses a diverse area for pharmacists to work within, and pharmacists working on general wards are increasingly coming into contact with critically ill patients. For the pharmacist who commits to a career in critical care, a competency framework describing various levels of specialist pharmacist practice has been drawn up and is published on the Department of Health's website.[1]

Tips, hints, and things you should bear in mind

Critical care can at first be a daunting area within which to work. Patients are on the extremes of the physiological spectra, often accompanied by a frightening array of equipment that bristles with buttons and gaudy displays, issuing all manner of warning squeaks, pips, and beeps. The patient is cared for by experienced efficient nurses and calm intelligent doctors, and can be surrounded by teams of personnel attending to various functions of care. An enormous variety and quantity of data are generated, with the patient's notes quickly expanding in size. All this activity is being watched by tense, tired, and often tearful relatives or carers, who are constantly looking for the slightest sign that their loved one's condition is getting either better or worse.

---

1 ℞ http://www.dh.gov.uk/en/Publicationsandstatistics/Publications/PublicationsPolicyAndGuidance/DH_084011

Put the patient first

In all your endeavours and work, you must put the patient first. If there are limited resources and you have several patient care responsibilities, then you must do the best you can for the patients who need you the most.

Not all patients are model citizens. They may have led very colourful lives, and this can complicate their medical management and their dealings with relatives, or affect your own personal feelings for them. You must put these aspects aside in order to do your best for them.

You will have to come to terms with the fact that a significant proportion of patients will die despite your best efforts. This of course reflects the severity of their illness, not your performance, and you will need to remind yourself of this from time to time.

Remember the relatives, carers, and friends

The patient is not always alone. Loved ones visit and stay by the bedside without restrictions on visiting hours. As a member of the team, you will be asked about various aspects of the patient's care. As a junior pharmacist, you should refer requests for information about progress or planning to a member of the medical team. This ensures that visitors receive consistent information. You may still need to talk to relatives to obtain information about medications, or possibly because you are asked to discuss a specific aspect of care with them by the medical team. When you do so, employ great sensitivity. Loved ones have a lot of time to think and dwell on the consequences of the illness that brings the patient to critical care, and as such can be extremely fragile. Remember that certain aspects of the patient may not be known to them and should not be divulged, sometimes at the specific request of the patient. This can give rise to some extraordinary circumstances, yet you must still employ strict patient confidentiality. Because of the situation they find themselves in, visitors may not take in everything you are saying. They may also make their own interpretation of any information you are giving them or asking of them. Be as clear and concise as you can. Note the key points of conversation in the patient's notes and, if possible, ensure that the patient's nurse is party to the conversation. As well as acting as a witness, they can dig you out of a hole.

Do not worry

You may not know the nuances and subtleties of various standard critical care interventions such as the use of vasopressors or sedation and analgesia. In fact you are unlikely to, unless you have committed to a career in critical care pharmacy. Fortunately, intensivists tend to know a fair bit about these agents and so you should be assured that, at more junior levels of practice, such in-depth knowledge is not necessary in order to contribute meaningfully to the team.

Nor will you be expected to know the function of every piece of kit available at the bedside, and no one will expect you to be able to interpret pressure waveforms or scan results. Your role is not the same as everyone else's. In time, you may understand the intricacies of the available monitoring and supporting equipment, but for now, concentrate on the area that you know best—basic clinical pharmacy.

Develop a methodical approach

Every critical care patient requires a high degree of pharmaceutical care/ medicines management. You must know the patient's medical history, drug history, allergy history, admitting complaint, progress, pharmacokinetic reserve, and prescription as a minimum dataset from which to work. Making professional notes is important in order to record all pertinent information and to aid in planning the patient care (including follow-up).

Do not become overloaded with the huge amount of information available. Always summarize trends and interpret where possible. It is usual to think in terms of individual body systems in order to avoid missing anything out, but of course these are interrelated and so you must always step back and consider the patient as a whole. Remember that medicines are only one of the tools that can be utilized in the care of a patient. Try to think beyond just drugs (e.g. there are mechanical methods for venous thrombus prophylaxis, as well as anticoagulants).

Draw on what you know . . .

Your broad generalist knowledge of medicine is a bonus. Critical care teams are highly specialist, and despite the broad case mix, many of the patients present to intensive care for the same sorts of reasons and require the same sorts of treatments. The fact that you know a bit about other medications found outside critical care is very useful to the team.

Despite the fact that the majority of critically ill patients have disturbances of organ function that necessitate adjustments of dose, route, or choice of agent, this area is often not consistently tackled by medical staff and is one area where you can make a major contribution. Examples include dose adjustment in renal dysfunction or changes in route of administration because of surgery.

Looking out for, or avoiding, adverse drug reactions/interactions is very important. This can sometimes be more about refuting that such a reaction has taken place rather than the more usual situation of avoiding problems that may arise.

. . . and say when you don't know

Knowing your limitations is something to be respected. Do not bluff your way through an issue—it is obvious when you do and nobody likes it. It can result in inappropriate interventions in the short term and appropriate advice or interventions being ignored or treated as suspect in the future.

Recognize others' expertise

Everyone has expertise: medics, surgeons, nurses, physiotherapists, dieticians, relatives, and loved ones—everyone. There will be overlaps as well as gaps in knowledge and differences in opinion. Learn to live with it and collaborate. Do not create conflict. This will not help the patient.

Be aware and utilize other resources

Liaise with pharmacists from the service that the patient came from. Critical care is a support service, treating the sickest patients from many other services. Obtaining valuable advice from pharmacists who routinely work in those services will greatly aid in the provision of appropriate care for the patient.

Critical care units do not work in isolation from each other. Each unit is part of a larger network or group of units that covers a distinct geographical location. This means that, within each network or group, there will be other critical care pharmacists whom you can talk to or draw support from. Find out who they are and introduce yourself to them (face to face, by telephone, or by email), before you need their advice in a crisis. Each network or group will have standards of practice and therapeutic protocols (often called care bundles). Obtain copies and be familiar with them.

Delirium/acute confusional state

Large numbers of patients become delirious in critical care. Some studies put the incidence as high as 80%, although it is probably nearer to 50% in a general ICU population in the UK. Delirium is important—it is associated with excess mortality, increased length of stay, new admissions to care home after leaving hospital, and increased likelihood of a long-term cognitive dysfunction (i.e. dementia).

Historically, delirium has been poorly recognized and treated. In particular, agitated delirium has been treated with sedation, which masks the condition without treating it, whilst non-agitated delirium goes unrecognized.

Detection

Detection should be through the routine use of a screening tool such as the Confusion Assessment Method modified for critically ill patients (CAM-ICU). Other tools also exist, such as the Intensive Care Delirium Screening Checklist (ISDSC) which some find easier to use. Routine screening increases recognition.

Prevention

Preventative measures are simple interventions such as avoiding dehydration, ensuring good sleep patterns and good nutrition, and normalizing the environment as much as possible. Humane attention to detail such as use of glasses and hearing aids make a difference, as well as interacting with the patient as much as possible.

Many medications may cause delirium. Good pharmaceutical care (reducing doses in renal failure and hepatic failure) and avoidance of precipitants such as drugs with anticholinergic activity, daily sedation breaks, and good sedative management all help.

Treatment

Pharmacological treatment options are based on a small evidence base. Antipsychotics are used at the lowest effective dose and withdrawn as the delirium clears. Specialist advice should be sought if delirium fails to clear after a week of therapy to rule out a more permanent decline in cognitive function (dementia). The aim of therapy is not to sedate the patient, but to clear the cognitive deficit. A sedative may be required in addition to keep a severely disturbed patient safe.

Haloperidol

Haloperidol is flexible; it has a wide dosing range and can be administered via a variety of routes (PO, NG, IV, IM). Typical doses are 1–5mg, depending on the degree of illness and age of the patient, given regularly every 6–8h.

Olanzapine

Olanzapine can be administered NG and IM. Typical doses are 2.5–10mg/day. It may be more effective in certain types of delirium and has fewer side effects than haloperidol.

Stress ulcer prophylaxis

Over three-quarters of ICU patients have endoscopic evidence of mucosal damage within 1–2 days of admission to intensive care, although in most cases the damage is superficial and will heal quickly. Clinical evidence for gastric bleeding occurs in up to a quarter of patients ('coffee grounds', malaena), and up to 6% of patients suffer clinically important bleeding that results in haemodynamic instability or a requirement for blood transfusions. The incidence of stress ulceration appears to be falling, probably because of general advances in the management of critically ill patients as well as specific prophylactic measures for stress ulceration.

Pathophysiology

It is thought that mucosal damage is brought about by a number of factors, such as disturbances in mucosal blood flow due to cardiovascular instability and hypoperfusion leading to a relative mucosal ischaemia, the presence of reduced gastric luminal pH, and altered mucosal protective mechanisms. At pH <4, the proteolytic enzyme pepsin destroys clots forming on damaged gastric mucosa, increasing the likelihood of bleeding and the extent of gastric damage.

Risk factors

A large number of risk factors have been identified for stress ulceration:
- >48 hours mechanical ventilation
- coagulopathy
- acute renal failure
- acute liver failure
- sepsis
- hypotension
- severe head injury
- history of GI bleeding
- burns covering >35% of body surface
- major surgery.

The two most important are mechanical ventilation for >48h and coagulopathy.

Aim of therapy

An increase in the gastric pH to >4 is thought to be sufficient to prevent superficial stress ulceration progressing to a more serious pathological state which is much more difficult to treat. Therefore the aim of therapy is to prevent further attack on already injured mucosa by reducing acidity and/or preventing proteolytic enzymes from attacking unprotected gastric mucosa. This can be differentiated from the aim of therapy for non-variceal upper GI bleeding where a higher pH is required (pH >6).

Methods of stress ulcer prophylaxis

Several large randomized placebo-controlled studies have been conducted, with conflicting results arising from each. The therapy of choice has changed a number of times over the years.

- H_2-receptor antagonists are usually used first line. Ranitidine 50mg given by bolus injection three times daily is common.
- PPI use is increasing, although there is at present no defining study that places this agent at the heart of stress ulcer prophylaxis therapy. Once-daily injections of omeprazole or pantoprazole have been used, and some centres use an extemporaneously prepared enteral formulation of omeprazole (simplified omeprazole suspension).
- The use of sucralfate has almost disappeared, and antacids are no longer used.

It is common practice to cease stress ulcer prophylaxis when NG feeding is established, although the limited evidence available suggests that feed is not an effective form of stress ulcer prophylaxis.

Some surgical procedures may result in a reduced acid secretory function through denervation of the stomach (e.g. oesophagectomy), but the effect this has on stress ulcer formation has not been studied.

Pharmacological stress ulcer prophylaxis is so routine in critical care that the prescribing of prophylaxis becomes an almost reflex response. Stopping acid suppression therapy in patients with a total gastrectomy can be a common pharmacist's intervention. Partial gastrectomy may still require stress ulcer prophylaxis if the acid secretory function remains intact (i.e. where the antrum of the stomach remains).

Unwanted effects of stress ulcer prophylaxis

- One large study found an increased incidence of nosocomial pneumonia in the ranitidine arm. This has largely been ignored since it was not found in subsequent studies, although an increased incidence of pneumonia in an ambulatory population taking acid suppressant therapy has also been reported.
- There is growing evidence that the use of acid suppressants increases *Clostridium difficile* acquisition rates. This effect may be greater with PPIs than with H_2 antagonists.
- The use of pH testing strips to confirm the correct placement of enteral tubes is unreliable where acid suppressant therapy is used.
- Ranitidine is associated with a number of side effects, including cardiac rhythm disturbance, but the evidence that it causes thrombocytopenia is very poor.

Motility stimulants

The provision of early enteral feed is an important goal in critically ill patients and has several advantages over parenteral feeding. Haemo-dynamic disturbance, pre-existing disease states, and drugs used in the critically ill patient (e.g. adrenergic agents, opiates) frequently result in failure of the patient to absorb enteral feed.

It is usual to use markers such as bowel sounds and gastric residue volume on aspiration to assess gut motility, although neither method is particularly reliable.

Metoclopramide

Metoclopramide is widely used to promote gut motility. However, the evidence base in the critically ill is very poor. This dopamine antagonist possibly works through blockade of dopaminergic neurons in the stomach and small bowel that would normally inhibit GI motility. It also increases lower oesophageal sphincter tone. A typical dose is 10mg three times daily.

Erythromycin

The evidence base for erythromycin is stronger than that for meto-clopramide and comes from several small-scale studies, but it is often reserved for second-line therapy after metoclopramide because of concerns about promoting antimicrobial resistance. Erythromycin acts as a motilin receptor agonist. The addition of erythromycin to a metoclopramide regime is not evidence based, although simultaneously targeting different motility pathways may prove beneficial.

Typical doses range from 250mg twice daily to 200mg three times daily intravenously. Doses as small as 70mg have been shown to have an effect in adults. It is believed that smaller doses are more effective than larger doses, and this is consistent with the well-known upper GI effects of antibiotic doses.

Neostigmine

Neostigmine infusions have been used to promote normal bowel function in the critically ill. Neostigmine directly stimulates acetylcholine release from nerve plexi within the gut wall. A continuous infusion of 0.4–0.8mg/h has found to be an effective prokinetic based on frequency of stool production.

Domperidone

There is no evidence to support or refute the usefulness of domperidone for gut motility. Activation of dopaminergic fibres found in the smooth muscle of the GI tract inhibit smooth muscle contraction and so blockade of these fibres by dopamine antagonists may encourage smooth muscle contraction. Therefore it is possible that a role for domperidone and other dopamine antagonists may be found in the future.

Mechanical ventilation

Mechanical respiratory support may be required in patients with a certain degree of respiratory failure. Typically such failure can be described in terms of a failure to oxygenate blood, such as during an acute asthma attack (type 1 respiratory failure), or a failure to ventilate the lungs resulting in carbon dioxide retention, such as in exacerbations of COPD (type 2 respiratory failure). Patients who do not protect their airway (e.g. through the consequences of acute head injury) may also require respiratory support.

Non-invasive ventilation

Selected patients may initially be managed using a form of tight-fitting facemask which acts as the interface between patient and ventilator. These come in a variety of shapes and sizes. An NG tube is usually *in situ* in order to decompress the stomach, which can frequently become inflated as a result of swallowing air.

Invasive ventilation

The more typical method for connecting a ventilator to a patient is through the insertion of a plastic pipe into the patient's trachea, placed either through the upper airways (nasal passages or mouth) or through a stoma in the patient's neck under the larynx. An inflatable cuff at the end of the tube secures it in the trachea. The ventilator is attached to the other end of the tube. The act of tube placement is known as intubation.

Drugs used to facilitate intubation

Feeding a large-diameter tube through the mouth or nose into the trachea generates all manner of physiological responses, none of which are described as 'pleasant'. Various agents are used to manage or attenuate such a noxious stimulus.

Rapid-sequence induction

This technique is used to secure the patient's airway rapidly whilst minimizing the risk of soiling the airways with stomach contents. A sedative agent such as thiopental 3–4mg/kg is used in combination with a muscle relaxant such as suxamethonium 1–1.5mg/kg to facilitate the technique. Other sedative agents used include propofol 2mg/kg, etomidate 0.1–0.4mg/kg or occasionally ketamine 1–2mg/kg. Alternative muscle relaxants include rocuronium 1mg/kg or vecuronium 80–100micrograms/kg.

Awake intubation

This is used to secure an airway where a difficult intubation is anticipated e.g. due to previous history or airway obstruction, unstable cervical spine fracture, or when anaesthetic induction is dangerous for the patient. Comfort for the patient is provided using topical anaesthetics such as lidocaine 4%, possibly with light sedation with an agent such as midazolam 1–2mg. Atropine 400–600micrograms or glycopyrronium bromide 200–400micrograms is given to dry up secretions.

Ventilation modes

A bewildering array of ventilation modes are used. The following is intended to be a brief overview of those most commonly used.

Continuous mandatory ventilation (CMV)

The ventilator controls movement of gas through the patient's lungs according to set parameters and takes no account of any residual breathing effort the patient may make. Set parameters can be volume-based, pressure-based, or a mixture of both.

Assist control ventilation (ACV)

The ventilator controls movement of gas through the patient's lungs according to set parameters either when the patient triggers a breath (assisted breaths) or at the set respiratory rate if the patient fails to trigger a breath (controlled breaths).

Intermittent mandatory ventilation (IMV)

The ventilator controls movement of gas through the patient's lungs according to the parameters set at a mandatory respiratory rate, but allows spontaneous breathing to occur between mandatory breaths.

Synchronous intermittent mandatory ventilation (SIMV)

The ventilator controls movement of gas through the patient's lungs according to the parameters set at a mandatory respiratory rate, but allows spontaneous breathing to occur between mandatory breaths. Assisted breaths are synchronized with spontaneous breaths when their timing is sufficiently close.

Pressure support ventilation (PSV)

The ventilator augments the flow of gas moving into the patient's lungs in order to maintain a preset pressure in the ventilator circuit during inspiration. When the flow rate falls below a set value, the expiration cycle begins. PSV may be combined with other modes of ventilation to support spontaneous breaths.

Continuous positive airway pressure (CPAP)

The ventilator maintains the ventilator circuit pressure at a constant value above ambient pressure during spontaneous breaths.

Positive end-expiratory pressure (PEEP)

The ventilator maintains the ventilator circuit pressure at a constant value above ambient pressure during ventilator-generated breaths.

Bilevel positive airway pressure (BiPAP)

The ventilator maintains the ventilator circuit pressure at one value above ambient pressure during inspiration and at a lower value (still above ambient pressure) during expiration.

Vasoactive agents

A variety of agents can be used to manipulate the cardiovascular system in critical care. These agents should only be used after the patient has been adequately fluid resuscitated. Terminology is often used incorrectly and interchangeably.

- Inotropes—affect the force of contraction of the heart
- Chronotropes—affect the heart rate
- Vasopressors—increase blood pressure

Charts of receptor activity are widely available. However, they can be tricky to use as different activities predominate at different infusion rates.

Adrenaline (epinephrine) (α_1^{+++}, β_1^{+++}, β_2^{++}, D_1^0, D_2^0)

Dose range effects

- Low doses (<0.01micrograms/kg/min)—predominant β_2 stimulation leads to dilatation of skeletal vasculature resulting in a fall in blood pressure.
- Medium doses (0.04–0.1 micrograms/kg/min)—predominant β_1 stimulation leads to an increase in heart rate, stroke volume, and cardiac output.
- Large doses (0.1–0.3micrograms/kg/min)—α_1 stimulation predominates leading to vasoconstriction which increases systemic vascular resistance and therefore increases blood pressure.
- Larger doses (>0.3micrograms/kg/min)—increased α_1 stimulation causes reduced renal blood flow and reduced splanchnic vascular bed perfusion. GI motility and pyloric tone are also reduced.

Uses

Anaphylactic shock, severe congestive cardiac failure, septic shock, status asthmaticus.

Other effects

Infusions of adrenaline can lead to arrhythmias, hyperglycaemia, and metabolic acidosis.

Noradrenaline (norepinephrine) (α_1^{+++}, β_1^{+}, β_2^0, D_1^0, D_2^0)

Dose range effects

- Low doses (<2micrograms/min)—predominant β_1 stimulation leads to an increase in heart rate, stroke volume, and cardiac output.
- Higher doses (>4micrograms/min)—predominant α_1 stimulation leads to vasoconstriction. Baroreceptor-mediated bradycardia is possible.

Uses

Increase the mean arterial pressure e.g. in septic shock, in severe head injury.

Other effects

Infusions of noradrenaline can lead to arrhythmias, hyperglycaemia, and metabolic acidosis. Not useful for cardiogenic shock because of increased afterload.

Dopamine (α_1^{++}, β_1^{++}, β_2^{++}, D_1^{+++}, D_2^{+++})

Dose range effects

- Low doses (<2micrograms/kg/min)—predominant D_1 stimulation leads to increased renal, mesenteric, and coronary perfusion.
- Medium doses (2–5micrograms/kg/min)—predominant β_1 stimulation leads to an increase in heart rate, stroke volume, and cardiac output.
- Large doses (>6micrograms/kg/min)—predominant α_1 stimulation leads to vasoconstriction which increases systemic vascular resistance and therefore increases blood pressure.

Uses

Cardiogenic shock. Should not be used as a 'reno-protective' agent, except occasionally when used it is used as a vasopressor on general wards to support blood pressure (and hence improves renal perfusion).

Other effects

Infusions of dopamine can lead to arrhythmias, hyperglycaemia, and metabolic acidosis.

Dobutamine (α_1^{+}, β_1^{++}, β_2^{+}, D_1^{0}, D_2^{0})

Dose range effects

- Usual dose (2.5–10micrograms/kg/min)—predominant β_1 stimulation leads to increased cardiac output.

Uses

Cardiogenic shock.

Other effects

Blood pressure may fall in hypovolaemic patients.

Dopexamine (α_1^{0}, β_1^{+}, β_2^{+++}, D_1^{++}, D_2^{++})

Dose range effects

- Usual dose (0.5–6micrograms/kg/min)—strong β_2 stimulation leads to vaso-dilatation. D_1 leads to increased renal perfusion. Splanchnic perfusion may also be increased.

Uses

May be useful to improve splanchnic perfusion.

Other effects

Heart rate increases in a dose-dependent manner.

Phosphodiesterase inhibitors (non-receptor-mediated effect)

Pharmacology

Inhibits phosphodiesterase, causing an intracellular excess of cAMP which causes a calcium ion influx. This causes increased myocardial contractility and smooth muscle relaxation.

Uses

Cardiac failure.

Other effects

Hypotension due to vasodilatation.

Renal replacement therapy

Acute renal failure is a common feature of critical illness. Renal function will recover in the majority of patients, although a proportion will go on to require chronic renal support. During the period of time it takes for the kidneys to recover, renal replacement therapy will be required to undertake some of the functions that the healthy kidneys would perform.

Terminology

Confusion often arises over the various techniques used for renal replacement therapy. Abbreviations add to the confusion, but there are basically two main renal replacement modes (dialysis or filtration), with a hybrid of the two also being commonly employed (diafiltration). The process is usually continuous (C), but can be intermittent (I). Blood follows a pressure gradient that is generated either by taking blood from an artery and returning it to a vein (arteriovenous or AV) or by taking blood from a vein and using the machine to generate the pressure gradient required before returning the blood to a vein (venovenous or VV). Putting the various abbreviations together with the mode of renal replacement gives the appropriate abbreviation for the technique (e.g. CVVHDF = **C**ontinuous **V**eno**V**enous **H**aemo**D**ia**F**iltration).

Haemodialysis (HD)

Not normally used in critical care, but may be used in a stable or pre-existing chronic renal failure patient.

Blood is pushed through thousands of small tubes made of a semi-permeable membrane (Fig. 28.1) Clearance of small (<2000Da), water-soluble molecules occurs by diffusion through a semipermeable membrane into dialysis fluid that bathes the tubes. Water may also be drawn off by altering the concentration of glucose in the dialysis fluid.

Clean fluid can be infused back into the patient if required, although this is unusual for this form of renal replacement.

Haemofiltration (HF)

Blood passes through thousands of small tubes made of a membrane full of small holes (typically 20 000Da in diameter). A pressure gradient pushes the patient's plasma through the holes (filtration) and this eluent is discarded. (Fig. 28.2).

Clean fluid is infused back into the patient.

Haemodiafiltration (HDF)

This is a hybrid form which adds a dialysis element to haemofiltration by allowing dialysis fluid to be added to the eluent generated from the filter, thus diluting it and causing an additional diffusion process to occur.

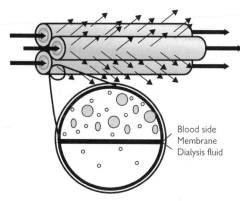

Fig. 28.1 Haemodialysis.

Blood side
Membrane
Dialysis fluid

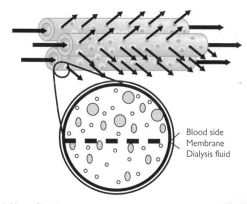

Fig 28.2 Haemofiltration.

Blood side
Membrane
Dialysis fluid

Buffer

Whichever technique is employed, vast quantities of fluid are required for the process to take place. One of the many small molecules that are cleared is bicarbonate. Bicarbonate is central to the acid–base balance of the human body, and its steady removal in renal replacement therapy without replacement would lead to increasing acidosis and ultimately to the patient's death.

Initial stability difficulties precluded manufacturers from simply adding bicarbonate to the dialysis or replacement fluids (although this has now been overcome). Therefore a buffer was added to the fluids in the form of either lactate or acetate, both of which are converted to bicarbonate by the patient. This may become problematic if the patient cannot utilize the buffer.

Anticoagulation

The passage of blood through the extracorporeal circuit activates clotting pathways (Fig. 28.3). The resulting coagulation clogs the filter circuit reducing its efficiency and ultimately destroying its patency.

Anticoagulants are employed to maintain circuit patency, unless the patient is particularly coagulopathic.

Heparin

Heparin has long been used to maintain filter patency through its inhibitory effects on the enzyme cascade. It can be infused into the circuit or the patient to maintain an APTT of 1–2 times normal. Heparin is poorly cleared by renal replacement therapy. Attempts have been made to neutralize heparin with protamine before it is returned to the patient, but the technique is tricky and not widely used.

Epoprostenol

Prostaglandins produced by the endothelial lining of the vasculature inhibit the effect of thromboxane on platelet activation. This activity is lost in the artificial environment of an extracorporeal circuit. Epoprostenol can be infused into the circuit as a substitute at 1–5ng/kg/min, and occasionally at even higher doses. Hypotension is a problematic side effect. The combination of heparin and epoprostenol has been shown to be synergistic.

Citrate

Citrate has been used to bind up ionized calcium in the circuit, thus inhibiting several calcium-dependent steps in the clotting cascade and inhibiting calcium influx into platelets, preventing platelet activation. Large quantities of citrate are needed, and this results in a large solute load and metabolic alkalosis. Specialized fluids are required and sourcing citrate can be problematic. This technique, whilst promising, is not widely used.

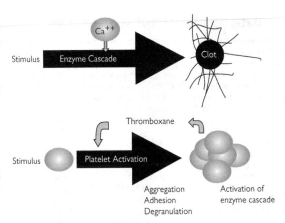

Fig. 28.3 Activation of the clotting cascade.

Treatment of alcohol withdrawal

Alcohol withdrawal syndrome is characterized by a range of symptoms including tremor, paroxysmal sweats, nausea and vomiting, anxiety, agitation, headache, and perceptual disturbances. Seizures are occasionally observed. Half of patients who experience a seizure only suffer a single fit. Some patients with severe withdrawal will progress to delirium tremens. Symptoms usually appear within 6–24h of the last consumption of alcohol and typically persist for 72h, but can last for several weeks.

Many alcohol-dependent people require no medication when withdrawing from alcohol. Supportive care, including information on the withdrawal syndrome, monitoring, reassurance, and a low-stimulus environment, are effective in ↓ withdrawal severity. Many alcohol-dependent patients might not be obvious 'alcoholics'.

If medication is required, a benzodiazepine loading dose technique is usually employed. The patient is given repeated doses until symptoms have diminished to an acceptable level. Chlordiazepoxide or diazepam are effective in the prevention and treatment of acute alcohol withdrawal seizures. Because of the relatively large doses usually given, and the long half-lives, it might not be necessary to give any further medication for withdrawal relief. However, if symptoms reappear, further doses should be administered, titrated according to symptom severity.

Suggested withdrawal regimen

Therapy should be started as soon as the patient can tolerate oral medication. Patients should be sedated on admission with chlordiazepoxide 20mg four times daily for 1–2 days, followed by rapid tailing-off over the subsequent 3–4 days.

- Day 1—20mg four times daily + 10mg when required up to a maximum of 200mg daily.
- Day 2—20mg four times daily + 10mg when required up to a maximum of 200mg daily.
- Day 3—20mg three times daily.
- Day 4—20mg twice daily.
- Day 5—10mg twice daily.
- Day 6—STOP.

Review dose daily and titrate on individual patient basis

There is a clinical opinion that patients given the recommended maximum dose and still suffering symptoms of withdrawal should be given further doses every 2h until symptoms are controlled or they are obviously too drowsy to swallow any more!

Cautions

- Patients might experience seizures as the dose of benzodiazepine is tailed off.
- Patients who are sedated for too long might develop a chest infection.
- The dose should be adjusted to provide effective sedative and anticonvulsant endpoints while preventing oversedation, respiratory depression, and hypotension.

- ❶ Benzodiazepines can cause temporary cognitive slowing and may interfere with learning and planning. This, and the need to avoid benzodiazepine dependence, are reasons for keeping the length of treatment to a maximum of 5 days.
- Doses of benzodiazepine should be reduced in severe liver dysfunction. Alternatively, a shorter-acting benzodiazepine (e.g. lorazepam) can be used (seek specialist advice). Patients with chronic liver disease should have their dose assessed twice daily to avoid oversedation.
- A maximum 24h dose (10mg twice daily) should only be prescribed on discharge from hospital if necessary.
- Clomethiazole, although historically used for the treatment in alcohol withdrawal of in-patients, has the potential for life-threatening respiratory depression if the patient continues to drink alcohol, which precludes its use.

Thiamine and vitamin supplements

Poor nutrition is common in patients who drink for the following reasons.
- Inadequate intake of food.
- Associated chronic liver disease.
- Chronic pancreatitis.
- Malabsorption (water-soluble and fat-soluble vitamins should be replaced and severely malnourished patients should be considered for enteral feeding).

Thiamine

Thiamine deficiency leads to polyneuritis with motor and sensory defects. Ophthalmoplegia (paralysis of the eye muscles), nystagmus, and ataxia are associated with Wernicke's encephalopathy, in which learning and memory are impaired; there is an estimated 10–20% mortality. Korsakoff's psychosis is characterized by confabulations (the patient invents material to fill memory blanks) and is less likely to be reversible once established.

IV thiamine replacement

There is no licensed IV thiamine preparation in the UK. One pair of Pabrinex® IV high-potency (vitamin B and C injection BPC) ampoules contain 250mg of thiamine. IV Pabrinex® should be given initially to those with severe withdrawal symptoms.

Dose

One pair of ampoules should be added to 100mL sodium chloride 0.9% solution or glucose 5% solution and administered intravenously over at least 10min once daily for 3 days or until the patient can take oral thiamine. In established Wernicke's encephalopathy higher doses are needed (consult product literature).

Oral thiamine replacement

If symptoms of withdrawal are not severe the following regimen is recommended.

- Oral thiamine 100mg should be given four times daily until withdrawal is complete. Then reduce the dose to 100mg twice daily.

Other vitamins

- Forceval® (or locally approved multivitamin product)—one capsule daily.
- Folic acid 5mg once daily (if folate deficient).

At discharge

Oral supplements should be continued at discharge in patients who are malnourished or have inadequate diets. Thiamine should be continued long term if there is cognitive impairment or peripheral neuropathy (100mg twice daily).

Consideration should also be given to the setting in which withdrawal occurs. Careful monitoring of withdrawal severity is essential in all cases, and more severe withdrawal requires in-patient care. Specialist alcohol treatment services and most hospitals can provide charts to be used in the monitoring of symptom severity.

Recommendations on the prevention of relapse in alcohol dependence

Acamprosate and supervised oral disulfiram are treatment options recommended as adjuncts to psychosocial interventions.

Further reading

SIGN (2003). *SIGN Guideline 74 The Management of Harmful Drinking and Alcohol Dependence in Primary Care:* http://www.sign.ac.uk/guidelines/fulltext/74/index.html

Dealing with poisoning enquiries

Poisoning incidents can be caused by the following means.
- Accidental poisoning—e.g. small children eating tablets or berries.
- Non-accidental—e.g. Munchausen's syndrome by proxy (in this syndrome one person creates symptoms in another by, for example, administering drugs).
- Deliberate self-poisoning—e.g. tablets or chemicals are ingested intentionally, sometimes to manipulate family or friends and, rarely, with the intention of (successful) suicide.

Any enquiry regarding a possible acute poisoning incident should be treated as potentially serious and urgent. Questioning can quickly establish if there is little possibility of harm, but if there is any doubt the patient should be referred to the nearest A&E department and/or a poisons information centre should be contacted for advice.

Some misconceptions

Members of the public might not be aware of the following.
- Alcohol poisoning can be potentially fatal, especially in children and adolescents. In children, if there are any signs of intoxication the patient should be referred to an A&E department.
- Some forms of poisoning might not cause symptoms initially—e.g. paracetamol overdose, ingestion of sustained release tablets and capsules. This can create the impression that there is no intoxication. Referral to an A&E department should be made if sufficient tablets have been taken, even in the absence of symptoms.

Be aware that some over-the-counter preparations might have similar brand names, e.g. Piriton® and Piriteze® and, Anadin® and Anadin®-paracetamol. Ensure that you and other healthcare professionals are clear what product is involved.

Sources of information

TICTAC

TICTAC is a computerized tablet and capsule identification system used by medicines information and poisons information centres. Information required to identify a tablet or capsule using TICTAC includes the following.
- Shape—straight, rounded, or bevelled edge for tablets.
- Colour—cap, body, and contents for capsules.
- Markings—including whether half or quarter scored.
- Coating—film, sugar, or uncoated.
- Length and width (in millimetres)—at longest/widest point.
- Weight.

Toxbase[1]

Toxbase is an online poisons information database which covers drugs (including over-the-counter medication), plants, household, industrial and agricultural chemicals, and snake and insect bites. Details of probable toxic

---

1 ⌂ http://www.toxbase.org

effects and appropriate management are provided. Toxbase is password-protected. Medicines information and poisons information centres have access to Toxbase, and NHS pharmacy departments can apply for a password through the website.

Poisons information centres

Poisons information centres provide 24h telephone advice. If there is any cause for concern in an acute poisoning incident, a poisons information centre should be contacted immediately. It is inappropriate to cause unnecessary delay in what might be a life-threatening situation by looking elsewhere for information. The doctor dealing with an acute incident should contact the poisons information centre direct so that first-hand information is given and received. Advise the doctor of the sort of information the poisons information centre might require. For a non-acute or general enquiry, it is appropriate for a pharmacist to contact the centre.

Information required to deal with a poisoning enquiry

Eliciting as much information as possible about a poisoning incident can facilitate speedy management. It is especially important to have the relevant information available when contacting a poisons information centre.

- Identity—brand name and active ingredients.
- Timing—when did the incident occur relative to the time of the enquiry.
- Quantity—number of tablets and volume of liquid. An estimate is better than no information. Checking the quantity left in a container versus its full contents at least gives an estimate of the maximum quantity ingested.
- If tablets or capsules—are these sustained release?
- Age and weight of the patient—especially if a child.
- Any relevant PMH—e.g. renal impairment.
- Any signs and symptoms observed.
- If the patient has vomited—any sign of the poison (e.g. coloured liquid, undigested plant material, tablet fragments).
- Any treatments or first aid already administered and the outcome.

If attendance at an A&E department is recommended, the enquirer should be advised to take any containers or plant material with them that could help with identification (taking suitable precautions to avoid contamination of skin or clothing with the poison).

First aid for poisoning incidents
- Do not induce vomiting.
- If fully conscious, give sips of water or milk.
- If unconscious, check ABC. As needed, perform the following.
  - Perform cardiopulmonary resuscitation, but not mouth-to-mouth except with a face shield (because of the risk of contaminating the first aider).
  - Place patient in the recovery position.
  - Call emergency services.
- Take the patient to an A&E department or phone the emergency services.

Further reading

Dines A et al. (2007) Poisoning: an overview of treatment. *Hospital Pharmacist* **14**: 7–9.
Dines A et al. (2007) Poisoning: antidotes and their use. *Hospital Pharmacist* **14**: 10–14.

Drug desensitization

Patients with drug hypersensitivity can usually be treated with an alternative agent. However, on rare occasions if there is no suitable alternative, drug desensitization might be appropriate. Drug desensitization is potentially hazardous and should never be attempted in patients who have had a severe allergic reaction, such as bronchospasm, facial swelling, or anaphylaxis. However, it can be attempted in those who have had a rash provided that this was not a severe skin reaction, such as Stevens–Johnson syndrome.

Desensitization schedules using both oral and parenteral administration have been developed for a variety of drugs, but mostly for antibacterials (notably penicillins) and some chemotherapy drugs. Examples of these are listed at the end of this topic as further reading.

Drug desensitization is potentially hazardous because there is always a risk of anaphylaxis. Thus, when attempting the procedure, the following precautions should be observed.

- The patient is informed of the potential risks (it is advisable that they give written consent to the procedure).
- The patient must be reasonably well (i.e. no active disease other than the current infection).
- The patient's drug history should be reviewed and any drugs known to exacerbate allergic reactions stopped—notably β-blockers and NSAIDs.
- Desensitization should be carried out as an in-patient or closely monitored day-case procedure.
- A doctor or appropriately trained nurse with authority to administer emergency drugs should be present throughout.
- Drugs and equipment required for treatment of anaphylaxis should be available.
- The patient should have an IV cannula placed for administration of emergency drugs before starting the procedure.
- Prophylactic antihistamines, adrenaline, or steroids should not usually be given as these can mask a reaction:
- Patient monitoring should be carried out before each dose and every 30min (if the dose interval is longer), and should include:
  - temperature, pulse, and BP
  - respiratory signs, including peak flow measurement
  - observation and direct questioning of the patient for signs and symptoms of allergic reaction (e.g. skin flushing, rash, itching, wheeze, shortness of breath, and tingling lips or tongue).
- Patients should continue to be monitored for at least 1h after the final dose of the desensitization schedule.
- Observations and details of drug administration should be documented in the patient's medical notes.

It is important to ensure that the desensitization schedule is followed as rigorously as possible.

- Measure doses accurately—e.g. using an oral syringe.
- The patient should rinse their mouth with water and swallow after oral doses.
- Doses should be administered at exactly the specified time intervals.

Because of the requirement for direct medical observation throughout the procedure, most schedules involve rapid desensitization. However, some longer schedules have been used, in which case the procedure is carried out on an out-patient basis. The patient's GP should be informed that out-patient desensitization is planned.

It is important that patients performing drug desensitization at home are carefully selected and that the patient agrees to the following.
- Undertakes never to be on their own throughout the procedure.
- Understands the risks and what action to take if a reaction occurs. Ideally, another responsible person in the home should also be informed.
- Should have access to a telephone and contact numbers for the physician supervising the procedure.
- Has access to suitable transport so that they can attend the hospital in the event of a minor reaction (the patient should call emergency services if there is a major reaction).
- Lives reasonably close to the hospital, and certainly not in a remote area with difficult access.

After the schedule is complete and treatment doses of the drug are being administered without adverse effects, a treatment course of the drug can be given. Desensitization is usually lost within 1–2 days of stopping the drug. If it is probable that further courses of the drug will be needed, low doses should be administered until the next course is required. It is important that patients understand that drug desensitization is only temporary.

Further reading

Examples of drug desensitization schedules

Sullivan TJ et al. (1982). Desensitisation of patients allergic to penicillin using orally administered beta-lactam antibiotics. *Journal of Allergy and Immunology* **69**: 275–82.

Kalanadhabhatta V et al. (2004). Successful oral desensitisation to trimethoprimsulpha-methoxazole in acquired immune deficiency syndrome. *Annals of Allergy, Asthma and Immunology* **92**: 409–13.

Confino-Cohen R et al. (2005). Successful carboplatin desensitisation in patients with proven carboplatin allergy. *Cancer* **104**: 640–3.

Eapen SS et al. (2005). A successful rapid desensitisation protocol in a loop diuretic allergic patient. *Journal of Cardiac Failure* **11**: 481.

Drug interference with laboratory tests

Drugs can interfere with laboratory tests through a pharmacological, toxic effect or through actual chemical interference with the testing process.

A pharmacological or toxic effect on the laboratory value is often expected and reflects what is happening within the body—e.g. steroids causing hyperglycaemia or diuretics effecting electrolyte concentrations. An example of the toxic effect is elevated LFTs (e.g. elevated transaminase, bilirubin levels, and clotting factors) subsequent to paracetamol overdose.

An analytical interference differs in that the true laboratory value is not measured accurately. The result is inaccurate because of a problem with *in vitro* laboratory test procedure, or occurs when a substance or process falsely alters an assay result. This may lead to inappropriate further tests, incorrect diagnoses, and treatments with potentially unfavourable outcomes for the patient.

Drug interference may be (1) chemical where the parent drug, metabolites, or additives cross-react, (2) where drugs or additives act as accelerators or inhibitors of the assay, or (3) photometric where the parent drug, metabolites, or additives may have similar absorption peaks to that of the measured chromogen.

Table 28.1 is in no way intended to be comprehensive but to highlight to practitioners examples of analytical interference from drugs or their metabolites.

Table 28.1 Drug–laboratory interferences are usually overlooked

Laboratory test	Increased by	Decreased by
Blood, serum, plasma		
Creatinine	Ascorbic acid, flucytosine, furosemide, levodopa, nitrofurantoin	
Glucose	Cefotaxime, dextran, methyldopa	Isoniazid, levodopa
Iron	Citrate salts, ferrous salts, rifampicin	Heparin, desferrioxamine
Magnesium	Calcium salts, cefotaxime	Cefotaxime, phosphate salts.
Potassium	Iodine salts	
Thyroxine	Heparin	Danazol, heparin
Uric acid	Paracetamol, caffeine, hydralazine, isoniazid, theophylline	Levodopa, methyldopa, ascorbic acid, rasburicase
Drug assay		
Serum lithium levels	Inadvertent use of lithium–heparin collection tube leads to spuriously high serum lithium determination	
Digoxin assay	Spironolactone	Interferes with certain specific digoxin assays
		Refer to biochemistry department for type of assay used locally
Plasma cortisol levels (Synacthen® test)	Metabolites of spironolactone fluoresce, which interferes when fluorometric analysis is used for tests	
	Erroneously ↑ cortisol levels	
Urine		
Ketones	Ifosfamide, levodopa, mesna, aspirin	
Protein test (bromophenol blue reagent, sulfosalicylic acid)	Carbonic anhydrase inhibitors (IV)	
	False positive	

Therapeutic drug monitoring (TDM) in adults

Dosage requirements of certain drugs in individual patients can vary significantly, particularly if the drug has a narrow therapeutic window. Although an estimate of the apparent volume of distribution and clearance of a drug can be made from population values, these should only be used as a guide when commencing treatment. Measured plasma/blood levels will enable a more accurate idea of the pharmacokinetic values in specific patients. This will result in a reduction in the risk of toxicity and/or optimization of the effectiveness of the drug regimen.

Sample collection

Drug concentrations can be measured in blood, plasma, saliva, CNS fluid, and urine. The timing of the sample (relative to the previous dose and method of administration) influences the interpretation of a drug concentration measurement. For most drugs there is a relationship between response and concentration which is based on steady state samples taken at specific times after the dose.

Trough concentrations taken at the end of the dose interval are commonly used for anticonvulsant drugs. Peak concentration measurements are useful for some antimicrobials, although a relationship between concentration by time over a threshold value (e.g. MIC) is sometimes determined. Responses to some anticancer drugs and immunosuppressant's have been related to the overall exposure to a drug, as measured by the area under the concentration–time curve (AUC).

Patient/drug characteristics

The appropriate use of TDM requires more than simply measuring the concentration of a drug and comparing it with a target range. It starts at the point when the drug is first prescribed and involves determining an initial dosage regimen that is appropriate for the clinical condition being treated, the patient's clinical characteristics, and the drug's characteristics.

- Age, weight, gender, nicotine exposure, renal function, concomitant drug therapy.
- Clinical issues that might effect bioavailability of oral drug forms—e.g. diarrhoea, short gut anomalies.
- Dosage form, administration rate, first-pass metabolism, protein binding, volume of distribution, loading dose.

When interpreting concentration measurements, the following factors need consideration.
- The sampling time in relation to the dose.
- Dosage history (whether or not the result represents steady state).
- Patient's response and desired clinical targets.
- Missed doses.

This information is to provide an assessment of the drug concentration that will assist in achieving rapid, safe, and optimum treatment.

TDM is generally of value in the following situations.
- Good correlation between blood concentration and effect.
- Wide variations in metabolism.
- High risk of side effects.
- Narrow therapeutic index.

Routine measurements might be warranted, for example, in determining adequate concentrations post-organ transplantation or more commonly ordered to add evidence to a specific clinical problem—e.g. investigate handling a patient with concurrent disease or confirm excessive dosing correlating with signs of toxicity. Table 28.2 covers common drugs and Table 28.3 covers antibiotics. However, other drugs, such as those used to treat HIV., might also benefit from TDM.
- For antibiotic assays, doses should ideally be timed for convenience, e.g. 10.00am. For pre-dose levels, a sample should be taken and the dose administered.
- For dosage adjustment, sampling at steady state is essential, except for suspicion of toxic concentrations.
- Sampling is taken at an appropriate time during a dose interval. You must coordinate when, or if, your pathology department can undertake the test or coordinate with another centre.
- Concentrations can be affected by various factors, such as age, drug interactions, protein binding, metabolism, and organ dysfunction.
- The pharmacist has a very important role in interpreting results from TDM.
  - Advice on what to do if there is an unexpectedly high/low result— e.g. check that dose was given, timing of sample in relation to dose or sampling technique.
  - Advice on whether or not another dose should be given if awaiting result.
  - Dose adjustment—most drugs follow linear kinetics (i.e. doubling the dose will double the level), but certain drugs (e.g. phenytoin) exhibit non-linear kinetics and require small incremental dose adjustments.
  - Timing of sampling if there is a suspicion of drug interaction from the introduction of new therapies.

Table 28.2 Common drugs

Drug	Therapeutic range (standard units)	Ideal sampling time	Comments and SI units	Type of sample required
Carbamazepine	4–12mg/L	Trough measurement before dose	Therapeutic ranges: adults, 34–51 Units: mmol/L Ranges desired from pre-dose specimens	Serum or plasma—SST (orange) or PST heparin (green)
Ciclosporin	Varies with indication	Trough measurement before dose	Therapeutic range depends on disorder/clinical situation being treated	Whole blood—EDTA (lavender)
Digoxin	0.8–2micrograms/L Reference range is valid for specimens taken 6–8h post-dose.	Sampling 8–24h after last dose	Adults, 1.0–2.0 Units: nmol/L	Serum or plasma—SST (orange) or PST heparin (green)
Lithium	Minimum effective concentration in mania prophylaxis is 0.5–1.2mmol/L Toxic conc. >1.5mmol/L	12h post-dose	Therapeutic range: 0.5–0.8 Toxicity: >1.0 Units: mmol/L Not in lithium heparin tube Please measure maintenance range 12h after last dose.	Serum–SST (orange)

Drug	Level	Timing	Therapeutic	Specimen
Phenytoin	10–20mg/L	Trough measurement before dose	Therapeutic levels (pre-dose specimen): 40–80 Units: mmol/L	Serum or plasma—SST (orange) or PST heparin (green)
Phenobarbital	15–40mg/L	Trough measurement before dose	Therapeutic range desired from pre-dose specimens: adults, 65–170 Units: μmol/L	Serum or plasma—SST (orange) or PST heparin (green)
Theophylline/ aminophylline	5–15mg/L	1) During a continuous infusion, preferably at 6h and 18h 2) SR preparation— pre-dose	28–85 Units: μmol/L.	Serum or plasma—SST (orange) or PST heparin (green)
Tacrolimus	5–15ng/mL	Trough measurement before dose	NA	Blood—EDTA (lavender)

Table 28.3 Antibiotics

Drug	Therapeutic range (mg/L)	Ideal sampling time	Comments	Type of sample required
Gentamicin, once daily	20	Trough level 18–24h after the first dose (ideal <1.0mg/L).	Not necessary to do a postdose level	Blood SST (orange)
Gentamicin, conventional dosing	Trough <2 Peak 5–10	Trough Peak—1h post-dose	Peak for endocarditits if having synergistic therapy 3–5mg/L	Blood SST (orange)
Amikacin	Trough <10 Peak 20–30	Trough Peak–1h post administration	Further usually twice weekly pre-dose levels if no dose changes and normal renal function	Blood SST
Vancomycin	Trough 5–10	Pre-dose before fourth dose	Further monitoring usually twice weekly	Blood SST (orange)
Teicoplanin	Trough 10–20	Trough	>20mg/L (<60mg/L) for deep seated infection	Blood SST (orange).
Tobramcyin	Trough <2 Peak 5–10	Trough 1h post-administration	Samples should to the fourth dose, depending on renal function	Blood SST

Supplementary data

Sodium content of parenteral drugs 628
Pathology ranges and interpretation 632
Normal ranges 639
Paediatric normal laboratory values 640
Drug interference with laboratory tests 644
Useful websites 646

Sodium content of parenteral drugs

A number of parenteral formulations contain a significant amount of sodium ions (Table A1). This sodium load is unlikely to be important in most patients, but could be clinically significant for some patient groups (e.g. neonates and patients with significant liver impairment). Table A1 is not exhaustive but lists the sodium content of more frequently used drugs or drugs in which the sodium level is paticularly high. The absence of drug from the table does not necessarily mean that it has a low sodium content—check additional sources. If a drug is reconstituted or infused with sodium chloride 0.9% solution, this further ↑ the sodium load (by 15mmol sodium for each 100mL of sodium chloride 0.9% solution). Note that some oral preparations, especially soluble tablets, can have high sodium levels.

Other sources that quote the sodium content of parenteral formulations

Royal College of Paediatrics and Child Health and the Neonatal Paediatric Pharmacists Group (2003). *Medicines for Children*. London: RCPCH Publications.

Barber N, Wilson A (1999). *A Clinical Pharmacy Survival Guide*. Edinburgh: Churchill Livingstone.

Shulman R et al (ed) (1998). *Injectable Drug Administration Guide*. Oxford: Blackwell.

Summaries of product characteristics

Table A1 Sodium content of parenteral drugs

Name	Vial/ampoule size	Sodium content per vial (mmol)
Acetylcysteine	2g	12.78
Aciclovir	250mg	1
Addiphos®	20mL	30
Amoxicillin	250mg	0.7
Ampicillin	250mg	0.7
Amphotericin lipid complex		
(Abelcet®)	100mg	3.13
Amphotericin liposomal		
(Ambisome®)	50mg	<0.5
Atenolol	5mg	1.3–1.8
Benzylpenicillin	600mg	1.68
Cefotaxime	500mg	1.1
Ceftazidime	500mg	1.2
Ceftriaxone	1g	3.6
Cefuroxime	50mg	1.8

Table A1 (Contd.)

Name	Vial/ampoule size	Sodium content per vial (mmol)
Chloramphenicol sodium succinate	1g	3.14
Clomethiazole	500mL	15–16
Ciprofloxacin	200mg	15.4
Co-amoxiclav	600mg	1.6
Co-trimoxazole	480mg	1.7
Desmopressin	4micrograms	0.15
Diazoxide	300mg	15
Disodium hydrogen phosphate	10mL	12
Ertapenem	1g	6
Flucloxacillin	250mg	0.5
Fluconazole	200mg	15
Flucytosine	2.5g	34.44
Folinic acid	15mg	0.2
Foscarnet	1g	15.6
Furosemide	250mg	1
Ganciclovir	500mg	2
Granisetron	3mg	1.17
Heparin	25000IU/mL	0.625–0.8
Human albumin solution (all concentrations)	100mL	100–160 (check label for exact amount)
Hydrocortisone:		
sodium phosphate	100mg	0.66
sodium succinate	100mg	0.37
Imipenem	500mg	1.72
Levofloxacin	500mg	15.4
Meropenem	1g	3.9

(continued)

Table A1 (*Contd.*)

Name	Vial/ampoule size	Sodium content per vial (mmol)
Metoclopramide	10mg	0.27
Metronidazole	500mg	13–14.55
Ofloxacin	200mg	15.4
Pamidronate:		
dry powder	15mg	0.1
	30mg	0.2
	90mg	0.3
solution	15mg	1.1
	30mg	1.1
Phenytoin	250mg	1.1
Piperacillin + tazobactam	4.5g	9.4
Rifampicin	300mg	<0.5
	600mg	< 0.5
Sodium bicarbonate	1.26%	150/L
	4.2%	500/L
	8.4%	1000/L
Sodium chloride	0.9%	150/L
Sodium nitroprusside	50mg	0.34
Sodium valproate	400mg	2.41
Sotalol	40mg	0.5
Teicoplanin	200mg	<0.5
	400mg	<0.5
Terbutaline	500micrograms	0.15
Thiopental sodium	500mg	23.26
Ticarcillin + clavulanic acid	3.2g	16
Verapamil	5mg	0.3
Vitamins B and C		
Pabrinex® high-potency IV	1+2 ampoules	2.95
Pabrinex® high-potency IM	1+2 ampoules	2.92

Pathology ranges and interpretation (Table A2)

Table A2 Pathology ranges and interpretation

	Levels ↑ by	Levels ↓ by	Comments
Sodium (Na⁺) 135–145mmol/L	Water depletion, nephrogenic diabetes insipidus, (e.g. lithium toxicity), mineralocorticoid excess (e.g. Cushing's syndrome), corticosteroids, 2° aldosteronism (e.g. CCF), nephritic syndrome, hepatic cirrhosis, and uraemia *Symptoms: dry skin, postural hypotension, oliguria. Cerebral dehydration → thirst, confusion, and eventually coma*	Water excess, mineralocorticoid deficiency (e.g. Addison's, thyroid deficiency), thiazide and loop diuretics, burns, SIADH, excess sweating, diarrhoea, vomiting, aspiration, atypical pneumonia, haemodilution caused by cardiac, hepatic or renal failure, oedema, infection, and carcinoma *Symptoms: headache, nausea, hypertension, cardiac failure, cramps, confusion, convulsions, and overhydration*	Regulated by aldosterone (ADH)
Potassium (K⁺) 3.5–5.0mmol/L	Mineralocorticoid deficiency (e.g. Addison's thyroid deficiency) ACE inhibitors, K⁺ sparing diuretics, renal failure, severe tissue damage (e.g. burns), hypoaldosteronism, diabetic ketoacidosis, excess K⁺ therapy, NSAIDs, β-blockers, heparin infusions, and sodium depletion (very rare) *Symptoms: muscle weakness and abnormal cardiac conduction (e.g. ventricular fibrillation, and asystole)*	Thiazide and loop diuretics, vomiting, diarrhoea, ileostomy, fistula, steroids, mineralocorticoid excess (e.g. Cushing's syndrome), β-agonists, aspiration and metabolic alkalosis *Symptoms: hypotonia, cardiac arrhythmias, muscle weakness, and paralytic ileus*	Regulated by aldosterone, insulin/glucose. For hypokalaemia, if on diuretics, then ↑ bicarbonate is the best indication that hypokalaemia is likely to be longstanding. Magnesium might be low and hypokalaemia is often difficult to correct until magnesium is normalized
Chloride (Cl⁻) 95–105mol/L	Excess ingestion and dehydration *Symptoms: non-specific*	Vomiting, diarrhoea, diuretics, dehydration and nephropathy	Cl⁻ follows Na⁺ movement

Analyte	Causes	Notes
Bicarbonate (HCO_3^-) 24–30mmol/L	Excessive antacid use, thiazide and loop diuretics, metabolic alkalosis, bicarb, hypokalaemia, vomiting, and Cushing's syndrome *Symptoms: vomiting*	Diarrhoea, renal failure, diabetes mellitus, metabolic acidosis, respiratory alkalosis, and hyperventilation *Symptoms: headache, drowsiness, and coma in severe acidosis*	Reflects renal, metabolic, and respiratory functions
Glucose 3.0–8.0mmol/L	Diabetes mellitus, severe stress, occasionally after CVA, corticosteroids, thiazides, relative insulin deficiency caused by ↑ growth hormone, ↑ glucocorticoids or placental lactogen during pregnancy (glucagonaemia) *Symptoms: polyuria, polydipsia and ketoacidosis*	Insulin overdose, sulphonylureas especially in the elderly, insulinoma, alcohol, and hepatic failure *Symptoms: dizziness, lethargy, sweating, tachycardia, agitation, and coma*	
Magnesium (Mg^{2+}) 0.70–1.10mmol/L	Renal failure and excessive antacids *Symptoms: loss of muscle tone, lethargy and respiratory depression*	Severe diarrhoea, fistula, alcohol abuse, diuretics, diabetes mellitus, TPN, hyper-aldosteronism, hepatic cirrhosis, and mal-absorption *Symptoms: tetany, paraethesiae, cramps, arrhythmias, neuro-muscular excitability, and hypoparathyroidism*	Deficiency can exacerbate digitalis toxicity and Mg^{2+} is excreted by the kidneys
Zinc (Zn^{2+}) 11–24μ	Zinc therapy	Cirrhosis, diarrhoea, alcoholism, drugs, parenteral nutrition, inadequate diet, steroids, diuretics, malabsorption syndrome, and rarely genetic *Symptoms: poor wound healing and growth, alopecia, infertility, and poor resistance to infection*	

(continued)

Table A2 (Contd.)

	Levels ↑ by	Levels ↓ by	Comments
Calcium (Ca²⁺) 2.20–2.60mmol/L (Beware to determine correct calcium level in hypoalbuminaemia and hyperalbuminaemia)	Paget's disease, vitamin A overdose, hyper-parathyroidism, vitamin D overdose, thiazides, oestrogen, lithium, tamoxifen, excess milk ingestion, excess calcium absorption, Hodgkin's disease, and myeloma _Symptoms: nausea, vomiting, constipation, abdominal pain, renal stones, cardiac arrhythmias, headache, depression, mental fatigue, and psychosis_	Thyroid surgery, hypoparathyroidism, alkalosis, renal failure, osteomalacia, vitamin D deficiency and acute pancreatitis _Symptoms: ↑ nervous excitability, tetany, convulsions, muscle cramps, spasms, tingling, numbness of fingers, and ECG changes_	Apparent hypocalcaemia might be caused by hypo-albuminaemia. Regulated by parathyroid hormone calcitonin (1,25-dihydroxychole-calciferol)
Phosphate (PO₄³⁻) 0.8–1.4mmol/L	Renal failure, hypoparathyroidism, diabetic ketoacidosis and ↑ vitamin D	Osteomalacia (starvation), hyperparathyroidism, alcohol abuse, ↓ vitamin D Al(OH)₃ therapy, and septicaemia	Ca²⁺ and PO₄³⁻ metabolism closely linked
Urea 2.5–7.0mmol/L	Renal failure, elderly (caused by ↓ renal function), urinary tract obstruction, CCF, dehydration, cortico-steroids, high-protein diet, ↑ catabolism (e.g. starvation), sepsis, and GI bleed	↑ GFR, pregnancy, excessive IV infusion, low protein intake, anabolic states or synthesis, liver failure, diabetes insipidus, diuresis, and overhydration.	Derived from amino-acid metabolism in the liver; indicator of kidney function
Creatinine 20–110μmol/L (Cr/Cl) 80–139mL/min (not considered impaired unless <50mL/min)	Dehydration, renal failure, ↓ GFR, urinary tract obstruction, and ↑ meat/vitamin C	Pregnancy and chronic muscle wasting	Derived from muscle mass, determined by lean body mass, and indication of glomerular insufficiency

Alkaline phosphatase <125IU/L	Renal failure, cholestasis, liver cell damage, osteomalacia and bone disease, hyper-parathyroidism (e.g. Paget's disease) and metastases. Also during third trimester of pregnancy, post menopause, carcinoma of liver/ prostrate, and drug-induced (e.g. chlorpromazine)	Hypothyroidism and growth retardation	~50% bone-related, ~50% hepatic fraction, and ~ 2–3% intestinal fraction
Creatine kinase 32–184IU/L	MI, skeletal muscle damage (even IM injection), muscular dystrophy, acute psychotic episodes, head injury, surgery, hypothyroidism, alcoholism, and neonates		Found in heart, skeletal and smooth muscle, and brain
Haemoglobin ♂: 13.5–18g/dL ♀: 11.5–16g/dL	Polycythaemia and dehydration	Sickle cell disease, thalassaemia, GI bleed, haemorrhage (acute/chronic) deficient RBC production, iron deficiency, marrow depression, renal failure, ↓ haemolysis and chronic liver disease	
White cell count 4.0–11.0×10⁹/L	Drugs (e.g. steroids), infection, septicaemia, malignancy, sulphonamides bacterial infection, alcohol hepatitis, and cholecystitis	Drugs, bacterial infections, HIV, hypersensitivity reactions, surgery, trauma, burns, haemorrhage, leukaemia, radiation, cytotoxics, ↓ vitamin B₁₂ and ↓ folate	Produced in bone marrow and stimulated by GSF
Haematocrit or packed cell volume ♂: 0.4–5.0 ♀: 0.37–0.47	Addison's thyroid deficiency, dehydration, polycythaemia and pregnancy	Anaemia and haemorrhage	Relative measure of cells in blood and packed cell volume

(continued)

Table A2 (Contd.)

	Levels ↑ by	Levels ↓ by	Comments
Platelets 150–400×10⁹/L	Inflammatory disorders, bleeding, malignancy, splenectomy, and polycythaemia	↓ production: bone-marrow failure/suppression, leukaemia, drugs (notably cytotoxic drugs), megaloblastic anaemia, SLE. Heparin. ↑ consumption: DIC, splenomegaly, furosemide, gold, idiopathic thrombocytopenia, and HIV drugs.	Derived from megakaryocytes in bone marrow and destroyed in spleen
Prothrombin time 10–14s INR—0.8-1.2	Severe liver damage, cholestasis causing malabsorption of vitamin K and warfarin		Used to monitor anticoagulant therapy and assess liver function
Thrombin time 12–15s	Heparin and DIC		
APPT	Heparin, haemophilia, and liver failure		Used to monitor heparin therapy
Fibrinogen 1.7–4.1g/L	Nephrotic syndrome, Hodgkin's and PE	DIC and massive blood transfusion	
Total protein 60–80g/L	Mineralocorticoid deficiency (e.g. Addison's thyroid deficiency) and myeloma	Catabolic states (e.g. septicaemia)	

Albumin 35–50g/L $t_{1/2}$=20–26days	Dehydration and shock	Lost through skin (e.g. burns and psoriasis) liver disease, mal-nutrition, septicaemia, nephrotic syndrome, and late pregnancy *Symptoms: oedema and toxic effects of drugs normally bound to albumin (e.g. calcium, bilirubin and phenytoin)*
Bilirubin—total <17μmol/L Bilirubin— conjugated (bound to albumin) <4μmol/L	Hepatocellular damage (e.g. viral hepatitis—inability to conjugate bilirubin), cholestasis (e.g. by phenothiazines and flucloxacillin) gallstones, inflammation, malignancy, Gilbert's syndrome, haemolysis, methyldopa, GI bleed, extensive bruising, and sulphonamides (displace bilirubin from albumin) *Symptoms: jaundice*	Derives from breakdown of red blood cells by monocyte macrophage system
γ-glutamyl transpeptidase ♂: 11–51IU/L ♀: 7–33IU/L	Cholestasis (e.g. carcinoma of pancreas or biliary tract), liver cell damage (e.g. hepatitis and cirrhosis). Enzyme inducers (e.g. alcohol, phenytoin, and phenobarbital) and alcoholism	Found in liver, kidneys, pancreas and prostrate; released by tissue damage
Aspartate transaminase 5–35IU/L	Hepatocellular damage, cirrhosis, viral hepatitis, severe haemolytic anaemia, myocardial injury (e.g. MI), cholestasis, trauma, or surgery	Found in liver, heart, kidneys, skeletal muscle, and erythrocytes
	Renal failure and vitamin B deficiency	

(continued)

Table A2 (Contd.)

	Levels ↑ by	Levels ↓ by	Comments
Amylase <180U/dL random urine <650IU/L	Acute pancreatitis, abdominal trauma, diabetic ketoacidosis, chronic renal failure, cholecystitis, intestinal obstruction, mumps, ruptured ectopic pregnancy, post-MI ruptured DU, and morphine	Hepatitis and pancreatic insufficiency	Found in parotoid glands and pancreas. Smaller amounts in ovaries, intestine, and skeletal muscle
Fibrin degradation products <10microgram/mL	DIC and adult respiratory distress syndrome		
Cholesterol 3.9–6mmol/L	Diabetes mellitus, familial hypercholesterolaemia excess alcohol, hypo-thyroidism, and hepatic and renal diseases	Severe illness, severe weight loss and MI (during first 2wks)	Treatment will depend on other risk factors
pH 7.35–7.45	Vomiting, K⁺ loss, burns, hyper-ventilation, stroke, SAH, anxiety, hyperthyroidism, excess antacids, aspirin overdose, fever, and uncompensated alkalosis	Respiratory failure, hypoventilation, diarrhoea, renal failure, ketoacidosis, trauma, shock, high plasma lactate (e.g. liver failure), hypoxia, anaemia, and uncompensated acidosis	Reflects ratio of acid to base and not absolute concentration. ∴ it might mask a defect for which the body has compensated
PaO₂ >10.6kPa	Artificial over-ventilation with O₂	COAD, respiratory failure, ARDS, and cardiogenic pulmonary oedema	
PaCO₂ 4.7–6.0kPa Total CO₂ 24–30mmol	COAD, hypo-ventilation, respiratory acidosis and ARDS-compensated metabolic alkalosis	Hyperventilation, respiratory alkalosis, anxiety, aspirin overdose, compensated metabolic acidosis, pulmonary embolism, and non-cardiogenic ARDS	CVA, Indicator of respiratory function

Normal ranges (Table A3)

Table A3 Normal ranges

Sodium	135–145mmol/L	White cell count	4.0–11×10⁹/L
Potassium	3.5–5.0mmol/L	PCV/haematocrit	♂=0.4–0.54
Chloride	95–105mmol/L	PCV/haematocrit	♀=0.37–0.47
Bicarbonate	24–30mmol/L	Platelets	150–400×10⁹/L
Glucose (fasting)	3.5–5.5mmol/L	INR	0.8–1.2
Magnesium	0.75–1.05mmol/L	KCR	0.8–1.2
Phosphate	0.8–1.4mmol/L	Thrombin time	Ratio <1.2
Zinc	11–24µmol/L	Fibrinogen	1.7–4.1g/L
Calcium	2.12–2.65mmol/L	Albumin	35–50g/L
FDP	<10microgram/mL	Total protein	60–80g/L
Urea	2.5–6.7mmol/L	Bilirubin(total)	3–17µmol/L
Creatinine	70–150µmol/L	Bilirubin-(conjugated)	<4µmol/L
Cr/Cl	80–139mL/min	GGT	♂: 11–40IU/L
			♀: 7–33IU/L
Alk phos	<150IU/L	AST	5–35IU/L
Creatine kinase	♂: 25–195IU/L		
	♀: 25–170IU/L		
Haemoglobin	♂=13.5–18g/dL	Amylase	<180IU/L
Haemoglobin	♀=11.5–16g/dL	Amylase (random urine)	<650IU/L
Cholesterol	3.9–6mmol/L	PaO₂	>10.6kPa
pH	7.35–7.45	PaCO₂	4.7–6.0kPa

Paediatric normal laboratory values

The values given in Tables A4 to A10 are a guide; local laboratories may differ. Check normal values with the laboratory you use.

Table A4 Biochemistry

Alanine aminotransferase	Newborn–1 month		≤70IU/L
	Infants and children		15–55IU/L
Albumin	Preterm		25–45g/L
	Newborn (term)		25–50g/L
	1–3 months		30–42g/L
	3–12 months		27–50g/L
	1–15yrs		32–50g/L
Alkaline phosphatase	Newborn		150–600U/L
	6 months–9yrs		250–800U/L
Amylase			70–300IU/L
Aspartate amino-transferase			<45IU/L
Bilirubin	Full term	Day 1	<65µmol/L
		Day 2	<115µmol/L
		Days 3–5	<155µmol/L
		>1 month	<10µmol/L
Calcium	Preterm		1.5–2.5mmol/L
	Infants		2.25–2.75mmol/L
	>1yr		2.25–2.6mmol/L
Chloride			95–105mmol/L
Creatine kinase	Newborn		<600IU/L
	1month		<400IU/L
	1yr		<30IU/L
	Children	♂	<190IU/L
		♀	<130IU/L
Creatinine	0–2yrs		20–50µmol/L
	2–6yrs		25–60µmol/L
	6–12yrs		30–80µmol/L
	>12yrs	♂	65–120µmol/L
		♀	50–110µmol/L

Table A4 (*Contd.*)

Creatinine clearance	<37wks gestation	<15mL/min/m^2
	Neonate	10–20mL/min/m^2
	1–2wks	20–35mL/min/m^2
	2–4 months	35–45mL/min/m^2
	6–125 months	45–60mL/min/m^2
	12 months to adult	50–85mL/min/m^2
C-reactive protein		<20mg/L
γ-glutaryl transferase	Newborn	<200IU/L
	1 month–1yr	<150IU/L
	>1yr	<30IU/L
Glucose	Newborn to 3 days	2–5mmol/L
	>1wk	2.5–5mmol/L
Lactate		0.7–1.8mmol/L
Magnesium	Newborn	0.7–1.2mmol/L
	Child	0.7–1mmol/L
Phosphate	Pre-term first month	1.4–3.4mmol/L
	Full-term newborn	1.2–2.9mmol/L
	1yr	1.2–2.2mmol/L
	2–10yrs	1–1.8mmol/L
	>10yrs	0.7–1.6mmol/L
Potassium	0–2wks	3.7–6mmol/L
	2wks–3 months	3.7–5.7mmol/L
	>3 months	3.5–5mmol/L
Protein (total)	1 month	50–70g/L
	1yr	60–80g/L
	1–9yrs	60–81g/L
Sodium		135–145mmol/L
Urea	0–1yr	2.5–7.5mmol/L
	1–7yrs	3.3–6.5mmol/L
	7–16yrs ♂	2.6–6.7mmol/L
	♀	2.5–6mmol/L

Table A5 Haematology

Age	Hb (g/dL) Mean (range)		MCV (fl) Mean (range)		WBC (x10⁹/L) range	Reticulocyte (%) range
Birth	18.5	(14.5–21.5)	108	(95–116)	5–26	3–7
1 month	14	(10–16.5)	104	(85–108)	6–15	0–1
6 months	11	(8.5–13.5)	88	(80–96)	6–15	0–1
1yr	12	(10.5–13.5)	78	(70–86)	6–15	0–1
6yrs	12.5	(11.5–14)	81	(75–88)	6–15	0–1
12yrs	13.5	(11.5–14.5)	86	(77–94)	5–15	0–1

Note: an artefactual high neonate WBC may be reported because automatic cell counters may wrongly include in the WBC the many normoblasts (red cell precursors) in the neonate.

Table A6 Respiratory rate

Newborn	30–60 breaths/min	Heart rate is usually four times the respiratory rate
6 months	30–45 breaths/min	
1–2yrs	25–35 breaths/min	
3–6yrs	20–30 breaths/min	
>7yrs	20–25 breaths/min	

Table A7 Blood pressure

	Mean (mmHg)	
	Systolic BP	Diastolic BP
Newborn to 2yrs	95	55
3–6yrs	100	65
7–10yrs	105	70
11–15yrs	115	70

Table A8 Urinary output

	mL/day
Infant	250–600
Child	500–1000
Adolescents	500–1500
Adult	500–2000

Table A9 Hypoglycaemia

	Serum glucose
Pre-term	<1.4mmol/L
Term	<2.0mmol/L
Child	<2.5mmol/L

Table A10 Electrolyte requirements

Na^+	2–4mmol/kg body weight/24h
K^+	1–3mmol/kg body weight/24h
Cl^-	3–5mmol/kg body weight/24h
Ca^{2+}	1mmol/kg body weight/24h
Mg^{2+}	0.15mmol/kg body weight/24h

Drug interference with laboratory tests

Drugs interfere with laboratory diagnostics (Table A11), which can lead to wrong diagnoses or treatments and unnecessary further tests.

Table A11 Drug–laboratory interferences are usually overlooked

Drug	Laboratory test	↑/↓	Mechanism of action
Acetazolamide		Leads to spurious ↑ of theophylline levels	Interferes with certain HPLC assays for theophylline
Amiloride	Creatinine	Leads to falsely high measurements of serum creatinine and ↓ creatinine clearance	Does not alter renal function, but blocks tubular secretion of creatinine
Amiodarone	T_4		Amiodarone inhibits peripheral conversion to T_3
Ascorbic acid	Urine sugar	(false + and −)	Clinitest
Oestrogens	Dexamethasone suppression	(false +)	Caused by ↑ corticosteroid binding globulin
Ketamine	Alk phos, GGT, ALT		Mechanism unknown
Levodopa	Urinary glucose	False +	
	Urinary ketones	False +	
Lithium	Serum lithium levels		Inadvertent use of lithium–heparin collection tube leads to spuriously high serum lithium determination
Oral contraceptives	Glucose		Alters glucose tolerance test
Spironolactone	Digoxin assay	↓ true level, i.e. can mask test confirmation of digoxin toxicity	Interferes with certain specific digoxin assays. Refer to biochemistry department for type of assay used locally
	Plasma cortisol levels (Synacthen® test)	Erroneously ↑ cortisol levels	Metabolites of spironolactone fluoresce, which interferes when fluorometric analysis is used for tests

Useful websites

Description	Web address (URL)
American Society of Clinical Oncology (ASCO)	http://www.asco.org
American Society of Hematology (ASH)	http://www.hematology.org
American Society of Health-System Pharmacists	http://www.ashp.org
Annals of Internal Medicine	http://www.annals.org
Australian Therapeutic Goods Administration	http://www.tga.gov.au
Bandolier 'Evidence-based thinking about healthcare'	http://www.medicine.ox.ac.uk/bandolier/
BNF	http://www.bnf.org
British Committee for Standards in Haematology (BCSH) guidelines	http://www.bcshguidelines.com
British Medical Journal (BMJ)	http://www.bmj.com
British Oncology Pharmacy Association (BOPA)	http://www.bopawebsite.org
British Society for Haematology (BSH)	http://www.b-s-h.org.uk
Canadian Health Technology Assessment Programme	http://www.nlm.nih.gov/hsrinfo/evidence_based_practice.html
Cancer Improvement	http://www.improvement.nhs.uk/cancer
Cancer Research UK	http://www.cancerresearchuk.org
Cancerline UK	http://www.cancerlineuk.net
COREC	http://www.corec.org.uk
Counterfeit drugs	http://www.pharmacistscombatcounterfeiting.org
CPD for Pharmacists	http://www.uptodate.org.uk
Cytotoxic guidelines	http://www.marchguidelines.com
Department of Health	http://www.dh.gov.uk
Drugs in breast milk	http://www.ukmicentral.nhs.uk
Drugs of porcine origin-downloadable booklet	http://www.mcb.org.uk/uploads/PBEnglish.pdf
Electronic Medicines Compendium	http://www.medicines.org.uk/emc